BIOLOGICAL AGING MEASUREMENT

CLINICAL APPLICATIONS

by

Ward Dean, M.D.

edited by
Paul C. Anacker, J.D.,
Richard C. Kaufman, Ph.D.,
and
Hans U. Weber, Ph.D.,

This book is unique and unparalleled in many ways. It is the first compendium of biological aging measurement systems ever published. It describes systems used by scientists around the world to accurately assess physiological changes in humans with age. Sufficient details are provided enabling clinicians and researchers to use these tests in laboratories and physicians' offices.

A special feature of the book is an extensive appendix illustrating the changes with age in nearly 300 physiological, biochemical, psychological and anthropometric parameters. These data have never before been published in a single volume, and their inclusion alone makes this an invaluable reference work for all gerontologists.

THE CENTER FOR BIO-GERONTOLOGY

jacket design by Glenn Braswell

BIOLOGICAL AGING MEASUREMENT

CLINICAL APPLICATIONS

by

Ward Dean, M.D.

edited by
Paul C. Anacker, J.D.,
Richard C. Kaufman, Ph.D.,
and
Hans U. Weber, Ph.D.,

The Center for Bio-Gerontology
Los Angeles, California

Copyright ©1988 by Ward Dean, M.D.

All rights reserved. No part of this book may be reproduced or transmitted in any form or by any means, electronic or mechanical, including photocopying, recording or by any information storage and retrieval system without written permission from the author, except for the inclusion of brief quotations in a review.

Second Edition

ISBN: 0-937777-00-5

Library of Congress Catalog Card Number: 85-63822

Published by: The Center for Bio-Gerontology, Los Angeles, California

BIOLOGICAL AGING MEASUREMENT
Clinical Applications

Foreword
   I. Johan Bjorksten, Ph.D. vii
   II. William Regelson, M.D. viii
Preface
   A. How to use this book ix
   B. A note to my professional colleagues x
Acknowledgments xii
Introduction xiii

Part I — Preliminary Evaluation

  1 BIOLOGICAL AGE 3
  2 HEALTH HAZARD APPRAISAL 11
  3 PERIODIC PHYSICAL EXAMINATIONS 15
  4 ADULT GROWTH EXAMINATION 33

Part II — Multiple Regression Analysis

  5 CLINICAL TEST BATTERIES 49
  6 AMERICAN TEST BATTERY — Harvard University 53
  7 DUTCH TEST BATTERIES — Institute for Preventive Medicine 59
  8 AUSTRALIAN TEST BATTERIES — University of New South Wales 71
  9 JAPANESE TEST BATTERIES — University of Osaka 81
10 JAPANESE TEST BATTERIES — Radiation Effects Research Foundation 93
11 FINNISH TEST BATTERIES — University of Jyvaskyla 103
12 AMERICAN TEST BATTERY — Gerontology Research Center 129
13 JAPANESE TEST BATTERIES — University of Kyoto 133
14 SOVIET TEST BATTERY — Minsk Institute of Gerontology 147
15 SOVIET TEST BATTERIES — Kiev Institute of Gerontology — I 157
16 SOVIET TEST BATTERY — Kiev Institute of Gerontology — II 171
17 GERMAN TEST BATTERY — Karl Marx University, Leipzig (GDR) 175
18 JAPANESE TEST BATTERIES — University of Nagoya 189

Part III — Miscellaneous Systems and Future Prospects

19 WHOLE-BODY CALORIMETRY 205
20 NEUROENDOCRINE TEST BATTERIES — Petrov Research Institute, Lenningrad 211
21 THE H-SCAN COMPUTERIZED SYSTEM 227
22 PROSPECTIVE SYSTEMS 233

Part IV — Clinical Applications

23 SYSTEMS — SELECTION AND USE 255

Appendices

A EQUIPMENT 271
B BIOMARKER SUB-TESTS — with age-adjusted normal values 297
C RECORD KEEPING — Calculation Sheet and Chart 409
D RECOMMENDED READING 411
E SUPPLEMENTAL BIBLIOGRAPHY 415

Index 421

Foreword

I. Johan Bjorksten, Ph.D.

Dr. Dean has singlehandedly done enough research and compiled enough information for several books, each of which should rightfully be the project of an entire department or institution.

First, he provides a compendium of all human biological aging measurement systems that have been published in the scientific literature over the past 30 years. This includes extensive personal correspondence with all of the scientists who conducted the original studies, and numerous photos. This gives the book historical as well as immediate practical value. Significantly, it is the first time that anyone has seriously proposed the use of these systems as the author suggests, to measure the short-term effects of potential gerontotherapeutic agents designed to retard the aging process.

Separate appendices give useful details of construction of the equipment discussed, describe the equipment required, where to obtain it, and how to conduct the tests. This is the only single source (based on personal correspondence) for this information.

Moreover, one of Dr. Dean's appendices includes charts depicting the normal age-adjusted values for numerous parameters used in the various aging measurement systems. This may well be the most detailed compilation of changes with aging that has ever been published.

Clearly, this book is a classic in clinical short range changes with aging and should be of great help to clinical workers and researchers in this area. It will be a valuable reference book in institutional libraries and in the personal libraries of workers in this field.

Johan Bjorksten, Ph.D.
President
Bjorksten Research Foundation
Houston, Texas
February 19, 1987

II. William Regelson, M.D.

This text is the first concise effort to summarize and provide in an ordered fashion a review of clinical methods for the bioquantitation of aging. These methods are readily applicable to clinical practice and provide convenient, cost conscious approaches to quantitating the physiology of aging in man.

It is obvious that before one can evaluate programs of intervention in aging, one must be able to conveniently and accurately measure aging in clinical studies.

Until methods and centers for bioquantitation of aging are readily available, we cannot expect the effective entry of the pharmaceutical industry into the search for anti-aging drugs because of the cost, time and uncertainty involved.

The insurance industry is finally recognizing that the efficient use of age-quantitated biomarkers will revolutionize the character of their actuarial risk pool that governs current insurance programs. It can be expected, in the near future, that health insurance salesmen will be competing with each other to provide age bioquantitation with readjustment of premium costs to meet true physiologic age and life expectation based on performance rather than chronology.

Efforts to accurately quantitate aging are the first step in programs that can be developed to prevent debility and dependency, which often accompany a longer life expectancy. The beneficial claims for high dose multivitamin, antioxidant, nutritional and exercise programs can only be legitimized by before-and-after performance standards related to physiologic measurements.

Centers of excellence for the bioquantitation of aging are a first step for the development of rational interventions to provide options for changing the crippling social and economic effects of an aging process that destroys the quality of our later years.

This text provides an organized review and manual for the growing number of practicing clinicians and gerontologists as well as the educated public who realize that intervention can only be meaningful if effective and economic assessment of physiologic age becomes readily available to all of us concerned with preventing the debility of aging.

William Regelson, M.D.
Professor of Medicine
Medical College of Virginia
February 18, 1986

Preface

A. How to use this book

For those without a background in bio-medical gerontology, reading this book from cover to cover like a novel may be mind-boggling because of the unfamiliar subject matter and mass of technical information. Before wading into the intricacies of the subject, I recommend obtaining an over-all perspective and general understanding of biological aging measurement by briefly reviewing a few of the book's highlights.

Chapter 1, *Biological Age*, defines the concept of biological age, and explains why it is essential for clinical gerontologists to conduct biological aging assessments.

Chapter 5, *Clinical Test Batteries*, the introductory chapter for Part II, discusses the technique of using a battery of physiological, biochemical and neuropsychological tests to calculate a composite biological age, using multiple regression analysis.

Chapter 23, *Systems — Selection and Use*, gives an over-all view of "where we're going." This chapter aids in the selection of one or more of the aging measurement systems presented in the book. It also explains how to use biological ages to determine aging rates, monitor the effectiveness of experimental age-retarding or health optimization programs, and adjust them when required.

All equipment and tests are fully described in Appendices A and B; this saves repetitive descriptions in various chapters. Details concerning equipment or test methods are mentioned in the body of the book only if they differ from the description in the Appendices. Names and addresses of manufacturers and distributors are provided in Appendix A, so that all necessary equipment and instruments can be obtained.

Appendix B contains charts that graphically portray the changes with age of various anthropometric, physiological, neuropsychological and biochemical tests that are included in the test batteries. These charts denote normal age-adjusted values. Because of biochemical and physiological individuality, what is normal for one person may be above or below the mean value. Despite this individual variability of absolute values, the rate of change with age of most variables will generally be the same as depicted in the charts. The goal is to restore and maintain values of each parameter at youthful (i.e., those of a healthy 25 year-old) levels. Individual values for these tests should be plotted on corresponding graphs in Appendix B each time they are measured.

Aging measurements should be plotted longitudinally on a copy of the chart provided in Appendix C, using a separate chart for each measurement system used.

Graphically displaying these changes longitudinally on charts (as opposed to the usual practice of collecting a periodic mass of unorganized data) is a unique aspect of the approach of this book. This will enable clinical gerontologists to assess rates of overall decline and to identify specifically where efforts should be directed to improve the values on which biological ages are based, guard against continued deterioration, improve health and possibly slow the rate of aging.

This book is intended for a broad audience, consisting of health care professionals, research scientists, and anyone interested in improving their health and extending their active lifespans.

B. A note to my professional colleagues

Sound and rational techniques for potential intervention in the human aging process have recently been advanced by bio-medical and clinical gerontologists. Appendix D lists a number of books, journals and newsletters that discuss and propose various techniques to potentially retard human aging. Most of these aging-intervention recommendations are based on the results of animal studies. Many of our patients already are conducting what amounts to self-experimentation by applying insights gained from these studies to themselves. These range from conservative measures such as stopping smoking, exercising moderately, and reducing the consumption of fats and refined carbohydrates, to more unconventional regimens as ingesting certain vitamins, chemicals, and drugs that may have age-retarding properties.

A shortcoming in all popular "life extension" books is the lack of specific guidance for physicians, despite the nearly unanimous recommendation for physician-monitoring of the various programs. Worse yet, the books do not recommend means to evaluate the efficacy of the proposed experimental age-retarding programs. Gerontologists have been accused of being the only scientists who are unable to measure the object of their research — aging. For those of us who consider the aging process itself a disease (for more on this subject, see Chapter 3), we must have some means to assess the progression of the disease and the effectiveness of therapeutic regimens.

This book should fill this void, and can be used as a physician's office manual. It provides step-by-step instructions to clinically evaluate biological age and aging rates. Most routine physical examinations produce an amorphous mass of usually meaningless data within the normal range. The aging measurement systems described in this book make it possible to put these data into a structured format, obtain a longitudinal perspective, and objectively measure age changes from one examination to another. Readers interested in the mathematical intricacies involved in the development of these systems should consult the original papers; such details are intentionally not discussed.

This is a compendium of all aging measurement systems published in the scientific literature within the past 25 years. Most of the original studies were incomplete, deficient in details that would enable them to be duplicated and verified by other scientists. Also, with one exception, no recommendations have been made for the practical use of these measurement systems in the clinical assessment of experimental gerontotherapeutic (age-retarding) regimens.

To obtain additional details and to invite opinions regarding the clinical application of these systems, I contacted all surviving scientists who conducted the original studies. They were generally supportive, and provided a great deal of data from their files (some over 20 years old).

This book includes the missing details, and proposes rational guidelines to evaluate health improvement and experimental age-retarding programs. Many of these tests can be incorporated into routine periodic exams as explained in Chapter 3. Chapter 23 gives recommendations for testing frequency.

Obviously, no unqualified recommendations can be made at this time regarding the most accurate system, nor optimum interval for testing. However, as many people are already haphazardly dosing themselves with large amounts of vitamins, drugs and chemicals in a relatively unsupervised, unstudied fashion, it would seem prudent to adopt the best tools available to evaluate this vast human experiment, and to provide our life extension experimenter-patients with the best professional guidance and assessment of which we are capable.

Since the science of biological aging measurement is still in the developmental stage, I welcome comments, questions and suggestions. I will attempt to answer inquiries personally, and will consider incorporating recommendations in future revisions.

Acknowledgments

With any enterprise, the end result is due to contributions and cooperation of others. This book is no exception. First, utmost thanks to those pioneering scientists on whose work this book is based—not only for conducting the research in the first place, but for their generous continuing support and helpful comments and criticisms throughout the writing of the book.

Mrs. Dorothy Walker, Cecelia Edwards, and Jennifer Gilmore—librarians at the Fort Bragg, NC, U.S. Army Hospital Medical Library—performed numerous administrative miracles in obtaining essential references from many obscure books and journals.

Hans Weber, Ph.D., patiently assisted in the preparation of the preliminary manuscript. Richard C. Kaufman, Ph.D., performed a second blood-letting nearly as severe as Dr. Weber's. Paul Anacker, J.D., put on the final polish—translating disks from CP/M Valdocs to DOS MS-Word format (Valdocs programmers said it couldn't be done!), making stylistic improvements, doing further editing, typesetting, and assisting with the publishing.

Others whose contributions were less direct, but equally significant, were: Nathan Shock, Ph.D., pioneered the field of aging measurement and spearheaded the formation of the NIA's Baltimore Longitudinal Study of Aging. This study should provide a valuable data base for future aging measurement research; Ed Schneider, M.D., former Deputy Director of the NIA, co-authored a previous work on the subject, *Biological Markers of Aging*. This book remains a landmark in its field. It is equaled only by the two-volume *Interventions in the Aging Process* by William Regelson, M.D. and Marrot Sinex, Ph.D.

Scientists and writers who reviewed preliminary versions and made helpful recommendations for change that were incorporated in the final version were: Lou Acheson, Ph.D.; Paul Anacker; Jon Archer, Ph.D.; Lord Lee-Benner, M.D.; Richard G. Cutler, Ph.D.; David Harrison, Ph.D.; John Mann; Durk Pearson and Sandy Shaw; William Regelson, M.D.; and Roy Walford, M.D.

The following people also contributed significantly in various ways to the project: Jack Campbell, Ph.D., Mike Perry, Ph.D., and Paul Anacker, wrote the computer programs enabling the validation of most of the equations; Lou Acheson and Paul Anacker did a final review of the mathematical integrity of the book.

Special thanks to Sherm, Jesse, Bucky, and especially Chuck—under whose auspices most of the research for the book was conducted—who provided me with the intellectual latitude to pursue this project; Rick Noe kept the alligators away; Dan Mathers introduced me to word processing (hate to think where I'd be without a computer); Richard Dokey and Jon Pearce tried to teach me to write; my patients, whose interest and confidence in our research made the preliminary comparative clinical studies possible.

Finally, special appreciation to my wife Kum-Ja, who provided support through five years of research and writing.

Introduction

People have been writing about aging retardation and rejuvenation since the beginning of recorded history. Recent advances in medical intelligence and technology gradually improve the feasibility of controlling the aging process. This is reflected not only by the recent proliferation of "how-to" life extension books from bio-medical gerontologists and science writers with specific proposals for retarding the aging process in humans, but also by the growing number of serious academic books relating to this subject written for the professional gerontological community. See Appendix D for a list of some of these books.

All of the popular life extension books advise their readers to consult their physicians before embarking on an experimental life extension program. However, few physicians have any training in clinical gerontology or gerontotherapeutics ("therapeutic management designed to retard aging and increase the healthy lifespan"). Therefore, most physicians tend to be reluctant to encourage their patients to pursue such programs. Even the relatively few sympathetic physicians willing to cooperate may not know what advice to give, nor have any idea of an effective means to reliably evaluate an experimental age-retarding program.

The lack of a method to assess the efficacy (or inefficacy) of the proposed anti-aging regimens has been a glaring and almost universal shortcoming in all of the popular life extension books. What is needed is a system of health measurement capable of quantitatively assessing biological age and health status, with sufficient accuracy and sensitivity to reflect aging changes over a relatively short period of time.

Without such a system, the only way to evaluate the effectiveness of potential anti-aging drugs and chemicals on humans is to perform human life-span studies using various combinations of these substances. After 40 or 50 years, scientists will be able to determine if those using the drugs lived longer than those who did not. Unfortunately, by the time the results are obtained, the information will be of little practical use to those of us now living.

Despite growing interest in finding a means to measure biological age, a standardized system has not yet been developed nor accepted by the scientific community.

The purpose of this book is to:

1. Propose methods of evaluating age-retarding or health improvement programs by measuring biological ages and rates of aging.

2. Refine the aging measurement system and thereby reduce the costs of diagnosis and treatment. The testing program itself costs time and money. Therefore, it is important to determine which are the most accurate and cost-effective systems, as well as the optimum frequency for testing. Obviously, it is foolish to continue investing time and money in an ineffective or harmful program.

This book presents a number of aging measurement systems developed by gerontologists around the world, and explains for the first time anywhere how these systems may be used by clinical gerontologists to evaluate age-retarding programs.

It should become apparent that it is essential for anyone embarking on an age retarding program to conduct periodic evaluations of biological age to determine the efficacy of the program and to identify any adverse or toxic effects the program may cause. As the measurement systems themselves become more accurate and refined, the various age retarding protocols in use also should become more effective.

Some of these systems use non-standard tests and units of measurement. These tests are included primarily for the benefit of physicians who wish to obtain the equipment or school themselves in the procedures and include them as a part of their routine office protocols. Other systems consist of various combinations of standard laboratory tests.

In order to encourage and facilitate the clinical use of these test batteries, conversion factors have been determined and included where appropriate for obsolescent or non-standard tests and results that varied due to anthropometric or ethnic differences.

To obtain the names of clinical gerontologists who may be equipped to conduct biological aging measurements, contact:

The MegaHealth Society, PO Box 60637, Palo Alto, CA 94306 (415/949-0919);

The Age Reduction Corporation, PO Box 85152, San Diego, CA 92138 (800/621-0852 ext. 585); or

The Center for Bio-Gerontology, 9061 Keith Avenue, Suite 103, Los Angeles, CA 90069 (213/275-9616).

Part I

Preliminary Evaluation

Chapter 1

BIOLOGICAL AGE

Biological age, (sometimes referred to as *physiological age* or *functional age*), is *the objective assessment of a person's health status*. Theoretically, a "normal" person's biological age—in terms of appearance, performance and functional capacity—should be the same as his chronological age.

It is not uncommon to encounter people who do not "look their age"—who appear either much younger or much older than their chronological age. The results of many measurements of biological age indicate that most older-appearing individuals are indeed older biologically than their chronological ages. Likewise, those who appear younger than their ages are usually *really* younger in biological terms (Borkan; Furukawa; Nakamura; Webster). In these studies—described in detail in subsequent chapters—those who appeared older or had hypertension, diabetes, or other chronic health conditions related to aging usually scored significantly older than their chronological ages. Also, in several long-term follow-up studies, *those who scored the oldest biologically died the soonest*.

THE IMPORTANCE OF MEASURING BIOLOGICAL AGE

In order to assess the efficacy (if any) of an age retarding protocol, it is essential to accurately measure biological age and aging rates. Otherwise, there is no way to know whether the program works or not.

While routine clinical lab tests are very useful for diagnosing clinical disease, they are almost useless in evaluating biological age or experimental age-retarding programs *when presented as they usually are as a mass of unrelated data*. This book provides a structured framework for organizing much of this heretofore random data into a single objective quantitation of biological age, as well as a means of longitudinally evaluating individual parameters.

CRITERIA FOR SELECTION OF AGING MEASUREMENT TESTS

A sophisticated aging measurement system should: (1) include values known to change with age; (2) be capable of evaluating one's health status and aging rate, and (3) detect subtle changes in the aging rate — either positive or negative.

Other criteria proposed by various scientists are: (1) the tests should cause minimal trauma (i.e., be relatively non-invasive); (2) the tests should provide highly reproducible results and reflect physiological age; (3) the clinical function being measured should display a significant alteration over a relatively short period of time; (4) the clinical function being measured should be crucial to the maintenance of health and prevention of disease in man (Reff and Schneider); (5) the degree of aging assayed should correlate with longevity (Harrison); (6) the markers should be easily assayed; and (7) the set of markers should be nonredundant (Sekuler).

DECLINE OF PHYSIOLOGICAL FUNCTION WITH AGE

The aging process is very subtle and results in only minor decrements in functional capacity and appearance from year to year (*Fig. 1-1*). Healthy individuals in their 80's or 90's score within the normal range for many routine laboratory tests. For example, there is essentially no change in the red and white blood cell counts, hemoglobin, and some blood tests between the healthy elderly and the young.

A normal healthy person, with a reasonably good genetic background, average diet, who exercises moderately and doesn't smoke, should have a biological age that coincides with his chronological age, and which should increase at the same rate. In other words, for every year of chronological age, the biological age should also increase one year (*Fig. 1-2*).

A sedentary person who smokes, regularly drinks more than two alcoholic drinks per day, thrives on "junk-burgers" (and who probably has one or more chronic illnesses as a result of his lifestyle), would probably score older biologically than his chronological age, and would probably age biologically faster than one year for each additional year of chronological age (Snowdon, D. A.) (*Fig. 1-3*).

If this same person saw the error of his ways and began to exercise regularly, eat more complex carbohydrates and less sugar and fat, take nutritional supplements and quit smoking, he would probably significantly slow his rapid aging rate and restore his biological age to normal (Snowdon) (*Fig. 1-4*).

Biological Age   **Chapter 1**

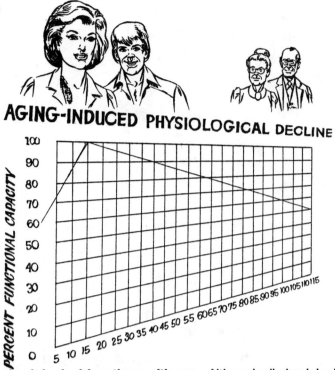

Fig. 1-1. **Decline of physiological functions with age.** Although all physiological functions decline with age, they decrease at varying rates. This graph is representative of the linear manner in which the functional capacity of most organs and organ systems is lost with age. (Art by Wayne Boring).

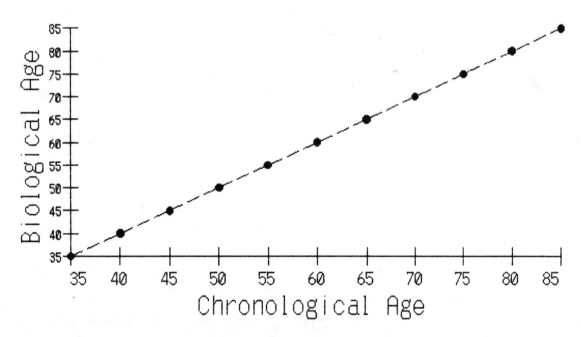

Fig. 1-2. **Normal aging.** Note that the biological age normally increases by one year for each year of chronological age.

Chapter 1 — Biological Age

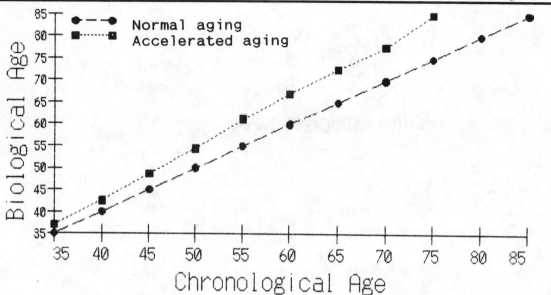

Fig. 1-3. **Accelerated aging.** Accelerated aging may be caused by environmental insults such as poor diet, smoking, excess drinking, or inadequate exercise. Note that the biological age is increasing more than one year for each year of chronological age.

Health enthusiasts practicing primitive but potentially successful age-retarding protocols like those proposed in the sources in Appendix D, may attain biological ages lower than their chronological ages, and the rates of change may be less than "normal". In other words, for each year of chronological age, the biological age should increase less than one year (*Fig. 1-5*). The more successful the program, the less the increase in biological age. Ideally, on a completely successful program, the rate of change should approach zero (indicating essentially no aging) (*Fig. 1-6*) or even be *negative* (indicating true *rejuvenation*) (*Fig. 1-7*).

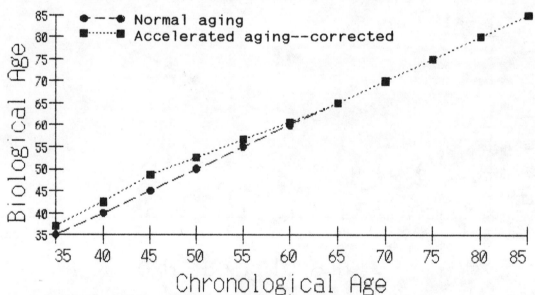

Fig. 1-4. **Corrected accelerated aging.** After the rapidly aging person in *Fig. 1-3* improved his lifestyle, the aging rate returned to near "normal".

Biological Age   **Chapter 1**

Aging-reversal—even more than aging retardation—remains in the theoretical realm. True reversal of aging requires the identification of the genetic loci that control the aging process, and the manipulation of these genes by genetic engineering techniques. This should cause the DNA to restore "old" cells to an optimal state, and essentially rejuvenate the organism. It should be noted that the only really "old" cells in an elderly person are the non-dividing cells in the brain, heart, and other organs. Even these cells are constantly undergoing regeneration of their molecular constituents. All other cells in an elderly person's body are not much older than those of a young person, but may be of poorer quality.

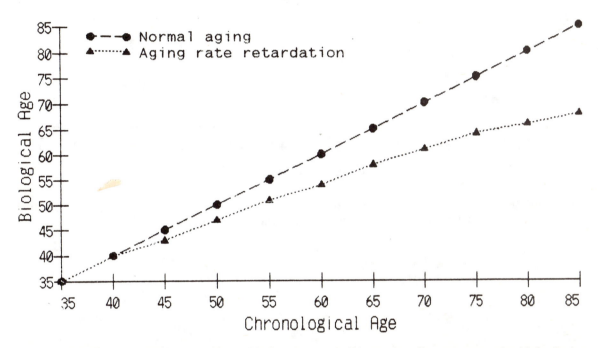

Fig. 1-5. **Aging rate retardation**. After initiating a successful age retarding program, the biological age should increase less than one year for each year of chronological age (as opposed to "normal aging", *Fig. 1-2*, in which the biological age increases a full year for each year of chronological age).

While aging reversal by genetic engineering is a theoretical possibility, the knowledge and technology to accomplish this are not currently known. In the meantime, we must endeavor to take advantage of current "state-of-the-art" aging intervention techniques, such as avoidance of risk factors, optimum nutrition, adequate exercise, caloric restriction, anti-oxidant therapy, immune restoration, hormonal manipulation, and other potential techniques discussed in the books listed in Appendix D.

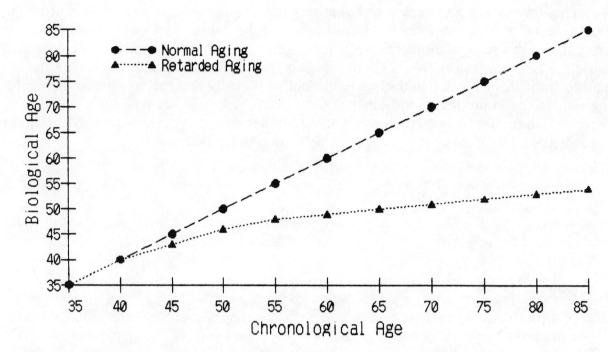

Fig. 1-6. **Highly effective age-retarding program.** There is an almost negligible increase in biological age for each year of chronological age. An extended maximum life span may result.

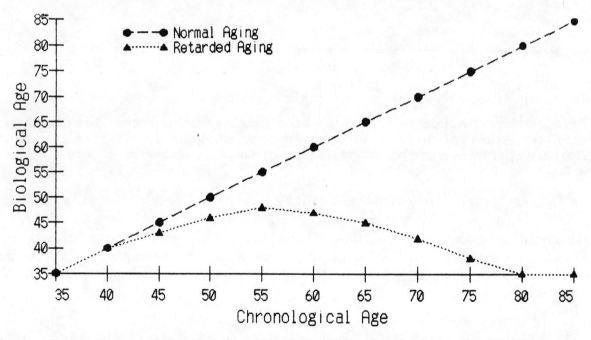

Fig. 1-7. **Optimum age-retarding program.** In this case, physiological and neuropsychological values and functional capacities have returned to more youthful levels. True rejuvenation has taken place. Although aging reversal is speculative at this time, it is theoretically possible and is the ultimate goal of gerontological research.

AGING MEASUREMENT SYSTEMS

Many attempts to measure biological age have been made during the past 20 years by scientists throughout the world. In most cases, the researchers studied large population samples and attempted to find physiological or biochemical variables correlated with chronological age. The results were combined into a system or an equation to calculate biological age.

The major problem with most of the proposed aging measurement systems is that — with a few notable exceptions — they were "one-shot" studies. That is, the experimenters studied large numbers of people, calculated their measurement systems, published the results, and then abandoned their research for other projects. Few researchers meticulously followed up on their own or others' measurement systems in comprehensive longitudinal or comparitive evaluations. Consequently, there is still no universally recognized standard for measuring biological age.

This book presents all of the measurement systems developed by responsible research scientists around the world that have been described in scientific books or journals. The tests are clearly explained in Appendix B, enabling physicians to conduct biological aging measurements in their offices — thus moving these studies from the research institute to the clinician's office. Appendix A lists sources of equipment required to conduct the tests.

STARTING OUT

Ideally, aging rates should be evaluated prior to embarking on an experimental age retarding program. In this way, changes (if any) from a successful protocol can be observed. Many people are already on such programs of their own design, developed without consulting a clinical gerontologist or measuring their biological age.

Once a person's aging status has been fairly well established, the effect of further alterations in the program will be reflected by changes in the aging rate. Aging measurements should be made whenever the program is altered, and at periodic intervals as recommended in Chapters 3 and 23.

If adjustments in an age retarding program (such as changes in dosage, or additions/deletions of various vitamins, minerals, drugs or chemicals) cause an apparent decrease in the rate of aging, the changes are probably beneficial. If the aging rate increases, the changes may be harmful, and the new program should be reevaluated.

Test results should be submitted to a data collection center. Evaluation of scores from thousands of people will enable the measurement systems to be refined, decrease the number of tests, increase the accuracy of the system, and reduce the costs.

Data can be submitted to:

> The Center for Bio-Gerontology
> 9061 Keith Ave., Suite 103
> Los Angeles, CA 90069.

REFERENCES

Borkan, G. Assessment of biological age using a profile of physical parameters. *J Geront*, 1980, Vol 35, No 3, pp. 177-184.

Furukawa, T., et al. Assessment of biological age by multiple regression analysis. *J Geront*, 1975, Vol 30, No 4, pp. 422-434.

Harrison, D. Experience with developing assays of physiological age, in: *Biological Markers of Aging*, by Reff, M.E., and Schneider, E. L. (eds). NIH Publication No. 82-2221, 1982.

Maranto, G. Aging—Can we slow the inevitable? *Discover*, December 1984, pp. 17-21.

Nakamura, E. The aged people and its physiological ages in relation to work capacity. *Kyoiku Igaku*, (1982), 28: 2-11.

Reff, M. E., and Schneider, E. L. *Biological Markers of Aging*, NIH Publication No. 82-2221, 1982.

Sekuler, R. Vision as a source of simple and reliable markers for aging, in: *Biological Markers of Aging*, Reff, M.E., and Schneider, E. L. (eds). NIH Publication No. 82-2221, 1982.

Snowdon, D.A. Epidemiology of aging: Seventh Day Adventists—A bellwether for future progress. In: *Intervention in the Aging Process, Part A: Quantitation, Epidemiology and Clinical Research*, Regelson, W. and Sinex, F. M. (eds.), New York, Alan R. Liss, 1983, pp. 141-149.

Webster, I.W. Subjective good health and biological impairments in female subjects. *Community Health Studies*, 1982, Vol VI, No 2, pp. 39-46.

Chapter 2

HEALTH HAZARD APPRAISAL

In an age-retarding program, it is obvious that every potentially hazardous habit or action should be identified and eliminated. While there is no proof that any of the theoretical life-extending protocols and techniques currently being followed by many people will keep their promise, there are many well-known life-shortening habits—smoking cigarettes, not wearing seat belts, overeating, abusing drugs and alcohol, and inadequate exercise. Clearly, it is absurd to waste money and energy on a life extension program if a life-shortening lifestyle is indulged—especially one that is largely correctable.

There is a practical means of identifying and quantifying life-shortening habits. It uses a computerized system known as *Health Hazard Appraisal, Health Risk Index, Health Risk Profile* or other similar terms (depending upon the organization which prepares the report). These similar analytical systems are computerized or hand-calculated evaluations of environment and lifestyle which may have an adverse effect on life expectancy. The Health Hazard Appraisal (HHA) quantifies both the life-shortening effect of these detrimental habits, and the increased life expectancy attainable if the habit is eliminated.

The concept of Health Hazard Appraisal was developed in the early 1960s by Drs. Lewis C. Robbins and Jack Hall at the Methodist Hospital of Indiana in Indianapolis. It is based on statistics derived from the monumental Framingham Study in Massachusetts, in which Dr. Robbins was a participant. In this ongoing study, medical teams monitor the health and lifestyle of some 5,000 residents of Framingham, Massachusetts. They carefully record weight, serum cholesterol, blood pressure, and other factors. When members of the community die of heart disease, stroke, and other ailments, the medical teams analyze the relationships between living habits and causes of death.

The study clearly shows that cigarette smoking, elevated cholesterol, and high blood pressure are linked with heart disease and stroke. The computer analysis also gives numerical values for the influence of each factor. It shows, for example, that someone with a systolic blood pressure of 160 is four times more likely to have a heart attack than someone with a systolic blood pressure less than 120.

| Chapter 2 | Health Hazard Appraisal |

In 1970, Robbins and Hall published a book for physicians entitled *How to Practice Prospective Medicine*. Their program provided a means to determine the relative risk of dying from various diseases or accidents during each decade of chronological age. It highlights the 10 major causes of death for each decade, identifies lifestyle factors that contribute to increased risk, and calculates a relative risk age. The "risk age" is determined by comparing an individual's chances of dying with others in the same chronological age group based on identified risk factors.

Risk age is not related to biological age. Nevertheless, the identification and elimination of potential life-shortening hazards greatly improves the chances of achieving one's maximum life span. It seems only reasonable that those interested in extending their lives should be interested in avoiding behavior that might shorten them.

Mounting evidence indicates that the quantitative information and recommendations concerning personal health presented in an HHA dramatizes the dangers of unhealthful lifestyles, and motivates people to make positive changes. In summary, Health Hazard Appraisal tells what chances one is taking with his life, and how the odds of surviving the next 10 years can be improved.

USING THE HHA

The appraisal begins with a questionnaire that ascertains factors contributing most directly to personal risks:

1. Lifestyle factors — smoking, drinking, exercising, driving practices, etc.

2. Physical measurements — blood pressure, weight, blood analysis, etc.

3. Presence in or absence from a high risk group, as may have been revealed by a recent health screening — for example, examination for breast or cervical cancer.

4. Personal and family history of diseases — heart disease, cancer, diabetes, etc

5. Personal background — age, sex, ethnic background, etc.

Health Hazard Appraisal Chapter 2

The completed questionnaire is processed by hand or computer, and generates a health forecast with the following information:

1. Risk age — The statistical or actuarial dangers associated with individual habits, family history, and present symptoms.

2. Achievable age — The lowest risk age that can be attained if the recommended changes in living habits and physical condition are made, and a life span prediction based on this risk age.

3. A list of the major health hazards one faces, and specific recommendations to reduce or eliminate them.

SOURCES OF HHA QUESTIONNAIRES

The Society of Prospective Medicine is a professional society comprised of physicians and health care professionals concerned with the promotion of positive health through lifestyle improvement and avoidance of risk factors. They have been instrumental in the development, continuing refinement and improvement of health hazard appraisal systems. The Society's address is:

The Society of Prospective Medicine, 1101 Connecticut Ave #700, Washington DC, 20036 (202) 857-1199.

A list of organizations that have developed health hazard appraisal questionnaires and software is available from the National Health Information Clearinghouse, P.O. Box 1133, Washington, DC 20013-1133.

DO-IT-YOURSELF APPRAISALS

A risk age can be determined manually using a handheld calculator and a risk factor questionnaire in a recent book, *The Longevity Factor — A Revolutionary New System for Prolonging Your Life* (Simon and Schuster) by Walter McQuade and Ann Aikman. Sources for other versions of manual health hazard appraisals are cited in the previously-mentioned publications list from the National Health Information Clearinghouse. Although these questionnaires are not as sophisticated or detailed as the computerized versions, they should be adequate for most purposes.

REFERENCES

Breslow, L., Fielding, J., Afifi, A. A., Couldson, A., Kheifets, L., Valdiviezo, N., Goetz, A., McTyre, R., Peterson, K., and Dane, K. *Risk Factor Update Project*. Atlanta. U.S. Department of Health and Human Services, Centers for Disease Control, Center for Health Promotion and Education, 1985.

Hall, J.H., and Zwemer, J.D. *Prospective Medicine*. 1979. Methodist Hospital of Indiana, Indianapolis.

McQuade, Walter, and Aikman, Ann. *The Longevity Factor — A Revolutionary New System for Prolonging Your Life*. 1979. Simon and Schuster, New York.

Robbins, L., and Hall, J. H. *How to Practice Prospective Medicine*. Indianapolis, Methodist Hospital of Indiana, 1970.

Chapter 3

PERIODIC PHYSICAL EXAMINATIONS

In recent years, there has been a great deal of controversy about the value of routine annual physical examinations. Many physicians now think that the routine exam is a waste of time and money for a healthy, asymptomatic person. They believe that some tests not only may be unwarranted, but also may be potentially harmful—such as excess radiation from unneeded chest X-rays.

Most clinical gerontologists think periodic examinations are essential, due to the special nature of their patients and their unusual nutritional regimens. The examinations are recommended partly for their traditional limited value of identifying diseases at an early stage, when curative intervention is likely to be more effective. Clinical gerontologists conduct the tests not only to detect adverse effects from experimental anti-aging substances, but also to monitor values related to health and for aging measurement protocols.

WHAT TESTS SHOULD BE CONDUCTED?

This question is still unresolved within the medical community. The American Medical Association's Council on Scientific Affairs recommends that healthy adults have medical evaluations at five year intervals until age 40. For those over 40, they recommend periodic evaluations in one to three-year intervals depending on the individual's occupation, health status, and medical history.

Several comprehensive studies have been conducted to evaluate the cost-effectiveness of various tests that are often included in routine physical examinations (American Cancer Society; Breslow and Somers; Canadian Task Force on Periodic Health Examinations; and Frame and Carson). The recommendations from these studies are summarized in *Table 3-I*. It is obvious that these recommendations are conflicting, indicating that both doctors and patients should select examination procedures based on individual factors—such as the patient's age, sex, and health—rather than use a standard protocol for all patients.

Chapter 3 — Periodic Physical Examinations

Surprisingly, the routine electrocardiogram, chest X-ray, urinalysis, and blood test traditionally done in most screening examinations were not recommended in any of the studies. Note that these recommendations rest on the premise of doing routine exams mainly to detect overt disease at an early stage.

AGING — A DISEASE?

Disease is defined by Webster as "an alteration of a living body that impairs its function". The traditional concept that disease is pathological while aging is "normal" is beginning to be questioned by many scientists. Dr. Horton A. Johnson of the College of Physicians and Surgeons, Columbia University (1985), points out that "if one looks hard enough, he can find in every organ or tissue a time-dependent loss of structure and function". The late Dr. Robert Kohn (1985) also emphasized that "every physiological process involved in the maintenance of homeostasis becomes less effective with increasing age" (*Fig. 3-1*).

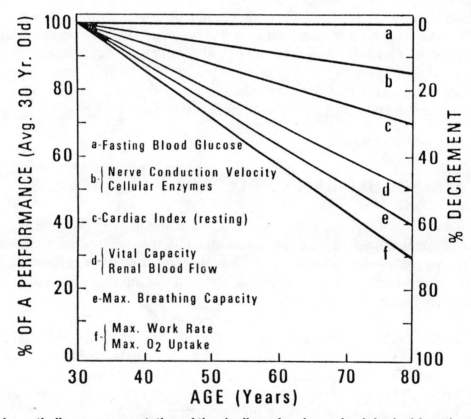

Fig. 3-1. **Schematic linear representation of the decline of various physiological functions with age** (Shock).

Periodic Physical Examinations   Chapter 3

It is a characteristic of biological systems that each has a certain redundancy of functional capacity or functional reserve. his concept is illustrated in *Fig. 3-2*. The vertical axis shows functional capacity. The line parallel to the X-axis is the death threshold. When vitality or functional capacity drop below this minimal level required to sustain life, death occurs. The level of the death threshold reflects the severity of the conditions to which the individual is exposed. If conditions are severe, the threshold will be higher, and the length of life will be shorter. The environmental challenges and stresses that individuals cope with are never completely constant, so the death threshold fluctuates around a mean value (Lamb). Although the decrease in functional capacity due to aging is shown here as a straight line, it is also likely that many factors that raise the death threshold may also accelerate the rate of aging.

As an example of the relationship between disease and the declining functional capacity due to aging and minimal functional capacity necessary to sustain life, consider that although atherosclerosis is present in many 30 year-olds, it may not cause symptomatic cardiovascular disease until age 50 or 60, when the arterial narrowing becomes so severe as to cause inadequate perfusion of some vital organ. Similarly, a pulmonary infection that would be insignificant in a younger person might prove fatal to an older person, due to the age-induced reduction in pulmonary function.

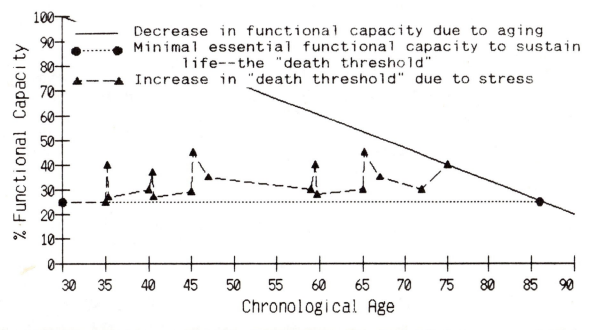

Fig. 3-2. **Relationship between decreasing functional capacity of physiological systems, minimal level required to sustain life, and increased functional requirements caused by stress, injury, disease, or exercise.** The "safety margin" between the minimum essential functional capacity for life and the decreasing functional capacity due to age becomes progressively smaller with age.

At some point these decrements ultimately become manifest in what is traditionally considered a full-blown disease. As mentioned, atherosclerosis is present in many individuals by the age of thirty. Some degree of brain atrophy is "normal" in old age and is not considered pathological. The point at which these conditions constitute disease is problematic, and is often one of semantics more than diagnostics. The distinction between aging and disease becomes progressively more arbitrary as one grows older (Johnson).

In addition to the universal decline of almost all physiological functions with age, the incidence of all diseases also increases with age (*Fig. 3-3*). Kohn (1978) pointed out that if atherosclerosis and cancer were abolished, the increase in life expectancy would be only 9-10 years. Other fatal processes would ultimately cause death--such as respiratory infections and accidents, which show very rapid increases in older individuals. This illustrates the futility of the orthodox treatment-of-individual-disease approach toward life extension. A more effective approach would obviously be to attack the aging process itself as a disease--the one disease suffered by everyone who lives beyond maturity.

Dilman (1981) lends support to this concept in his book *The Law of Deviation of Homeostasis and Diseases of Aging*. In this book, he painstakingly and convincingly points out that the *diseases of aging* (atherosclerosis, cancer, hypertension, diabetes, immune dysfunction, depression, increased body fat) are characterized by similar metabolic shifts. He argues that these metabolic shifts are caused by the aging process--triggered by the aging-induced increased resistance of the hypothalamus to feedback-inhibition. Thus, the symptoms of the *diseases of aging* can be considered to be various overt manifestations of the primary underlying disease — the aging process.

Harman (1984), who conceived the *free radical theory of aging*, has a related view based on his research into free radical pathology. He presents impressive evidence that endogenous free radical reactions cause (or contribute significantly to): cancer, atherosclerosis, hypertension, Alzheimer's disease, amyloidosis, immune deficiency, arthritis, diabetes and Parkinson's disease, among others.

Walford (1974) advances another approach with his *autoimmune theory of aging*. He proposes that many diseases of aging (cancer, autoimmune diseases, infections, and amyloidosis) result from the aging-induced decrease in immune competence.

Each of these theories are incomplete. Nevertheless, they are not mutually exclusive, and there is a great deal of overlap among them. Furthermore, they share the common characteristic of offering diverse yet complementary therapeutic approaches to the aging process.

Effective therapies based on Dilman's, Harman's or Walford's theories--that may be directed at the fundamental causes of aging--should not only alleviate (or prevent) the spectrum of age-related diseases, but may also alter the aging process itself.

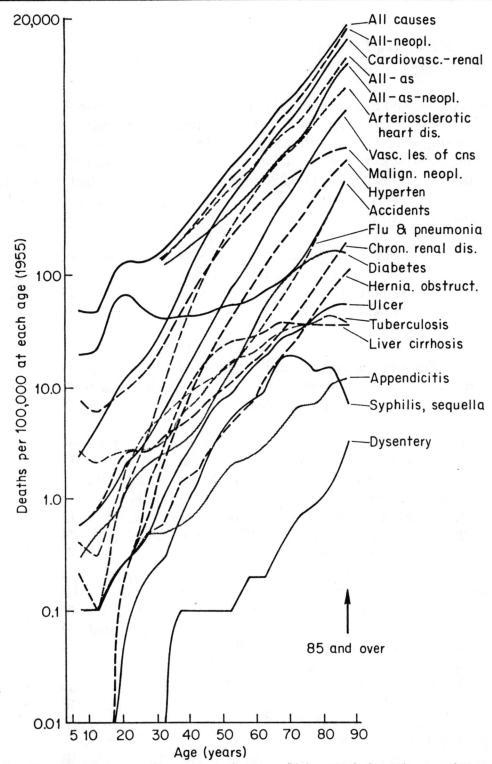

Fig. 3-3. **Age-specific death rates from selected causes** (Kohn, 1963). It can be seen that even if cancer and cardiovascular-related deaths were eliminated, the average life-expectancy would only increase by ten or eleven years. Those who are younger chronologically (and biologically) suffer from less disease.

| Chapter 3 | Periodic Physical Examinations |

WHY ALL AIRLINE PILOTS ARE UNDER 60 YEARS OLD

In 1959, the FAA decreed that commercial pilots could no longer be medically cleared to fly because of the risk of sudden incapacity. The FAA, implicitly recognizing aging as a disease--but lacking any way to diagnose it--arbitrarily picked the age of 60 as "too old" for a pilot to fly--while admitting in the same document that "the evidences of the aging process are so varied in different individuals that it is not possible to determine accurately with respect to any individual whether the presence or absence of any specific defect...led to or precluded a sudden incapacitating attack" (Pyle).

The problem with the routine physical examination is that it is unable to detect the disease of aging. Probably the best example of this is the rigorous flight physical examination which commercial airline pilots must undergo every 6 months. Surprising to many is the fact that this exam can be passed by a healthy 65 or 70-year old former pilot just as easily as by many 45 year-old active pilots.

Some former pilots who are physiologically young at 65 are unfairly prohibited from flying, while there are probably some biologically older 55 year-old pilots who may be risking the lives of their passengers by being allowed to continue to fly.

Clearly, the FAA, the Airline Pilots Association, and anyone who flies a commercial airline would seem to have a stake in aging measurement. In fact, in 1980, the Institute of Medicine of the National Academy of Sciences, formed a Committee to Study Scientific Evidence Relevant to Mandatory Age Retirement for Airline Pilots, to investigate whether the "age-60 rule" should be changed, abolished, or kept in place. The Committee published the results of their study in 1981 (Anonymous. Institute of Medicine).

The Commission was composed of representatives of the Aerospace Medical Association, Air Line Pilots Association, American Medical Association, Civil Aeromedical Institute, FAA, and many other distinguished organizations. Although they contacted a number of researchers from many prestigious institutes, incredibly, none of the scientists who developed the systems described in the rest of this book were consulted!

Of the contributing scientists, only Dr. Nathan Shock, of the NIA's Gerontology Research Center, had been a specialist in biological aging measurement, and only Dr. Stanley Mohler, former President of the Aerospace Medical Association, had any experience in evaluating the effects of age on pilot performance.

Mohler (1981, 1985) thinks that the "age 60 rule" is untenable scientifically--and that the only requirements a pilot should meet to continue flying beyond age 60 are that the aviator: (1) be free from impairing disease; (2) be capable of performing the job requirements; and

Periodic Physical Examinations   Chapter 3

(3) desire to continue flying (While I agree with him in principle, I think he overlooks that aging itself is an "impairing disease", and that it needs to be quantified by some means other than simple chronological age. This may be a semantic disagreement, as he concedes the requirement for the aviator to demonstrate the ability to perform the job, implying some means of objective evaluation).

The conclusions of this study (contrary to the recommendations of Shock and Mohler) were that biological age could not be measured, and that the age 60 rule should be retained without change. To the Committee's credit, a number of worthwhile suggestions were made for the development of functional age indices for pilots (that would have contributed to the development of biological aging measurement systems in general). However, no action has been taken on any of these recommendations by any of the organizations involved. The U.S. Navy has continued to pursue this line of research for active duty combat pilots, however (Braune and Wickens)--research that could easily be adapted to the commercial aviation environment.

The Air Line Pilots Association is no longer pushing to change the rule--they are more interested in retiring the older pilots, to allow younger pilots to be promoted. The Aerospace Medical Association is not studying the issue. The FAA has lost interest in the project (except for trying to discourage those who are trying to challenge the rule). And the NIA, the Department charged by Congress to develop a better understanding of biological age, has done remarkably little to accomplish this objective.

ROUTINE EXAMINATIONS FOR EXPERIMENTAL AGING RETARDATION

I recommend at least one examination per year be conducted, including tests from *Table 3-I*. In addition, although not generally recommended by the study groups, I also recommend that a sequential multiple analysis (SMA) be conducted, using some or all of the tests recommended by Pearson and Shaw (*Tables 3-II* and *3-III*). Although the diagnostic yield in terms of early disease detection is small for asymptomatic patients during routine examinations, the cost is quite reasonable. Also, as previously mentioned, the results from many tests in SMA panels are required for several aging measurement test systems.

Table 3-IV lists a battery of routine clinical laboratory tests used in one or more of the aging measurement systems in this book. Even if a clinical gerontologist who routinely assesses biological age is unavailable, by including these tests in periodic physical examinations, individuals will be able to accomplish several of these measurement systems. Other, more complicated tests are required for completion of many of the systems, however. Specific details for the incorporation of these tests into aging measurement calculations and utilization in the

Chapter 3	Periodic Physical Examinations

evaluation of life extension programs are provided in the particular chapters which describe each system. Recommendations for their use are summarized in Chapter 23.

In addition, I recommend the enzyme-linked immunosorbent assay (ELISA) be conducted for antibodies to the human immunodeficiency virus (HIV)--the etiologic agent for the acquired immunodeficiency syndrome (AIDS). Although AIDS remains largely restricted to several distinct populations (male homosexuals, illicit intravenous drug users, and hemophiliacs), I think this test should be considered for the following reasons: (1) the disease is 100% fatal; (2) all who have the disease are sero-positive for the HIV antibody; (3) all modes of transmission for the disease are not known for certain (a recent report hypothesizes that it could be transmitted by vectors such as mosquitoes and fleas [Branch]); (4) the incidence of the disease is still increasing geometrically--thus requiring increased surveillance; (5) the incubation period is not yet clearly defined. If an individual becomes sero-positive for the HIV antibody, tests for immune function (as described in Appendix B. 12) should be done with increased frequency--and if the individual demonstrates a decline in normal immune function and confirmatory tests for AIDS (i.e., Western Blot) are positive, immuno-stimulant therapy can be initiated early to delay the development of disease symptoms.

Periodic Physical Examinations — Chapter 3

TABLE 3-1. **Recommendations for frequency of routine diagnostic examinations**

Age	32	33	34	35	36	37	38	39	40	41	42	43	44	45	46	47	48	49	50	51	52	53
History & Physical			B						B					B					B			
M.D. Breast Exam	AF	F	AB	F					F AB	F AB	F AB		F AB		F AB		F AB	A	CF AB			
Pelvic Exam	AF	F	AB	F		AF			F AB	AF	A	A	AF	AF	AF	AF	AF	A	F AB	A	AF	A
Rectal Exam			B						AB	A	A	A	A	AB	A	A	A	A	AB	A		A
Hearing Test														B								
Tetanus-Diptheria					C				B						C				B			
Influenza Immunization																						
Blood pressure	CF	F	BC	CF		F			F BC	BF		F	F	BC	CF	BC	CF	C	F BC	BC	F BC	BC
Pap smear	F AC	F	C AB		F		AF		F BC	F BC	A		AF	BC	F	AB	F		CF AB		BF	A
Cholesterol	F	F	C AB	F					BF				F	B		F	F		B		F	
VDRL	F							F			F								F			
PPD																			F			
Stool for occult blood									BF	BF		F	F	BC	F	AB F	BC	CF	CF AB		BF	A
Sigmoidoscopy																		C		A		A
Mammography					A														C AB			

A = American Cancer Society C = Canadian Task Force on Periodic Heath Examinations
B = Breslow and Somers F = Frame and Carlson

Table 3-1. Recommended frequency of routine diagnostic examinations

Chapter 3 — Periodic Physical Examinations

Age	54	55	56	57	58	59	60	61	62	63	64	65	66	67	68	69	70	71	72	73	74	75
History & Physical	B						B						B				B		B		B	B
M.D. Breast Exam				CF AB			F AB						F AB				F AB					AB
Pelvic Exam	AF	AB	AF	A	AF	A	F AB	F AB	F AB	A	F AB	A	F AB	A	F AB	A	F AB	A	AB	A	AB	AB
Rectal Exam	A	AB	A			A	AB	A	AB	A	AB	A	AB	A	AB	A	AB	A	AB	A	AB	AB
Hearing Test	B						B															
Tetanus-Diptheria			C				B						C				B					
Influenza Immunization							B			B		BC	C				B					BC
Blood pressure	F BC	BC	F BC	BC	F BC	BC	F BC	BC	F BC	BC	F BC	BC	F BC	BC	F BC	BC	F BC	BC				BC
Pap smear	BF								F AB			C AB	F	AF			F BC	A	B	A	BC	
Cholesterol	B	F					BF					B		B			B					B
VDRL																						
PPD							F															
Stool for occult blood																	CF AB	C AB			C AB	
Sigmoidoscopy	A					A					A			A			A					A
Mammography					C AB	AB																AB

A = American Cancer Society   C = Canadian Task Force on Periodic Heath Examinations
B = Breslow and Somers   F = Frame and Carlson

Table 3-I. (cont'd) **Recommended frequency of routine diagnostic examinations**

Periodic Physical Examinations   Chapter 3

TABLE 3-II

CLINICAL LABORATORY TESTS--Short Screen for Toxic Effects

   HEMATOLOGY
- CBC (complete blood count): Red blood cell count, white blood cell count with differential, and hemoglobin level

   SERUM CHEMISTRY
- SGOT (serum glutamic oxaloacetic transaminase)
- SGPT (serum glutamic pyruvic transaminase)
  urate (uric acid)
- glucose
  sodium
  potassium
  bilirubin
- creatinine
- BUN (blood urea nitrogen)

   URINE
     sodium
     potassium
     cystine
     oxalate
     urate
     albumin
     occult blood

   MISCELLANEOUS
     stool guaiac
     bleeding time

- (Tests included in one or more aging measurement systems).

(From *Life Extension*, by Durk Pearson and Sandy Shaw. Courtesy, Warner Books).

TABLE 3-III

CLINICAL LABORATORY TESTS FOR DETERMINING TOXICITY AND METABOLIC EFFECTS OF EXPERIMENTAL AGE RETARDING NUTRIENTS

SERUM CHEMISTRY
- urate (uric acid)
- •glucose
- sodium
- potassium
- •cholesterol, total
- cholesterol, free
- cholesterol, esterified
- total lipids
- •phospholipids
- •triglycerides
- total fatty acids
- free fatty acids
- •albumin
- •alkaline phosphatase
- acid phosphatase
- amylase
- bilirubin, total and direct
- •BUN
- •creatinine
- CPK (creatinine phosphokinase)
- immunoglobulin electrophoresis (expensive option--tests some immune functions)
- LDH (lactic dehydrogenase)
- •lipoprotein electrophoresis (always desirable; essential if lipids are too high; this test gives the relative amounts of VLDL, LDL, and HDL)
- PBI (protein bound iodine)
- •SGOT
- •SGPT
- G6PD (Glucose-6-phosphate-dehydrogenase)
- •T-3
- •T-4
- •TSH (thyroid stimulating hormone)

URINE
- sodium
- potassium
- cystine

| **Periodic Physical Examinations** | Chapter 3 |

    oxalate
    urate (uric acid)
    albumin
    occult blood

MISCELLANEOUS
    stool guaiac test
    BSP
   •complete blood count, with white cell differential
   •hemoglobin level
    bleeding time
   •ESR (erythrocyte sedimentation rate)
    red blood cell osmotic fragility
    pulmonary macrophage sputum test (an immune assay)[*]

[*]A special sample mailing kit can be obtained from the following two laboratories:

Micronetic Laboratories
1420 Koll Circle
San Jose, CA 95112
(408) 297-7711.

California Micropathology Associates
16311 Ventura Blvd., Suite 860
Encino, CA 91436
(23) 995-7787

Micronet Laboratories provides a photomicrograph of the specimen as well as a pathologist's evaluation.

•(Tests included in one or more aging measurement systems).

(From *Life Extension*, by Durk Pearson and Sandy Shaw. Courtesy, Warner Books).

TABLE 3-IV

ROUTINE CLINICAL LABORATORY TESTS INCLUDED IN AGING MEASUREMENT SYSTEMS

SERUM CHEMISTRY
    cholesterol (total and HDL)
    glucose
    total protein
    BUN
    alkaline phosphatase
    SGOT, SGPT

HEMATOLOGY
    hemoglobin
    erythrocyte sedimentation rate

AUDIOMETRY
    hearing loss in decibels at 500, 1,000, 2,000, 4,000 and 6,000 Hz*

VISION
    near point of vision in cm, in, and diopters
    visual acuity

PULMONARY FUNCTIONS
    FEV_1*
    vital capacity*
    forced vital capacity*

CARDIOVASCULAR
    systolic and diastolic blood pressure
    maximal oxygen uptake*

DENTAL
    caries index
    periodontal index

Periodic Physical Examinations Chapter 3

ANTHROPOMETRIC
    height
    weight
    hand grip[*]
    triceps skinfold

NEUROPSYCHOLOGICAL
    O'Connor Pegboard test of finger dexterity[*]
    Purdue Pegboard test of finger dexterity[*]
    vibratory sensitivity[*]

MISCELLANEOUS
    oral glucose tolerance test (OGTT)
    creatinine clearance

[*](Although these are routine tests, they require diagnostic equipment that some general physicians may not have on hand).

REFERENCES

American Cancer Society: ACS report on the cancer-related health check-up. *CA* 30: 194, 1980.

Anonymous. *Airline Pilot Age, Health, and Performance*. Institute of Medicine, National Academy Press, Washington, D.C., 1981.

Branch, D. Insect vector in Florida AIDS cluster not confirmed. *Internal Medicine News*. (1985) 18:15, 3, 44.

Braune, R., and Wickens, C. D. Individual differences and age-related performance assessment in aviators. Part I: Battery development and assessment. Part II: Initial battery Validation. Technical Report EPL-83-7/NAMRL-83-2 and EPL-83-4/NAMRL-83-1. Naval Aerospace Medical Research Laboratory, Pensacola, FL.

Breslow, L., and Somers, A.R.: The lifetime health- monitoring program. A Practical approach to preventive medicine. *N Engl J Med*, 296: 601, 1977.

Brewer, L. M. The periodic health examination. Of what real value is it? *Postgraduate Medicine*, Vol. 74, No. 5, Nov 1983, 125-129.

Canadian Task Force on Periodic Health Examinations: The periodic health examination. *Can Med Assoc J* 121: 1193; 1979.

Council on Scientific Affairs, Division of Scientific Activities, American Medical Association. Chicago: Medical evaluations of healthy persons. *JAMA*, 249: 1626, 1983.

Delbanco, T. L., and Taylor, W. C.: The periodic health examination: 1980. *Ann Int Med* 92: 251, 1980.

Frame, P.S., and Carlson, S.J. A critical review of periodic health screening using specific screening criteria. *J Fam Pract*, 2: 29, 1975.

Harman, D. Free radical theory of aging: The "free radical" diseases. *J Am Aging Assn*. (1984) 7:4, 111-131.

Johnson, H.A. Is aging physiological or pathological? in: *Relations Between Normal Aging and Disease*, by H. A. Johnson (ed.). New York, Raven Press. 1985.

Kohn, R.R. Human aging and disease. *J Chron Disease* (1963). 16: 5-21.

Kohn, R.R. *Principles of Mammalian Aging*, 2d ed. (1978). Prentice Hall, Englewood Cliffs, pp. 151-152.

Kohn, R.R. Aging and age-related diseases: Normal processes, in: *Relations Between Normal Aging and Disease*, by H.A. Johnson (ed.). New York, Raven Press. 1985. Lamb, M.J. Biology of Aging (1977). Blackie, London, pp. 3-4.

Machol, L. Routine screening: Which patients, which tests, how often? *Diagnosis*, Dec. 1983, 40-61.

Medical Practice Committee, American College of Physicians: Periodic health examination: a guide for designing individualized preventive health care in the asymptomatic patient. *Ann Int Med* 95: 729, 1981.

Mohler, S.R. Functional aging: Present status of assessments regarding airline pilot retirement. *Aerospace Medicine*, (1973) 44: 9, 1062-1066.

Mohler, S.R. Reasons for eliminating the "age 60" regulation for airline pilots. *Aviation, Space, and Environmental Medicine*. (1981), 52:8, 445-454.

Mohler, S.R. Age and space flight. *Aviation, Space, and Environmental Medicine*. (1985), 56:7, 714-717.

Moskowitz, M.A., and Osband, M.E. *The Complete Book of Medical Tests*. W. W. Norton and Co., 1984.

Pearson, D., and Shaw, S. *Life Extension, A Practical Scientific Approach*. New York, Warner Books, 1982, pp. 441-453.

Pinckney, C., and Pinckney, E.R. *Do it Yourself Medical Testing*. 1983. New York, Facts on File.

Pyle, J.T. Maximum age limitations for pilots. Federal Register. Doc. 59-10304, filed 4 Dec. 1959. Civil Air Regulations Amendment 42-44, effective March 15, 1960.

Shock, N.W. Systems Integration, in: *Handbook of the Biology of Aging*, 1977, New York, Van Nostrand Reinhold Co.

Walford, R.L. The immunologic theory of aging, current status. *Fed Proc*, 1974, 33: 2020-2027.

Chapter 4

THE ADULT GROWTH EXAMINATION

Dr. Robert F. Morgan (*Fig. 4-1*), a clinical psychologist and specialist in applied gerontology, has been studying biological aging measurement systems for over 20 years. He was formerly the Dean for Academic and Professional Affairs at the California School of Professional Psychology in Fresno, California, and is now the Dean of Academic Affairs, Pacific Graduate School of Psychology, Menlo Park, California. He is also the Founding President of the International Association of Applied Psychology. While completing his doctorate degree in psychology at Michigan State University in the mid-1960s, he developed an aging measurement system called the Adult Growth Examination (AGE) (Morgan, 1968, 1972, 1977, 1981, 1986; Morgan and Wilson).

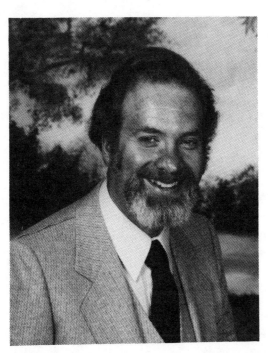

Fig. 4-1. Dr. Robert F. Morgan.

Chapter 4 — The Adult Growth Examination

AGE is a relatively easy test battery to administer, comprising three basic tests, and five supplementary tests. Since first developing AGE, Morgan has served on the faculties of several American and Canadian Universities, and has continued to refine and validate his system. While the system may lack the comprehensiveness and precision of most of the measurement systems described in Part II, it remains the simplest and most widely tested system currently available.

REQUIREMENTS FOR THE BASIC TESTS:

1. Sphygmomanometer and stethoscope (Appendix A, 1-1).
2. Audiometer (Appendix A, 3-1).
3. Equipment for measuring near vision (Appendix A, 4-1).

REQUIREMENTS FOR THE SUPPLEMENTARY TESTS:

1. Blood chemistry tests.
2. Dental exam.
3. O'Connor Pegboard Test Set (Appendix A, 5-1).

AGE BASIC TESTS:

1. Systolic blood pressure (Appendix B, 1-1) (sitting), in mm Hg. Three separate measurements are taken at intervals between the other tests. The average of the three readings is used.
2. Audiometric exam (Appendix B, 3-1), in decibel loss for best ear at 6,000 Hz.
3. Near vision (Appendix B, 4-1), in inches.

The Adult Growth Examination — Chapter 4

SUPPLEMENTARY TESTS:

1. Serum cholesterol (Appendix B, 9-1), in mg/100 ml, based on a random, non-fasting sample.
2. Oral glucose tolerance test at one hour (Appendix B, 11-1), in mg/100 ml. This protocol varies from the standard in that it is based on a non-fasting sample, one hour after ingestion of 50 gm of glucose.
3. Periodontal index (Appendix B, 7-1).
4. Caries index (Appendix B, 7-2).
5. Finger dexterity (Appendix B, 5-1) in number of holes filled in 4 minutes using the O'Connor Pegboard.

SCORING THE TEST:

Morgan bases his scores on a single point for each chronological year--forming a single line determined by the mean values from the studies on which his tests are based. It should be stressed that individual variability is extensive, and no one should be overly concerned if they score below average for their age on some tests. Of major importance--similar to all aging measurement tests--is the longitudinal change of each parameter from successive tests.

BASIC TESTS

Plot the score for each basic subtest on corresponding graphs in *Figs. 4-2* through *4-6*, and find the mean body age for that value. Some of these figures differ from graphs for the same tests in Appendix B. I have retained Morgan's values in this chapter.

Enter the raw score for each subtest (hearing, near vision, systolic blood pressure) and the equivalent age score on the calculation sheet at the end of the chapter. Then place these scores in order from highest to lowest. The middle score is the biological age. If one of the three basic subtests has not been done for any reason, the average of the other two age scores is the biological age.

Chapter 4 — The Adult Growth Examination

SUPPLEMENTARY TESTS

The supplementary tests are scored using *Figs. 4-7* through *4-14*. Morgan's values for cholesterol and glucose are for random non-fasting samples. If the results are based on fasting samples, the appropriate graphs in Appendix B should be used.

Morgan deemphasizes the importance of the supplementary tests, and feels that they should be used only to provide a rough correlation with the body age score from the Basic subtests. He stresses that the main emphasis of AGE should be on the three basic AGE tests of (1) blood pressure, (2) hearing, and (3) near vision.

CLINICAL USE OF THE ADULT GROWTH EXAMINATION (AGE):

AGE is one of the few aging measurement systems that has been used extensively. It has been used by Morgan to measure changes in biological age over time, and to assess the effectiveness of interventionist regimens designed to reduce biological age.

A study from the Departments of Biology and Psychology, Maharishi International University in Fairfield, Iowa, reported on the effects of transcendental meditation on biological age, using the Adult Growth Examination to quantify the results (Wallace, et al). The study reported a significant reduction in biological age for meditators compared to controls.

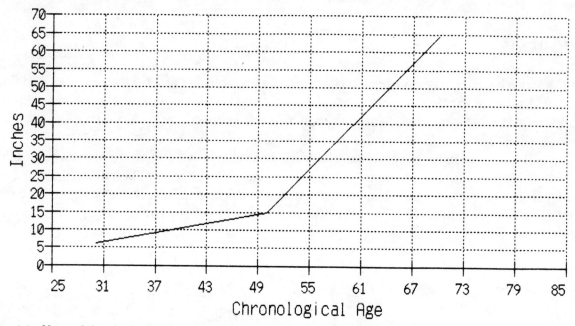

Fig. 4-2. **Near vision in inches--men and women** (Morgan and Wilson).

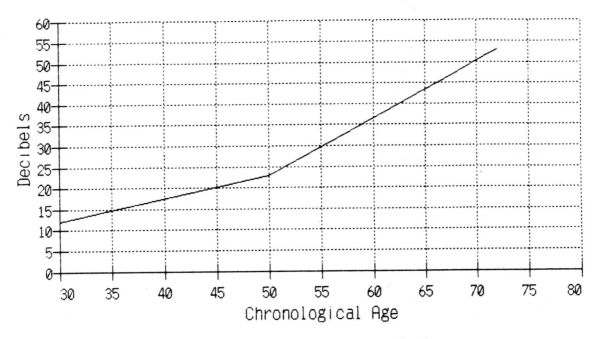

Fig. 4-3. **Hearing loss in decibels at 6,000 Hz--men** (Morgan and Wilson).

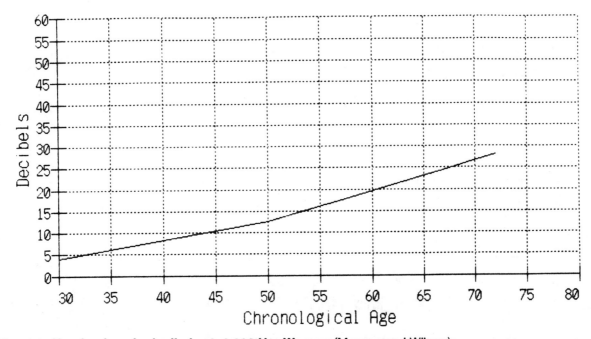

Fig. 4-4. **Hearing loss in decibels at 6,000 Hz--Women** (Morgan and Wilson).

Chapter 4 **The Adult Growth Examination**

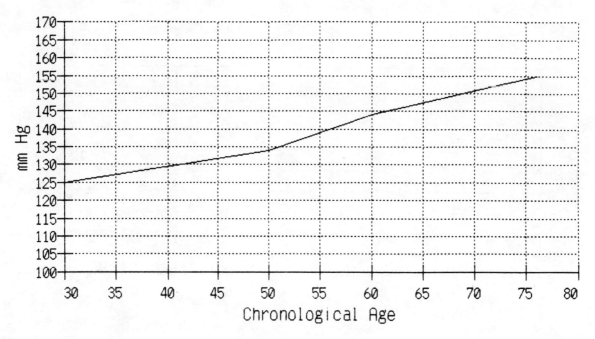

Fig. 4-5. **Systolic blood pressure--men** (Morgan and Wilson).

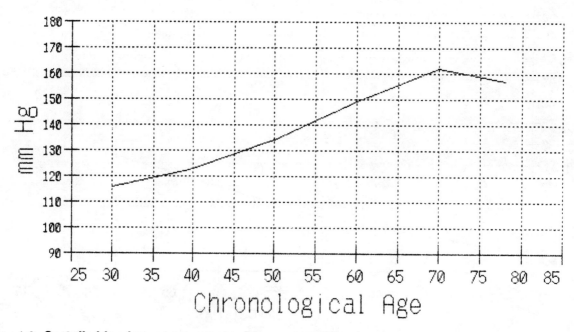

Fig. 4-6. **Systolic blood pressure--women** (Morgan and Wilson).

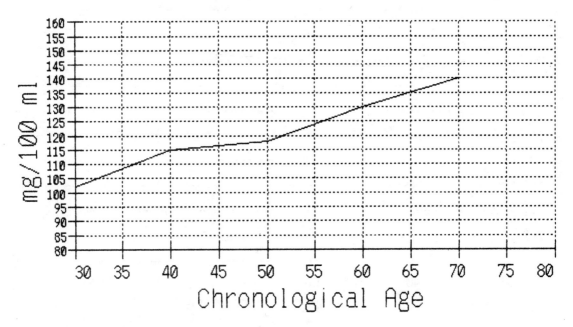

Fig. 4-7. **Oral glucose tolerance test at one hour--men** (Morgan and Wilson).

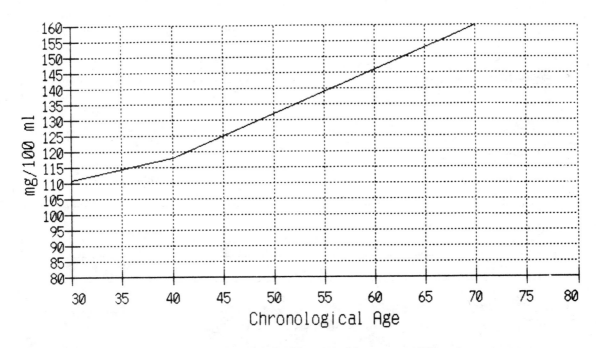

Fig. 4-8. **Oral glucose tolerance test at one hour--women** (Morgan and Wilson).

Chapter 4

The Adult Growth Examination

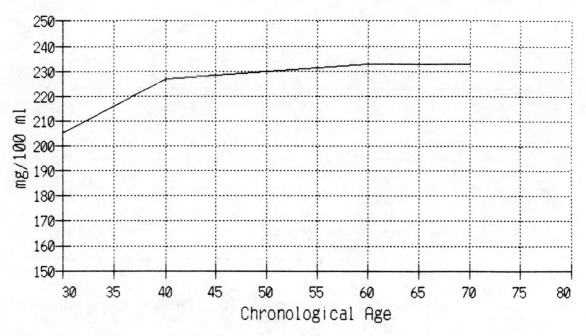

Fig. 4-9. **Serum cholesterol--men (non-fasting)** (Morgan and Wilson).

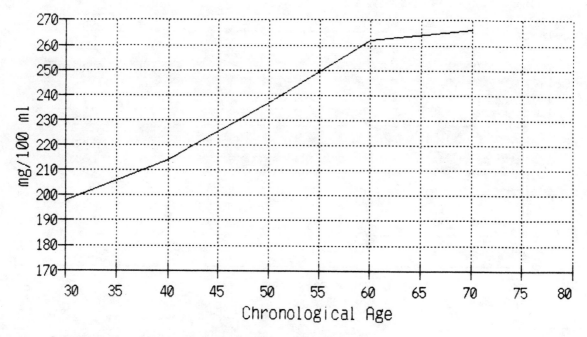

Fig. 4-10. **Serum cholesterol--women (non-fasting)** (Morgan and Wilson).

The Adult Growth Examination — Chapter 4

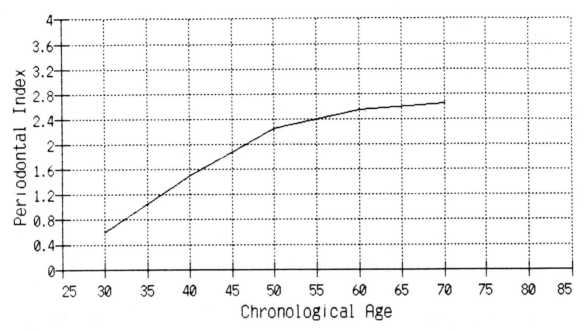

Fig. 4-11. **Periodontal index--men** (Morgan and Wilson).

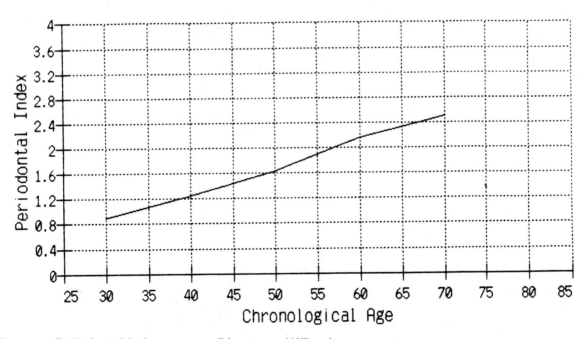

Fig. 4-12. **Periodontal index--women** (Morgan and Wilson).

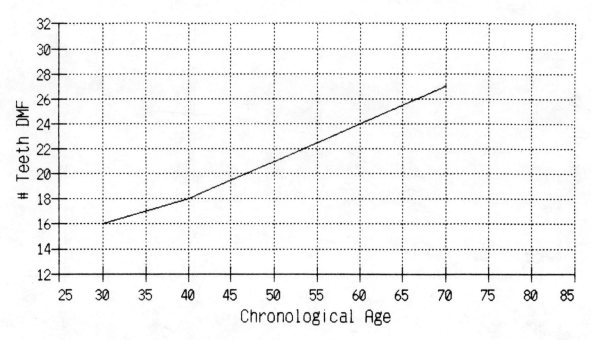

Fig. 4-13. **Caries index--men** (Morgan and Wilson).

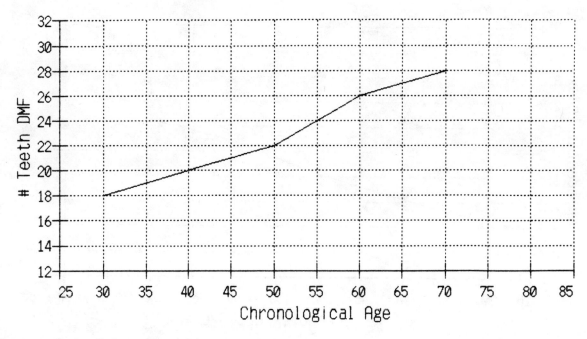

Fig. 4-14. **Caries index--women** (Morgan and Wilson).

The Adult Growth Examination — Chapter 4

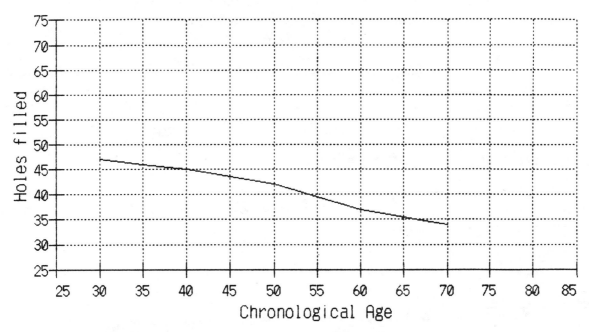

Fig. 4-15. **Finger dexterity--men and women** (Morgan and Wilson).

Chapter 4	The Adult Growth Examination

CALCULATION SHEET
ADULT GROWTH EXAMINATION (AGE)
FOR MEN AND WOMEN

Name: _____   Date of Exam : ___/___/___

　　　　　　　　　　　　　　　　　　Date of Birth: ___/___/___

　　　　　　　　　　　　　　　　　　Chronological Age: _____

<u>Systolic blood pressure in mm Hg</u>

   1st reading: _____
   2nd reading: _____   Average reading: _____
   3rd reading: _____

<u>Auditory acuity</u>
  Min. vol. (in db's heard) at 6,000 Hz: _____

<u>Near vision</u>
  Nearest point indicator in inches : _____

<u>CALCULATED AGES</u>　　　　　　　<u>PLACED IN ORDER (HIGH TO LOW)</u>

Blood pressure age : _____ 　　　　1. _____

Auditory acuity age: _____ 　　　　2. _____

Near vision age   : _____ 　　　　3. _____

The middle score is the biological age according to Morgan. If one or more of the three basic subtests are unable to be conducted, the average of the two scores obtained is the "AGE" biological age.

(Plot on a graph in Appendix C) "AGE" age: _____

<u>Supplementary Tests</u>　　　　<u>Body Age</u>

Finger dexterity : _____ 　　_____

Serum glucose   : _____ 　　_____

Serum cholesterol: _____ 　　_____

Periodontal index: _____ 　　_____

Caries index   : _____ 　　_____

REFERENCES

Morgan, R. F. The Adult Growth Examination: Preliminary comparisons of physical aging in adults by sex and race. *Perceptual and Motor Skills*, 1968, 27, 595-599.

Morgan, R. F. *Conquest of Aging: Modern Measurement and Intervention.* Pueblo, CO. Applied Gerontology Communications, 1977.

Morgan, R. F. *Measurement of Human Aging in Applied Gerontology.* Dubuque, Iowa. Kendall/Hunt, 1981 a.

Morgan, R.F. *Interventions in Applied Gerontology.* Toronto, Kendall/Hunt Publishing Company, 1981.

Morgan, R.F., and Wilson, J. *Growing Younger--Adding Years to Your Life by Measuring and Controlling Your Body Age.* New York, Methuen, 1982.

Morgan, R.F. Personal communications, 4 September, 1983, and 11 February, 1984.

Morgan, R. F. *The Adult Growth Examination Adult Body Age Test Manual.* Fresno, International Association of Applied Psychology, Division of Gerontological Psychology, 1986.

Morgan, R. F., and Fevens, S. K. Reliability of the Adult Growth Examination: A standardized test of individual aging. *Perceptual and Motor Skills*, 1972, 34, 415-419.

Wallace, R. K., Dillbeck, M. Jacobe, E., and Harrington, B. The effects of the Transcendental Meditation and TM-SIDHI program on the aging process. *Int J Neuroscience*, 1982, Vol 16, 53-58.

Part II

Multiple Regression Analysis

Chapter 5

CLINICAL TEST BATTERIES

One does not need to be a gerontologist to differentiate between an old and a young person. This is obvious, even to a child. However, the changes occurring from day to day and even from year to year are not so easy to observe. It is only after many years have passed, after wrinkles have appeared, hair has turned grey, and muscle tone has been lost, that aging changes are readily apparent. Age-related functional declines do not all start at the same time, nor do they proceed at the same rate (*Fig. 5-1*).

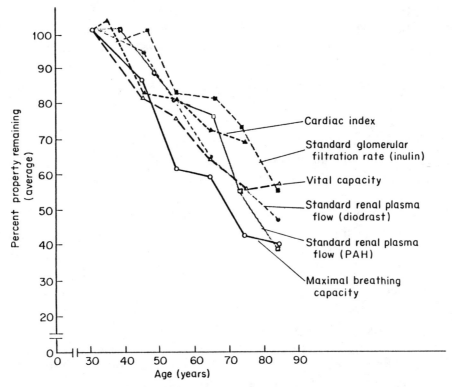

Fig. 5-1. **Variable rate of decline of many physiological functions** (Shock, 1960).

Chapter 5 — Clinical Test Batteries

Many gerontologists think that a test battery that measures a number of functions known to change significantly with age should give a good approximation of one's physiological age status, and should provide a more accurate estimate of biological age than is possible by simple observation and merely guessing at someone's age.

Dr. Nathan Shock, former Scientific Director of the National Institute on Aging, maintains that some combination of tests can be assembled to serve as an index of biological age, and that such a combination of tests should give more accurate predictions than would any single test (Shock, 1981). Important questions remain: How do we know which functions to test; and how do we determine the relative importance of each function?

One way to combine a series of diverse tests into a single value that correlates with chronological age is by multiple regression analysis. Mathematical linear regression is a statistical method for determining an equation which represents a straight line that best fits a set of two or more data pairs. The line generated by the solution of the equation gives a graphic portrayal of the relationship between the variables.

In applying this method to biological aging assessment, a number of physiological and biochemical measurements are made on a large number of people, and the relative correlation of each parameter with age is determined. Because most measurements which change with age do so in a linear fashion, an equation can be calculated based on the results of the test battery. Biological ages of individuals can be obtained by inserting an individual's own values into the equations and solving the equation. This gives a value close to the subject's biological age.

To determine individual biological ages using this method, it is obviously necessary to: (1) select one or more equations calculated by the research groups; (2) conduct the tests; (3) insert the values from the tests into the formulae; and (4) solve the equations.

The concept is complicated by the fact that many different equations have been calculated for both men and women using a variety of clinical laboratory tests. Unfortunately, few of the researchers attempted to validate any of the equations by repeating either their own, or anyone else's study. Instead, they usually used different combinations of tests, and calculated new equations for each set of studies.

In order to test the validity of the equations in Chapters 6-18, a computer program was designed by Dr. Jack Campbell, one of my associates. Using this program and standardized age-adjusted mean values for each variable (from Appendix B), we found that several of the equations as originally published gave aberrant biological ages. Inquiry was made to the scientists who conducted the studies, and in each case they found that a coefficient had been transposed, a decimal point misplaced, or the units of measurement had been incorrect in the

Clinical Test Batteries — Chapter 5

original published article. We made appropriate corrections so that each equation now gives estimated biological ages that appear to be reasonably accurate.

The equations have been tested for comparative accuracy by "dry-labbing" and by limited clinical studies. It is still not possible to state unequivocally which is the best or most accurate. This illustrates that much of what we do in clinical gerontology is guesswork. Dr. Roy Walford (*Fig. 5-2*), Professor of Pathology at UCLA (and author of *Maximum Life Span* and *The One Hundred and Twenty Year Diet*) says, however, that it is "educated guesswork" (1983). Since the equations in this book were generally calculated from large numbers of test subjects with standard statistical methods, they should give statistically reliable results that are both accurate and reproducible. At the present time, they are probably the best means at our disposal to measure biological age and aging rates.

Chapter 23 gives specific recommendations for test battery selection and use in biological aging measurement and age-retarding program evaluation and adjustment.

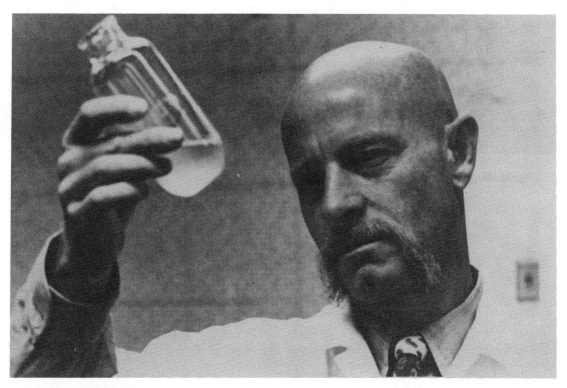

Fig. 5-2. **Dr. Roy Walford**.

REFERENCES

Shock, N.W. Indices of functional age, in: *Aging: A Challenge to Science and Society, Vol. 1, Biology*. Danon, D., Shock, N.W., and Marois, M. (eds). New York: Oxford University Press, 1981, pp. 270-286.

Shock, N. W. Discussion on mortality and measurement, in: Strehler, B. L., Ebert, J. D., Blass, H. B., and Shock, N. W. (eds) *The Biology of Aging*. American Institute of Biological Sciences, Wash. D.C. 1960.

Walford, R.L. *Maximum Life Span*. 1983. New York: W. W. Norton, Inc.

Chapter 6

AMERICAN TEST BATTERY
Harvard University

An interesting attempt to measure biological age by measuring the dimensions of various parts of the body was performed by the late Dr. Albert Damon of Harvard University (1972). Using standard anthropometric techniques (Hertzberg, et al), Damon and his colleagues measured 51 lengths, widths and girths of different body parts of 600 men, ranging in age from 25-75. He selected the ten measurements correlating most closely with chronological age, and used them to calculate an aging measurement equation.

BASIS FOR USING PHYSICAL MEASUREMENTS

While Damon's rationale may seem obscure, it is based on sound reasoning. Changes in physical appearance are one of the most obvious manifestations of the aging process (*Fig. 6-1*). Dr. Gary Borkan (1980)--whose work is described in chapter 12--asked physicians involved in aging measurement studies at the Veteran's Administration to make preliminary guesses of subjects' ages prior to their undergoing more sophisticated aging measurements. He found that those who were estimated to be older than their chronological ages (based solely on physical appearance) actually scored older biologically. Similarly, most of those who appeared younger also scored younger. Damon tried to establish a method to objectively quantify such subjective appraisals of appearance.

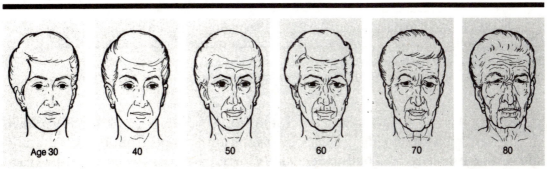

Fig. 6-1. **Sequence of facial changes that occur with age**. Courtesy, *Postgraduate Medicine*, April 1984,

The principle of using body measurements as an indicator of age is further exemplified by the ability of most pediatricians to make an accurate assessment of a child's age if sequential measurements of the child's height, weight, and head circumference are known. These data can be compared with one of several standard pediatric growth charts (*Fig. 6-2*) to determine age.

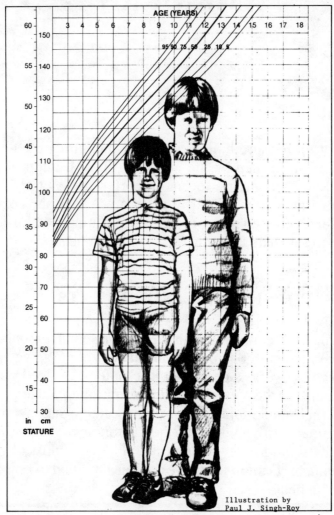

Fig. 6-2. **Pediatric Growth Chart** (Illustration by Paul J. Singh-Roy, abstracted with permission from *Patient Care*, September 30, 1984. Copyright 1984, Patient Care Communications, Inc., Darien, CT All rights reserved).

Although similar charts have not been developed for adults because skeletal growth has ceased, it is well known that changes in body composition result from aging. Alterations in bone and cartilage density, lean body mass, hair color and hair density occur as the years pass.

One may question the significance to aging measurement of such superficial observations as balding, grayness, and other obvious cosmetic changes, surmising that they are unrelated to loss of vitality or increased mortality. Although this question is certainly valid, another consideration is that these changes may be of some significance that we do not yet appreciate. Since these changes in appearance are due to changes in the tissues--ultimately resulting from age-related changes in cells--the loss of hair, reduction in hair pigmentation, decrease in muscle size and strength and other physical characteristics are direct reflections of cellular changes. Since superficial changes are directly related to more fundamental aging processes, the possibility exists that therapeutic regimens aimed at restoring youthful appearance may serendipitously affect primary aging processes as well.

For example, growth of hair has been demonstrated in some bald or balding men using the anti-hypertensive drug *minoxidil* (Upjohn), both orally and as a topical preparation. Although it has been hypothesized that the regrowth was due to vasodilation resulting in improved blood flow to the scalp, this has been questioned. It may be that minoxidil somehow restores the cells of the hair follicles to more youthful levels by an unknown action on these (and other?) cells.

ADVANTAGES, DISADVANTAGES AND SIGNIFICANCE OF DAMON'S METHOD

Determination of biological age from body measurements and observations may be one of the least sensitive and least accurate means of measuring *absolute* biological age, due to: (1) the gross measurements made; (2) the difficulty to accurately quantify the degree of grayness or baldness; (3) the slowness and (4) slight degree of change of most of the parameters. Finally--as mentioned above--some may question the significance of such measurements.

Nevertheless, this method is interesting and has several advantages over other more sophisticated test batteries. First, the results are highly reproducible, because the measured dimensions change slowly. Second, it is one of the least expensive methods. The amount of equipment needed for the tests is minimal and readily available. Third, the tests can be repeated as often as desired at little cost. Finally, while the significance of such superficial traits as baldness, grayness, and muscularity may be criticized, the importance of such characteristics to many people is demonstrated by the fact that a great deal of money is spent for hair coloring and hair restoring preparations, cosmetic surgery, body-shaping regimens, and other purely cosmetic procedures.

REQUIREMENTS FOR DAMON'S TEST BATTERY.

1. Anthropometric caliper (Appendix A. 6-2).
2. Sliding caliper (Appendix A. 6-3).
3. Skin fold caliper (Appendix A. 6-4).
4. Handgrip dynamometer (Appendix A. 6-1).
5. Tape measure.
6. Large draftsman's triangle.
7. Camera, for recording extent of baldness and grayness, for later comparisons.

TESTS IN DAMON'S TEST BATTERY:

1. Hair grayness (G) (Appendix B. 6-1).
2. Handgrip strength (HGS), dominant hand (Appendix B. 6-2), in kg.
3. Ear breadth (EB) (Appendix B. 6-3), in mm.
4. Sitting Height (SH) (Appendix B. 6-4), in mm.
5. Ear length (EL) (Appendix B. 6-5), in mm.
6. Nose breadth (NB) (Appendix B. 6-6), in mm.
7. Bideltoid breadth (BB) (shoulder breadth) (Appendix B. 6-7), in mm.
8. Abdominal depth (AD) (Appendix B. 6-8), in mm.
9. Triceps skinfold thickness (TSF) (Appendix B. 6-9), in mm.
10. Baldness (B) (Appendix B. 6-10).

DAMON'S EQUATION FOR BIOLOGICAL AGE:

Biological age = 50.56 years + 2.86 (G) - 0.08 (HGS) 0.36 (EB) - 0.03 (SH) + 0.28 (EL) + 0.37 (NB) - 0.09 (BB) + 0.08 (AD) - 0.21 (TSF) + 0.66 (B)

Harvard University Chapter 6

CALCULATION SHEET
AMERICAN TEST BATTERY
HARVARD UNIVERSITY

Name: _____ Date of Exam : ___/___/___

Date of Birth: ___/___/___

Chronological Age: _____

1. Hair grayness (none=0, slight=1,
   25%=2, 50%=3, 75%=4, complete=5): _____ x 2.86 = _____

2. Handgrip strength,
   dominant hand, in kg ....: _____ x 0.08 = _____

3. Ear breadth, in mm ....: _____ x 0.36 = _____

4. Sitting height, in mm ....: _____ x 0.03 = _____

5. Ear length, in mm ....: _____ x 0.28 = _____

6. Nose breadth, in mm ....: _____ x 0.37 = _____

7. Bideltoid breadth
   (shoulder breadth), in mm .....: _____ x 0.09 = _____

8. Abdominal depth, in mm ....: _____ x 0.08 = _____

9. Triceps skinfold thickness, in mm: _____ x 0.21 = _____

10. Baldness (none=0, slight=1,
    25%=2, 50%=3, 75%=4, complete=5): _____ x 0.66 = _____

Biological age = 50.56 + 1. _____ − 2. _____ + 3. _____

− 4. _____ + 5. _____ + 6. _____ − 7. _____ + 8. _____

− 9. _____ + 10. _____ .

(Plot on a graph--App. C)   Biological age = _____

REFERENCES

Borkan, G. Assessment of biological age using a profile of physical parameters. *J Geront*, 1980, Vol. 35, No. 2, 177-184.

Damon, Albert. Predicting age from body measurements and observations. (1972) *Aging and Human Development*, Vol. 3, No. 2, pp. 169-173.

Fuller, E. Growing up...and up...with hGH. (1984) *Patient Care*, Vol. 18 No. 16, pp. 18-39.

Larrabee, W., Caro, I. The aging face. (1984) *Postgraduate Medicine* 76 (Nov 15): 37-46.

Chapter 7

DUTCH TEST BATTERIES
Institute for Preventive Medicine

An early aging measurement study which remains a classic, and is still among the most comprehensive--was conducted by scientists from the Netherlands Institute for Preventive Medicine in Leiden. The team was led by Dr. Johan M. Dirken (*Fig. 7-1*), who is now Vice Chancellor, Delft University of Technology.

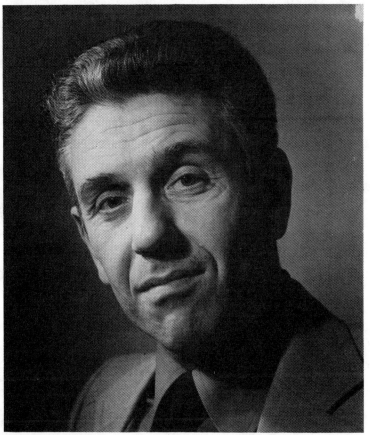

Fig. 7-1. **Professor Johan Maurits Dirken.**

The purpose of the study was to design prototype test batteries to measure the "functional age" of industrial workers, so management could determine the ability of older workers to perform their jobs. Like most other systems, there was little or no follow-up, and no practical use of these test batteries has ever been made.

Besides measuring a number of standard physiological parameters, these systems include many time-consuming neuro-psychological tests requiring non-standard equipment and techniques. Because it may be inconvenient to obtain the equipment for some of the tests, the Dutch test batteries may be less popular with clinical gerontologists than other test batteries requiring only standardized equipment and techniques.

Notwithstanding, these systems have some definite advantages. First, they may appeal to gerontological psychologists, who conduct these types of tests routinely (although generally utilizing slightly different tests and equipment) (*Fig. 7-2*). Second, they may become increasingly popular due to the growing appreciation of the importance of the functions of the brain and nervous system in aging. Third, they incorporate tests of functional capacity as determined by a sub-maximal exercise test on a bicycle ergometer. Many scientists feel that age indices based on this type of test provide the most accurate assessment of biological age (Bruce; Nakamura; Shock).

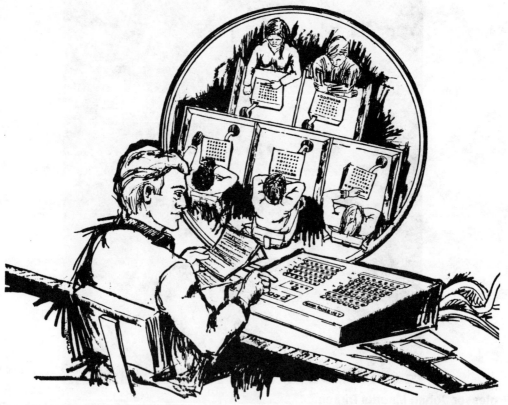

Fig. 7-2. **Multi-Stimulus Display Unit for neuropsychological tests** (Courtesy, Lafayette Instrument Co).

Institute for Preventive Medicine — Chapter 7

REQUIREMENTS FOR THE DUTCH TEST BATTERIES:

1. High frequency audiometer (Appendix A. 3-2).
2. Charts for measuring visual acuity (Appendix A. 4-2).
3. Spirometer (Appendix A. 2-1).
4. Bicycle ergometer (Appendix A. 1-2).
5. Sphygmomanometer and stethoscope (Appendix A. 1-1).
6. Heart rate monitor (Appendix A. 1-6).
7. Hand steadiness measuring device (Appendix A. 5-3).
8. Apparatus for measuring choice reaction times (Appendix A. 5-12).
9. Pack of 20 test cards for the Dutch intelligence test (Groninger intelligence test--GIT) (Appendix A. 5-4).
10. Bourdon-Wiersma test sheets (Appendix A. 5-5).
11. Semantic categorization test panel (Appendix A. 5-7).

TESTS IN THE DUTCH TEST BATTERIES:

1. High frequency audiometry (HFA), in kHz (Appendix B. 3-2).
2. Visual acuity (VA), as a decimal (Appendix B. 4-2).
3. Picture recognition (PR), in the number of GIT pictures correctly identified (Appendix B. 5-3).
4. Hand steadiness (HS), in the number of the last correctly performed hole (Appendix B. 5-2).
5. Concentration (CN), in the number of Bourdon lines completed in 4 minutes (Appendix B. 5-4. a.).
6. Categorization (CT), in the number of wrong answers (Appendix B. 5-5).
7. Four-choice reaction time (CRT4), in seconds (Appendix B. 5-13. a).
8. Forced expiratory volume in one second (FEV1), in liters (Appendix B. 2-1).

The following values are measured using a bicycle ergometer and the procedures described in Appendix B. 1-5. b. The heart rate is recorded from the heart rate monitor every minute. All other measurements are made over one-minute periods at loads immediately preceding

50-Watt increments, i.e., 40-50 Watts, 90-100 Watts, and so on, during the minutes immediately preceding exhaustion and at the end of the test.

9. Maximum systolic blood pressure (SBPmax), in mm Hg (Fig. B. 1-3). This is the highest systolic pressure attained during the last completed minute during the exercise test.

10. Maximum respiratory rate (RRmax), in breaths per minute (R) (Appendix B. 2-3) during the last minute of the exercise test.

11. Maximum heart rate (HRmax) (Appendix B. 1-6).

12. Maximum load (Lmax), in Watts (Appendix B. 1-7).

13. Maximum oxygen uptake (VO_2max) in ml/min (Appendix B. 1-5. b). This is calculated using the maximum heart rate, maximum load in Watts, and the nomogram (Fig. B. 1-11) and method described in Appendix B. 1-5.

DUTCH EQUATIONS:

I. Biological age = 93.96 - 1.57 (HFA) - 1.7 (VA) - 0.386 (PR) + 12.2 (CRT_4) - 0.475 (CT) - 0.144 (RRmax) - 0.006 (VO_2max) + 0.037 (SBPmax) - 0.004 (FEV_1)

II. Biological age = 88.56 - 1.62 (HFA) - 0.377 (PR) + 13.6 (CRT_4) - 0.499 (CT) - 0.008 (VO_2 max) + 0.046 (SBPmax) - 0.004 (FEV_1)

III. Biological age = 92.83 - 1.58 (HFA) - 0.398 (PR) + 13.3 (CRT_4) - 0.504 (CT) - 0.142 (RRmax) - 0.006 (VO_2max) + 0.039 (SBP) - 0.004 (FEV_1)

IV. Biological age = 83.05 - 1.53 (HFA) - 2.45 (VA) - 0.154 (HS) - 0.382 (CN) - 0.273 (PR) + 11.3 (CRT_4) - 0.081 (Lmax) + 0.038 (SBPmax) - 0.004 (FEV_1)

USE OF CORRECTION FACTORS

After calculating the equations, the results appeared to be slightly skewed. Younger people generally scored older than they should, and older people scored younger. To correct this artifactual deviation, a "fudge factor" was calculated that must be added to or subtracted from the calculated biological age to give a more accurate result. These correction factors are listed in *Table 7-II*.

Institute for Preventive Medicine Chapter 7

TABLE 7-I

ORDER AND CATEGORIZATION OF SEMANTIC STIMULI

	Professions	**Animals**	**Objects**	**Cities**
1				Detroit
2	Store clerk			
3		Reindeer		
4			Clothes pin	
5				Boise
6		Tiger		
7				Dayton
8	Lawyer			
9		Haddock		
10			Pincers	
11				Portland
12			Razor	
13		Monkey		
14	Waitress			
15			Pick-ax	
16				Camden
17			Soup bowl	
18	Pilot			
19			Wine glass	
20		Otter		
21	Farmer			
22				Phoenix
23		Rabbit		
24	Sailor			
25				Dallas
26			Glass jar	
27		Weasel		
28	Blacksmith			
29		Donkey		
30			Hand bag	
31	Typist			
32				Richmond

TABLE 7-II. **CORRECTION FACTORS**

Chronological Age	Equation Number			
	I	II	III	IV
30	-6.3	-6.6	-6.3	-6.6
31	-6.0	-6.2	-6.0	-6.3
32	-5.7	-5.9	-5.7	-5.9
33	-5.3	-5.6	-5.4	-5.6
34	-5.0	-5.2	-5.0	-5.3
35	-4.7	-4.9	-4.7	-4.9
36	-4.4	-4.5	-4.4	-4.6
37	-4.0	-4.2	-4.0	-4.2
38	-3.7	-3.9	-3.7	-3.9
39	-3.4	-3.5	-3.4	-3.6
40	-3.1	-3.2	-3.1	-3.2
41	-2.7	-2.8	-2.7	-2.9
42	-2.4	-2.5	-2.4	-2.5
43	-2.1	-2.2	-2.1	-2.2
44	-1.8	-1.8	-1.7	-1.8
45	-1.4	-1.5	-1.4	-1.5
46	-1.1	-1.1	-1.1	-1.2
47	-0.8	-0.8	-0.8	-0.8
48	-0.5	-0.5	-0.4	-0.5
49	-0.1	-0.1	-0.1	-0.1
50	+0.2	+0.2	+0.2	+0.2
51	+0.5	+0.6	+0.6	+0.6
52	+0.8	+0.9	+0.9	+0.9
53	+1.2	+1.2	+1.2	+1.2
54	+1.5	+1.6	+1.5	+1.6
55	+1.8	+1.9	+1.9	+1.9
56	+2.1	+2.3	+2.2	+2.3
57	+2.5	+2.6	+2.5	+2.6
58	+2.8	+2.9	+2.9	+3.0
59	+3.1	+3.3	+3.2	+3.3
60	+3.4	+3.6	+3.5	+3.6
61	+3.8	+4.0	+3.8	+4.0
62	+4.1	+4.3	+4.2	+4.3
63	+4.4	+4.6	+4.5	+4.7
64	+4.7	+5.0	+4.8	+5.0
65	+5.1	+5.3	+5.2	+5.4
66	+5.4	+5.7	+5.5	+5.7
67	+5.7	+6.0	+5.8	+6.0
68	+6.0	+6.7	+6.5	+6.7
69	+6.4	+6.7	+6.5	+6.7

Instructions for use of this table: After a *biological age* has been calculated using one or more of the Dutch equations, add or subtract the number of years obtained from the table above, in accordance with the chronological age of the subject and the equation that was used. This will provide a "corrected" biological age.

| Institute for Preventive Medicine | Chapter 7 |

CALCULATION SHEET
DUTCH TEST BATTERY FOR MEN
INSTITUTE FOR PREVENTIVE MEDICINE

Equation I

Name: _____   Date of Exam: ___/___/___

Date of Birth: ___/___/___

Chronological Age: _____

1. High frequency audiometry, in kHz: _____ x 1.57 = _____

2. Visual acuity, as a decimal .... : _____ x 1.7 = _____

3. Picture recognition,
   in no. of GIT pictures .... : _____ x 0.386 = _____

4. 4-choice reaction time, in sec : _____ x 12.2 = _____

5. Categorization, in no. of
   too-slow and incorrect reactions: _____ x 0.475 = _____

6. Maximum respiratory rate,
   in breaths per min .... : _____ x 0.144 = _____

7. Maximal oxygen uptake, in ml/min : _____ x 0.006 = _____

8. Maximum systolic blood
   pressure, in mm Hg .... : _____ x 0.037 = _____

9. Forced expiratory volume
   in 1 sec, in liters .... : _____ x 0.004 = _____

Biological age = 93.96 − 1. _____ − 2. _____ − 3. _____

+ 4. _____ − 5. _____ − 6. _____ − 7. _____ + 8. _____

− 9. _____

Biological age _____ + correction factor _____ (Table 7-II)

(Plot on a graph--App. C)   Corrected biological age _____

Chapter 7 | Institute for Preventive Medicine

CALCULATION SHEET
DUTCH TEST BATTERY FOR MEN
INSTITUTE FOR PREVENTIVE MEDICINE

Equation II

Name: _____ Date of Exam: ___/___/___

Date of Birth: ___/___/___

Chronological Age: _____

1. High frequency audiometry, in kHz: _____ x 1.62 = _____

2. Picture recognition,
   in no. of GIT pictures .... : _____ x 0.377 = _____

3. 4-choice reaction time, in sec : _____ x 13.6 = _____

4. Categorization, in no. of
   too-slow and incorrect reactions: _____ x 0.499 = _____

5. Maximal oxygen uptake, in ml/min : _____ x 0.008 = _____

6. Maximum systolic blood
   pressure, in mm Hg .... : _____ x 0.046 = _____

7. Forced expiratory volume
   in 1 sec, in liters .... : _____ x 0.004 = _____

Biological age = 88.56 - 1. _____ - 2. _____ + 3. _____
- 4. _____ - 5. _____ + 6. _____ - 7. _____

Biological age _____ + correction factor _____ (Table 7-II)

(Plot on a graph--App. C)   Corrected biological age _____

Institute for Preventive Medicine   **Chapter 7**

CALCULATION SHEET
DUTCH TEST BATTERY FOR MEN
INSTITUTE FOR PREVENTIVE MEDICINE

Equation III

Name: _____   Date of Exam : ___/___/___

                                                            Date of Birth: ___/___/___

                                                            Chronological Age: _____

1. High frequency audiometry, in kHz: _____ x 1.58 = _____

2. Picture recognition,
   in no. of GIT pictures .... : _____ x 0.398 = _____

3. 4-choice reaction time, in sec   : _____ x 13.3 = _____

4. Categorization, in no. of
   too-slow and incorrect reactions: _____ x 0.504 = _____

5. Maximum respiratory rate,
   in breaths per min .... : _____ x 0.142 = _____

6. Maximal oxygen uptake, in ml/min : _____ x 0.006 = _____

7. Systolic blood pressure, in mm Hg: _____ x 0.039 = _____

8. Forced expiratory volume
   in 1 sec, in liters .... : _____ x 0.004 = _____

Biological age = 92.83 - 1. _____ - 2. _____ + 3. _____

- 4. _____ - 5. _____ - 6. _____ + 7. _____ - 8. _____

Biological age _____ + correction factor _____ (Table 7-II)

(Plot on a graph--App. C)   Corrected biological age _____

Chapter 7   Institute for Preventive Medicine

CALCULATION SHEET
DUTCH TEST BATTERY FOR MEN
INSTITUTE FOR PREVENTIVE MEDICINE

Equation IV

Name: _____   Date of Exam : ___/___/___

                                                                          Date of Birth: ___/___/___

                                                                          Chronological Age: _____

1. High frequency audiometry, in kHz: _____ x 1.53 = _____

2. Visual acuity, as a decimal .... : _____ x 2.45 = _____

3. Hand steadiness, in no. of
    last correctly performed hole   : _____ x 0.154 = _____

4. Concentration,
    in no. of Bourdon lines .... : _____ x 0.382 = _____

5. Picture recognition,
    in no. of GIT pictures .... : _____ x 0.273 = _____

6. 4-choice reaction time, in sec   : _____ x 11.3   = _____

7. Maximum load on
    bicycle ergometer, in Watts ... : _____ x 0.081 = _____

8. Maximum systolic blood
    pressure, in mm Hg .... : _____ x 0.038 = _____

9. Forced expiratory volume
    in 1 sec, in liters .... : _____ x 0.004 = _____

Biological age = 83.05 - 1. _____ - 2. _____ - 3. _____

- 4. _____ - 5. _____ + 6. _____ - 7. _____ + 8. _____

- 9. _____

Biological age _____ + correction factor _____ (Table 7-II)

(Plot on a graph--App. C)   Corrected biological age _____

REFERENCES

Bruce, R. A. Exercise, functional aerobic capacity, and aging--another viewpoint. *Medicine and Science in Sports and Exercise*, 16:1, pp. 8-13, 1984.

Dirken, Johan Maurits. *Functional Age of Industrial Workers*, Wolters-Noordhoff Publishing, Groningen, 1972.

Dirken, Johan Maurits. *The development of a measuring device for determining the functional age of elderly industrial workers*. Netherlands Institute for Preventive Medicine. 22-6-1963.

Dirken, Johan Maurits, *Personal Communications*, 17 January 1984, and 6 August 1984.

Nakamura, E. The aged people and its physiological ages in relation to work capacity [author's translation]. *Kyoiku Igaku* (1982) 28: 2-11.

Shock, N. W. Indices of Functional Age, in: *Aging: A Challenge to Science and Society, Vol. 1. Biology*, Oxford University Press, New York, 1981. p. 282.

Chapter 8

AUSTRALIAN TEST BATTERIES
University of New South Wales

In 1976, Dr. Ian W. Webster, and Mr. Alexander R. Logie of the School of Community Medicine, University of New South Wales, Australia, calculated an aging measurement equation based on various physiological and biochemical measurements of 1,080 women, ranging in age from 21 to 83. Of the 37 values measured, six were included in the equation.

In the course of his study on women, Webster also collected data on 1,461 men. Although he has not previously published the results obtained from this study, he sent them to me for inclusion in this chapter (Webster, 6 Feb, 1984).

As mentioned in Chapter 5, one problem with most aging measurement systems is that few of them have been validated in longitudinal studies. The systems discussed here are no exception. However, after calculating the equations, the authors did attempt to validate them by comparing the biological ages of non-smokers who considered themselves to be in good health with those of others in the group who either smoked or felt that they were not in good health. As would be expected, the healthy non-smoking individuals scored younger than their chronologic ages, and the not-so-healthy smokers scored older. These findings support the concept, validity, and usefulness of these equations.

REQUIREMENTS FOR THE AUSTRALIAN TEST BATTERIES:

1. Standard clinical laboratory chemistry and hematological tests.
2. Spirometer (Appendix A. 2-1).
3. Sphygmomanometer and stethoscope (Appendix A. 1-1).

TESTS IN THE AUSTRALIAN EQUATIONS:

1. Blood urea nitrogen (BUN) (Appendix B. 9-5), in mg/100 ml.
2. Forced expiratory volume in 1 second (FEV_1), (Appendix B. 2-1) in liters.
3. Systolic blood pressure (SBP) (Appendix B. 1-1) (supine) in mm Hg.
4. Alkaline phosphatase (AP) (Appendix B. 9-6). Alkaline phosphatase is usually measured in I.U. per milliliter. Here it is expressed as the log_{10} of this value. This is a non-standard expression that can be easily determined using a hand-held calculator with a log function capability, or from the conversion table in this chapter (*Table 8-I*).
5. Erythrocyte sedimentation rate (ESR) (Appendix B. 8-1), measured in mm per hour, using the Westergren technique. It is also expressed as the log_{10} of the value, also obtainable from *Table 8-I*.
6. Cholesterol (C) (Appendix B. 9-1), in mg/100ml.

AUSTRALIAN EQUATION FOR WOMEN:

I. Biological age = 8.93 years + 0.71 (BUN) - 6.93 (FEV_1)
   + 0.12 (SBP) + 10.97 (log_{10} AP) + 2.38 (log_{10} ESR) + 0.05 (C)

AUSTRALIAN EQUATION FOR MEN:

II. Biological age = 47.00 + 0.42 (BUN) - 6.63 (FEV_1)
    + 0.10 (SBP) + 5.37 (log_{10} ESR)

ADDITIONAL AUSTRALIAN STUDIES

From 1974-1977, The Community Health and Anti-Tuberculosis Association in Australia used a mobile laboratory (*Fig. 8-1*) to carry out a number of health surveys in the Sydney Metropolitan area. The laboratory was equipped to measure pulmonary functions, blood pressure, height and weight, and to process blood and urine samples for biochemical analysis. Altogether, they studied over 12,000 apparently healthy subjects.

From this mass of data, Webster and his colleagues selected 5 measurements closely correlated with chronological age and again calculated equations for both men and women. These measurements are:

1. Forced vital capacity (FVC) (Appendix B. 2-2) in liters.
2. Systolic blood pressure (SBP) (Appendix B. 1-1) in mm Hg.
3. Blood urea nitrogen (BUN) (Appendix B. 9-5) in mg/100 ml.
4. Cholesterol (C) (Appendix B. 9-1) in mg/100 ml.
5. Calcium (CA) (Appendix B. 9-9), in mg/100 ml. Although most other studies have not shown calcium to change significantly with age, Webster (1985) assured me that (to his surprise as well) it did.

SECOND AUSTRALIAN EQUATION FOR WOMEN:

III. Biological age = 51.01 + 0.84 (BUN) - 5.53 (FEV_1) + 0.20 (SBP) + 0.093 (C) - 5.53 (CA)

SECOND AUSTRALIAN EQUATION FOR MEN:

IV. Biological age = 93.86 + 0.44 (BUN) - 4.92 (FEV1) + 0.19 (SBP) + 0.10 (C) - 9.01 (CA)

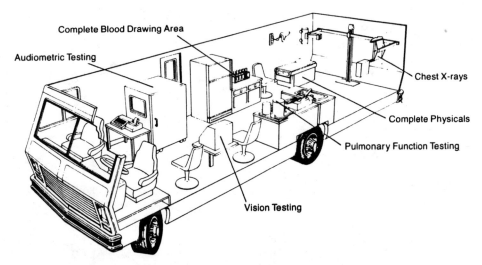

Fig. 8-1. **Mobile medical van of the type used by Webster**
(Courtesy, Mobile Medical Testing Service, Inc., Hartford, CT).

Chapter 8

TABLE 8-1. **LOGARITHMIC CONVERSION TABLE**

No.	$\log_{10}$	No.	$\log_{10}$	No.	$\log_{10}$
1	0	41	1.6128	81	1.9085
2	0.301	42	1.6232	82	1.9138
3	0.4771	43	1.6335	83	1.9191
4	0.6021	44	1.6435	84	1.9243
5	0.6990	45	1.6532	85	1.9294
6	0.7782	46	1.6628	86	1.9345
7	0.8451	47	1.6721	87	1.9395
8	0.9031	48	1.6812	88	1.9445
9	0.9542	49	1.6902	89	1.9494
10	1.00	50	1.6990	90	1.9542
11	1.0414	51	1.7076	91	1.9590
12	1.0792	52	1.7160	92	1.9638
13	1.1139	53	1.7243	93	1.9685
14	1.1461	54	1.7324	94	1.9731
15	1.1761	55	1.7404	95	1.9777
16	1.2041	56	1.7482	96	1.9823
17	1.2304	57	1.7559	97	1.9868
18	1.2553	58	1.7634	98	1.9912
19	1.2788	59	1.7709	99	1.9956
20	1.3010	60	1.7782	100	2.0000
21	1.3222	61	1.7853	101	2.0043
22	1.3424	62	1.7924	102	2.0086
23	1.3617	63	1.7993	103	2.0128
24	1.3802	64	1.8062	104	2.0170
25	1.3979	65	1.8129	105	2.0212
26	1.4150	66	1.8195	106	2.0253
27	1.4314	67	1.8261	107	2.0294
28	1.4472	68	1.8325	108	2.0334
29	1.4624	69	1.8388	109	2.0374
30	1.4771	70	1.8451	110	2.0414
31	1.4914	71	1.8513	111	2.0453
32	1.5051	72	1.8573	112	2.0492
33	1.5185	73	1.8633	113	2.0531
34	1.5315	74	1.8692	114	2.0569
35	1.5441	75	1.8751	115	2.0607
36	1.5563	76	1.8808	116	2.0645
37	1.5682	77	1.8865	117	2.0682
38	1.5798	78	1.8921	118	2.0719
39	1.5911	79	1.8976	119	2.0755
40	1.6128	80	1.9031	120	2.0792

University of New South Wales   Chapter 8

CALCULATION SHEET
AUSTRALIAN TEST BATTERY FOR WOMEN

Equation I

Name: _____   Date of Exam : ___/___/___

                                          Date of Birth: ___/___/___

                                          Chronological Age: _____

1. Blood urea nitrogen, in mg/100 ml   : _____ x 0.71 = _____

2. Forced expiratory volume
     in 1 sec, in liters ....   : _____ x 6.93 = _____

3. Systolic blood pressure, in mm Hg   : _____ x 0.12 = _____

4. Plasma alkaline phosphatase
     in IUs _____ = ($\log_{10}$ alk phos)   : _____ x 10.97 = _____

5. Erythrocyte sedimentation rate
     in mm/hr _____ = ($\log_{10}$ ESR) .... : _____ x 2.38 = _____

6. Cholesterol, in mg/100 ml ....   : _____ x 0.05 = _____

Biological age = 8.93 + 1. _____ - 2. _____ + 3. _____

+ 4. _____ + 5. _____ + 6. _____

(Plot on a graph--App. C)   Biological age _____

75

Chapter 8   University of New South Wales

CALCULATION SHEET
AUSTRALIAN TEST BATTERY FOR MEN

Equation II

Name: _____ Date of Exam : ___/___/___

                                        Date of Birth: ___/___/___

                                        Chronological Age: _____

1. Blood urea nitrogen, in mg/100 ml   : _____ x 0.42 = _____

2. Forced expiratory volume
   in 1 sec, in liters .... : _____ x 6.63 = _____

3. Systolic blood pressure, in mm Hg   : _____ x 0.10 = _____

4. Erythrocyte sedimentation rate
   in mm/hr _____ = ($\log_{10}$ ESR) .... : _____ x 5.37 = _____

Biological age = 47.00 + 1. _____ − 2. _____ + 3. _____

+ 4. _____

(Plot on a graph--App. C)   Biological age _____

University of New South Wales **Chapter 8**

CALCULATION SHEET
AUSTRALIAN TEST BATTERY FOR WOMEN

Equation III

Name: _____   Date of Exam : ___/___/___

Date of Birth: ___/___/___

Chronological Age: _____

1. Blood urea nitrogen, in mg/100 ml : _____ x 0.84 = _____
2. Forced vital capacity, in liters   : _____ x 5.53 = _____
3. Systolic blood pressure, in mm Hg : _____ x 0.20 = _____
4. Cholesterol, in mg/100 ml .... : _____ x 0.093 = _____
5. Calcium, in mg/100 ml .... : _____ x 5.53 = _____

Biological age = 51.01 + 1. _____ − 2. _____ + 3. _____

+ 4. _____ − 5. _____

(Plot on a graph--App. C)   Biological age _____

| Chapter 8 | University of New South Wales |

CALCULATION SHEET
AUSTRALIAN TEST BATTERY FOR MEN

Equation IV

Name: _____ Date of Exam : ___/___/___

Date of Birth: ___/___/___

Chronological Age: _____

1. Blood urea nitrogen, in mg/100 ml   : _____ x 0.44 = _____
2. Forced vital capacity, in liters   : _____ x 4.92 = _____
3. Systolic blood pressure, in mm Hg   : _____ x 0.19 = _____
4. Cholesterol, in mg/100 ml ....   : _____ x 0.10 = _____
5. Calcium, in mg/100 ml ....   : _____ x 9.01 = _____

Biological age = 93.86 + 1. _____ - 2. _____ + 3. _____

+ 4. _____ - 5. _____

(Plot on a graph--App. C)   Biological age _____

REFERENCES

Gibson, J.B., Adena, M.A., Craft, R.F., Rawson, G.K., and Webster, I.W. Human variation related to age in an urban population. *Proceedings of the Satellite Conference of the 11th Congress of the International Association of Gerontology*, Sydney, 10-13 August, 1978, pp. 107-109.

Webster, Ian W., and Logie, Alexander R. A relationship between functional age and health status in female subjects. *Journal of Gerontology*, 1976, 31:5, 546-550.

Webster, Ian W. *Personal communications*, 25 Nov, 1983; 6 Feb, 1984; 3 Aug, 1984; 21 Jan, 1985; and 20 Feb 1986.

Chapter 9

JAPANESE TEST BATTERIES
University of Osaka

In 1975, Dr. Toshiyuki Furukawa (*Fig. 9-1*) and his colleagues at the Osaka University Medical School conducted a meticulous study of 308 males. From these data they developed several equations for biological age. This chapter deals with the two most accurate of their equations, and includes a third equation recently calculated by Furukawa (29 August, 1985) especially for inclusion in this book. Furukawa is now a Professor on the Faculty of Medicine at the Institute of Medical Electronics, University of Tokyo.

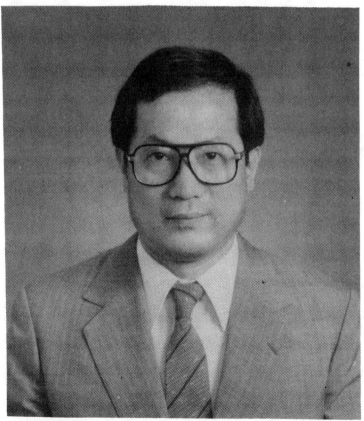

Fig. 9-1. **Professor Toshiyuki Furukawa.**

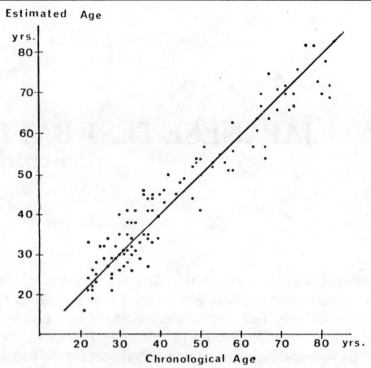

Fig. 9-2. **Comparison of chronological and biological ages--Equation I** (Furukawa, *J Geront*).

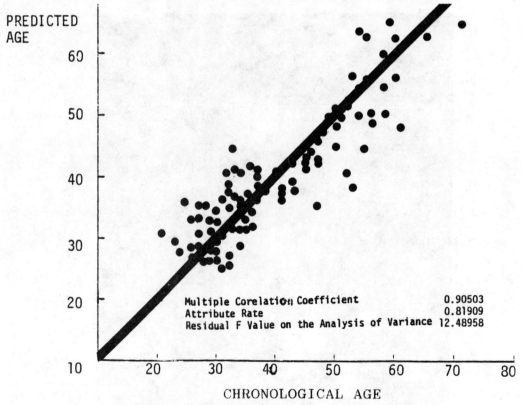

Fig. 9-3. **Comparison of chronological and biological ages--Equation III** (Furukawa, 29 Aug 1985).

An idea of the accuracy obtainable with Furukawa's equations may be appreciated by noting the comparison of biological and chronological ages illustrated in *Figs. 9-2* and *9-3*.

To validate the equations, Furukawa used a technique similar to that of Webster, described in the preceding chapter. Using Equation I, biological ages were calculated for a group of hypertensive subjects (*Fig. 9-4*) showing that the hypertensives were older biologically than chronologically. This confirms the generally held belief that hypertension contributes to accelerated aging (Anonymous, Modern Medicine).

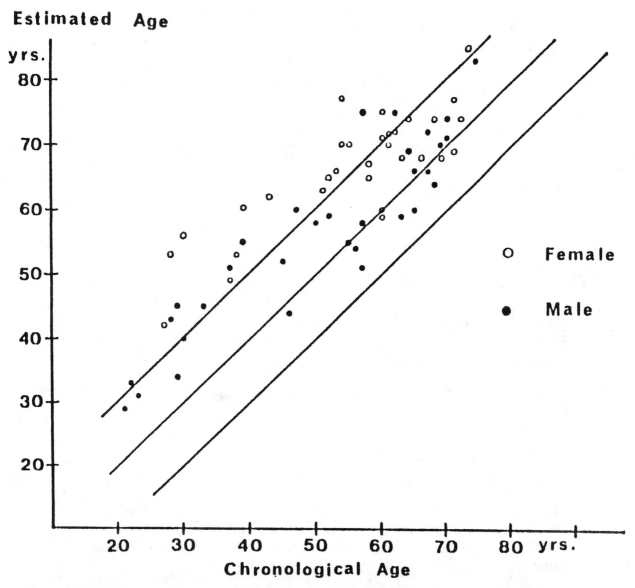

Fig. 9-4. **Biological ages of a group of hypertensive subjects, using Equation I.** Biological ages generally exceed chronological ages, confirming the hypertension contributes to accelerated aging (Anonymous, *Modern Medicine*) (Furukawa, *J Geront*).

REQUIREMENTS FOR THE OSAKA TEST BATTERY:

1. Standard clinical laboratory chemistry and hematological tests.
2. Sphygmomanometer and stethoscope (Appendix A. 1-1).
3. Body weight scale (in kg).
4. Tape measure.
5. Spirometer (Appendix A. 2-1).
6. Berens near-point indicator; or Krimsky-Prince rule (Appendix A. 4-1).
7. Vibrometer (Appendix A. 5-8).
8. Manual laboratory counter (Appendix A. 5-9).
9. Handgrip dynamometer (Appendix A. 6-1).
10. Goniometer (Appendix A. 6-8).
11. Master's 2-step staircase (Appendix A. 1-5).
12. Heart rate monitor (Appendix A. 1-6).

TESTS IN THE OSAKA TEST BATTERY:

1. Systolic blood pressure (SBP) (Appendix B. 1-1), recorded in a sitting position, and measured in mm Hg.
2. Diastolic blood pressure (DBP) (Appendix B. 1-2) in mm Hg.
3. Height (HT) (Appendix B. 6-13) in cm. Non-Asians should multiply their height by 0.94.
4. Weight (WT) (Appendix B. 6-14) in kg. Non-Asians should multiply their weight by 0.72.
5. Vital Capacity (VC) (Appendix B. 2-2) in ml.
6. Phenolsulfonphthalein test (PSP) (Appendix B. 10-1) in percentage of dye excreted in the urine after 15 minutes. This is a near-obsolete test of kidney function. Comparative values can be determined from creatinine clearance using the conversion scale in Appendix B. (Fig. B. 10-2).
7. Near vision (NV) (Appendix B. 4-1), in diopters.

8. Vibratory sensitivity (Appendix B. 5-6) of the right (VS_R) and left (VS_L) index fingers, measured using the vibrometer. Furukawa used a vibrometer that measured in decibels, but this device is no longer available. The measurement in volts (V) obtained with the vibrometer can be converted to decibels from *Fig. B. 5-9* in Appendix B.

9. Tapping rate (TR) with a laboratory counter, in taps per 30 seconds (Appendix B. 5-7. a).

10. Handgrip strength (HGS) (Appendix B. 6-2), in kg. The strength of the dominant hand is measured. If the test is conducted on a non-Asian, the conversion chart in Appendix B. should be used (*Fig. B. 6-3*).

11. Body flexibility (Appendix B. 6-11. a), recorded in degrees, by bending forewards (anteflexion--AF), sidewards (sideflexion--SF) and backwards (retroflexion-- RF).

12. Heart rate recovery after exercise (Appendix B. 1-8. a), based on the heart rate while resting (RHR), and 30 sec, 1 min, 1.5 min, 3 min and 4 min after exercise, respectively ($HR_{0.5}$, $HR_{1.5}$, HR_3, and HR_4).

OSAKA UNIVERSITY'S AGING MEASUREMENT EQUATIONS:

I. Biological age = 95.232 - 0.138 (HT) - 0.180 (WT) + 0.142 (SBP) - 0.072 (DBP) - 0.003 (VC) - 0.252 (PSP) - 1.433 (NV_R) - 0.816 (NV_L) + 0.262 (VS_R) + 0.315 (VS_L)

II. Biological age = 171.437 - 0.595 (HT) - 0.532 (WT) - 0.027 (SBP) + 0.445 (DBP - 0.318 (TR) - 0.180 (HGS) + 0.409 (AF) - 0.007 (RF) + 0.042 (SF) - 0.039 (RHR) - 1.162 ($HR_{0.5}$) + 0.773 (HR_1) + 0.007 ($HR_{1.5}$) - 0.342 (HR_2) + 0.777 (HR_3) + 0.004 (HR_4)

III. Age = 203.931 - 0.0016 $(HT)^2$ - 0.0070 $(WT)^2$ + 0.0113 $(SBP)^2$ - 2.534 (SBP) - 0.016 $(DBP)^2$ + 2.691 (DBP) - 0.0045 $(TR)^2$ + 0.675 (TR) + 0.012 $(HGS)^2$ - 0.958 (HGS) - 0.0067 $(AF)^2$ + 1.638 (AF) + 0.0006 $(RF)^2$ - 0.0001 $(SF)^2$ + 0.0321 $(RHR)^2$ - 4.723 (RHR) - 1.31 ($HR_{0.5}$) + 0.011 $(HR_1)^2$ - 1.632 (HR_1) - 0.107 (HR_2) + 0.0161 $(HR_3)^2$ - 0.016 (HR_3) + 0.0017 $(HR_4)^2$

Chapter 9 — University of Osaka

CALCULATION SHEET
JAPANESE TEST BATTERY FOR MEN
OSAKA UNIVERSITY
Equation I

Name: _____ Date of Exam : ___/___/___

Date of Birth: ___/___/___

Chronological Age: _____

1. Height, in cm (non-Asians:
   multiply by 0.94 first) .... : _____ x 0.138 = _____

2. Weight, in kg (non-Asians:
   multiply by 0.72 first) .... : _____ x 0.180 = _____

3. Systolic blood pressure
   (supine), in mm Hg .... : _____ x 0.142 = _____

4. Diastolic blood pressure
   (supine), in mm Hg .... : _____ x 0.072 = _____

5. Vital capacity, in ml .... : _____ x 0.003 = _____

6. *Phenolsulfonphthalein (PSP),
   % excretion in 15 min .... : _____ x 0.252 = _____

7. Near vision, right eye in diopters: _____ x 1.433 = _____

8. Near vision, left eye in diopters : _____ x 0.816 = _____

9. Vibratory sensitivity,
   right index finger, in dB ...... : _____ x 0.262 = _____

10. Vibratory sensitivity,
    left index finger, in dB .... : _____ x 0.315 = _____

*This can be determined from creatinine clearance by using the scale--Fig. B. 10-2.

Biological age = 95.232 - 1._____ + 2. _____ + 3. _____ - 4. _____

- 5. _____ - 6. _____ - 7. _____ - 8. _____ + 9. _____

+ 10. _____

(Plot on a graph--App. C)   Biological age _____

University of Osaka Chapter 9

**CALCULATION SHEET
JAPANESE TEST BATTERY FOR MEN
OSAKA UNIVERSITY
Equation II**

Name: _____   Date of Exam : ___/___/___

   Date of Birth: ___/___/___

   Chronological Age: _____

1. Height, in cm (non-Asians:
   multiply by 0.94 first) .... : _____ x 0.595 = _____

2. Weight, in kg (non-Asians:
   multiply by 0.72) .... : _____ x 0.532 = _____

3. Systolic blood pressure
   (supine), in mm Hg .... : _____ x 0.027 = _____

4. Diastolic blood pressure
   (supine), in mm Hg .... : _____ x 0.445 = _____

5. Tapping rate, in taps per 30 sec : _____ x 0.318 = _____

6. *Hand grip strength, in kg ...... : _____ x 0.180 = _____

7. Anteflexion, in degrees .... : _____ x 0.409 = _____

8. Retroflexion, in degrees .... : _____ x 0.007 = _____

9. Sideflexion, in degrees .... : _____ x 0.042 = _____

10. Resting heart rate,
    in beats per minute (BPM) ...... : _____ x 0.039 = _____

11. Heart rate, in BPM
    30 sec after exercise .... : _____ x 1.162 = _____

12. Heart rate, in BPM
    1 min after exercise .... : _____ x 0.773 = _____

13. Heart rate, in BPM
    1.5 min after exercise .... : _____ x 0.007 = _____

14. Heart rate, in BPM
    2 min after exercise .... : _____ x 0.342 = _____

15. Heart rate, in BPM
    3 min after exercise .... : _____ x 0.777 = _____

16. Heart rate, in BPM
    4 min after exercise .... : _____ x 0.004 = _____

*Non-Asian subjects should use the conversion scale in Fig. B. 6-3 to obtain an adjusted handgrip strength for this equation.

Biological age = 171.437 − 1. _____ − 2. _____ − 3. _____
+ 4. _____ − 5. _____ − 6. _____ + 7. _____ − 8. _____
+ 9. _____ − 10. _____ − 11. _____ + 12. _____ + 13. _____
− 14. _____ + 15. _____ + 16. _____

(Plot on a graph--App. C)   Biological Age _____

University of Osaka   Chapter 9

CALCULATION SHEET
JAPANESE TEST BATTERY FOR MEN
OSAKA UNIVERSITY
Equation III

Name: _____   Date of Exam : ___/___/___

                                                                             Date of Birth: ___/___/___

                                                                             Chronological Age: _____

1. $Height^2$, in $(cm)^2$ (non-Asians:
   before squaring multiply by 0.94): _____ x 0.0016 = _____

2. $Weight^2$, in $(kg)^2$ (non-Asians:
   before squaring multiply by 0.72): _____ x 0.0070 = _____

3. Systolic blood $pressure^2$
   (supine), in $(mm\ Hg)^2$ .... : _____ x 0.0113 = _____

4. Systolic blood pressure
   (supine), in mm Hg .... : _____ x 2.5340 = _____

5. Diastolic blood $pressure^2$
   (supine), in $(mm\ Hg)^2$ .... : _____ x 0.0160 = _____

6. Diastolic blood pressure
   (supine), in mm Hg .... : _____ x 2.6910 = _____

7. Tapping $rate^2$,
   in $(taps\ per\ 30\ sec)^2$ .... : _____ x 0.0045 = _____

8. Tapping rate, in 30 sec .... : _____ x 0.6750 = _____

9. *Handgrip $strength^2$, in $(kg)^2$ ... : _____ x 0.0120 = _____

10. *Handgrip strength, in kg .... : _____ x 0.9580 = _____

11. $Anteflexion^2$, in $(deg)^2$ .... : _____ x 0.0067 = _____

12. Anteflexion, in deg .... : _____ x 1.6380 = _____

13. $Retroflexion^2$, in $(deg)^2$ .... : _____ x 0.0006 = _____

14. $Sideflexion^2$, in $(deg)^2$ .... : _____ x 0.0001 = _____

15. Resting heart $rate^2$, in $(BPM)^2$: _____ x 0.0321 = _____

16. Resting heart rate, in BPM ...... : _____ x 4.723 = _____

17. Heart rate, in BPM
    30 sec after exercise ....: _____ x 1.3100 = _____

18. Heart rate^2, in (BPM)^2
    1 min after exercise ....: _____ x 0.0110 = _____

19. Heart rate, in BPM
    1 min after exercise ....: _____ x 1.6320 = _____

20. Heart rate, in BPM
    2 min after exercise ....: _____ x 0.1070 = _____

21. Heart rate^2, in (BPM)^2
    3 min after exercise ....: _____ x 0.0161 = _____

22. Heart rate, in BPM
    3 min after exercise ....: _____ x 0.0160 = _____

23. Heart rate^2, in (BPM)^2
    4 min after exercise ....: _____ x 0.0017 = _____

*Non-Asian subjects should use the conversion scale in Fig. B. 6-3 to obtain adjusted handgrip strength values for this equation.

Biological age = 203.931 - 1. _____ - 2. _____ + 3. _____
- 4. _____ - 5. _____ + 6. _____ - 7. _____ + 8. _____
- 9. _____ + 10. _____ - 11. _____ + 12. _____ - 13. _____
+ 14. _____ + 15. _____ - 16. _____ - 17. _____ + 18. _____
- 19. _____ - 20. _____ - 21. _____ - 22. _____ - 23. _____

(Plot on a graph--App. C)   Biological age _____

REFERENCES

Anonymous. Hypertensive diabetics a higher death risk. *Modern Medicine*, Nov 1984, pp. 37-41.

Furukawa,, T., Inoue, M., Kajiya, F., Inada, H., Takasugi, S., Fukui, S., Takeda, H., and Abe, H.. Assessment of biological age by multiple regression analysis. *Journal of Gerontology*, 1975, Vol. 30, No. 4, 422-434.

Furukawa, T. Personal communications, 17 April 1984; 21 June 1984; 13 February 1985; 19 April, 1985; and 29 Aug, 1985.

CHAPTER 10

JAPANESE TEST BATTERIES
Radiation Effects Research Foundation

One of the first aging measurement systems was developed in 1962-63 by a team of scientists from the Atomic Bomb Casualty Commission (ABCC), led by Dr. J. William Hollingsworth (*Fig. 10-1*) (Hollingsworth, et al). Most subsequent systems are based on this landmark study. The ABCC was a joint U.S-Japanese government-supported research agency created to study the effects of radiation on the survivors of the Hiroshima and Nagasaki A-Bombs.

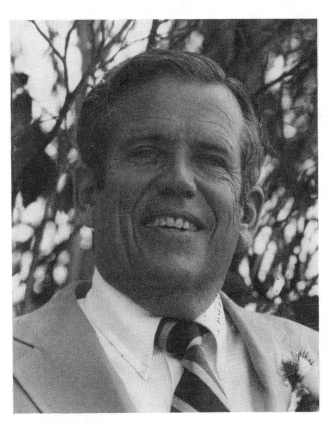

Fig. 10-1. **Dr. J. William Hollingsworth.**

Chapter 10 — Radiation Research Foundation

Gerontologists once believed that radiation exposure hastened the rate of aging (Curtis). One of the aims of the Hollingsworth study was to investigate whether the A-bomb survivors were physiologically older than their non-irradiated peers. The researchers planned to continue these studies throughout the lifespans of the subjects and compare the results and lifespans with normal non-irradiated people. Examinations of mortality data on a large sample of Japanese from 1950 to 1972 provided no support for the hypothesis that exposure to ionizing radiation accelerates aging (Shock, et al).

Hollingsworth is now Chief, Medical Services, U. of California, San Diego. Although he is no longer involved with aging measurement research, in recent correspondence (1985) he expressed his agreement that the time is near for the clinical application of biological aging measurement systems.

HOLLINGSWORTH'S ORIGINAL EQUATION LOST

The original equation and test battery were based on 17 physiological tests in 437 subjects. Data were obtained during their annual physical examinations in 1960. Of the 17 variables, 8 were eliminated for various reasons, and 9 were selected for inclusion in the equation. The tests used to determine the final equation were: skin elasticity, systolic blood pressure, vital capacity, handgrip strength, light extinction time, vibratory perception, visual acuity, auditory function, and serum cholesterol.

Although the method used to calculate the equation was outlined in the paper, for some reason the authors chose not to include the coefficients of the equation, precluding its use by others. Mr. Seymour Jablon, currently at the National Research Council Commission on Life Sciences, is the statistician who developed the equation. He recently wrote (1983), disclosing that the data used to formulate the equation were lost, and he did not keep the records with the complete equation. Also, since the data were analyzed by hand, he was not satisfied with the accuracy of the results (Jablon, 19 April 1984). Hollingsworth (1985) also did not retain records of the data.

STUDIES BY THE RADIATION EFFECTS RESEARCH FOUNDATION (RERF)

In 1978, a second study was conducted on the atomic bomb survivors by scientists from the Radiation Effects Research Foundation (RERF), the successor to the Atomic Bomb Casualty Commission (Belsky, et al). They used essentially the same tests as in the earlier study, and calculated several new equations. These equations are presented below.

Though these scientists agreed that a biological age could be derived from the results of age-related physiological and functional tests, they considered that their clinical use to estimate biological age would be premature if there was no longitudinal validation. Despite their reservations and recommendations for longitudinal tests, they apparently did not conduct further tests to confirm or reject their hypothesis. Jablon (19 Apr, 1984) agrees that the lack of continuous systematic analysis of the data obtained is a major fault of most government-supported longitudinal studies. These studies provide a tremendous untapped potential to design and validate accurate aging measurement systems.

The test battery is presented here for use by clinical gerontologists who ultimately may amass the necessary longitudinal data that the Radiation Effects Research Foundation scientists apparently failed to gather.

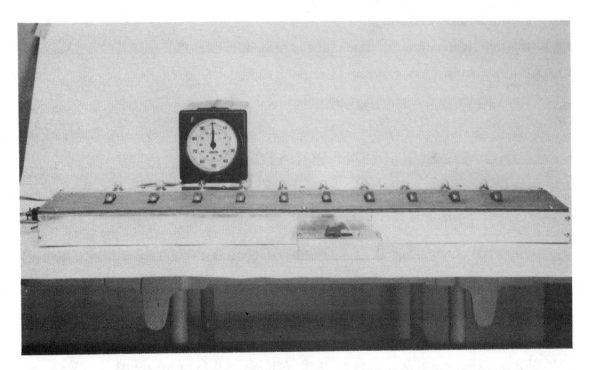

Fig. 10-2. **Photo of original Bogitch light extinction device used in the studies**, courtesy, Seymour Jablon.

REQUIREMENTS FOR THE RERF EQUATIONS:

1. Handgrip dynamometer (Appendix A. 6-1).
2. Skinfold calipers (Appendix A. 6-4).
3. Stopwatch, for use in the skin elasticity measurements.
4. Vibrometer (Appendix A. 5-8).
5. "Bogitch" light extinction device (Appendix A. 5-13).
6. Audiometer (Appendix A. 3-1).
7. Visual acuity charts (Appendix A. 4-2).

TESTS IN THE RERF TEST BATTERIES:

1. Handgrip strength (HGS) (Appendix B. 6-2), dominant hand, in kg. The maximum of 3 tries is recorded.
2. Skin elasticity (SE) (Appendix B. 6-12), in seconds.
3. Vibratory sensitivity (VS) (Appendix B. 5-6) of the left medial malleolus (left inner ankle), in volts.
4. "Bogitch" light extinction time (LET) (Appendix B. 5-13. b).
5. Auditory acuity (AA) (Appendix B. 3-1), right ear, in decibels.
6. Visual acuity, as a decimal (Appendix B. 4-2).

RERF AGING MEASUREMENT EQUATIONS

I. Men: Biological age = 51.9 - 0.155 (HGS) + 0.0457 (AA) + 0.141 (VS) + 3.57 (NV) + 1.17 (SE) - 2.39 (LET)

II. Women: Biological age = 45.8 - 0.160 (HGS) + 0.0677 (AA) + 0.166 (VS) + 3.36 (NV) + 2.57 (SE) - 1.52 (LET)

III. Men: Biological age = 60.2 - 0.327 (HGS) + 0.0949 (AA) + 0.258 (VS) - 3.06 (NV)

IV. Women: Biological age = 54.8 - 0.485 (HGS) + 0.141 (AA) + 0.329 (VS) - 2.19 (NV)

Radiation Research Foundation   **Chapter 10**

CALCULATION SHEET
JAPANESE TEST BATTERY FOR MEN
RADIATION EFFECTS RESEARCH FOUNDATION
Equation I

Name: _____   Date of Exam : ___/___/___

                                                                           Date of Birth: ___/___/___

                                                                           Chronological Age: _____

1. *Handgrip strength, dominant hand,
   in kg .... : _____ x 0.155   = _____

2. Audiometry, right ear,
   in dB at 4,000 hz .... : _____ x 0.0457 = _____

3. Vibratory sensitivity, left
   medial malleolus, in volts ...... : _____ x 0.141   = _____

4. Visual acuity (decimal) .... : _____ x 3.57   = _____

5. Skin elasticity, in sec .... : _____ x 1.17   = _____

6. Light extinction time, in sec ... : _____ x 2.39   = _____

*Non-Asian subjects should use the conversion scale in Fig. B. 6-3 to obtain an adjusted handgrip strength for this equation.

Biological age = 51.9 - 1. _____ + 2. _____ + 3. _____

+ 4. _____ + 5. _____ - 6. _____

(Plot on a graph--App. C)   Biological age _____

Chapter 10 Radiation Research Foundation

CALCULATION SHEET
JAPANESE TEST BATTERY FOR WOMEN
RADIATION EFFECTS RESEARCH FOUNDATION
Equation II

Name: _____   Date of Exam : ___/___/___

Date of Birth: ___/___/___

Chronological Age: _____

1. *Handgrip strength, dominant hand,
   in kg .... : _____ x 0.160 = _____

2. Audiometry, right ear,
   in dB at 4,000 hz .... : _____ x 0.0677 = _____

3. Vibratory sensitivity, left
   medial malleolus, in volts ...... : _____ x 0.166 = _____

4. Visual acuity (decimal) .... : _____ x 3.36   = _____

5. Skin elasticity, in sec .... : _____ x 2.57   = _____

6. Light extinction time, in sec .... : _____ x 1.52   = _____

*Non-Asian subjects should use the conversion scale in Fig. B. 6-3 to obtain an adjusted handgrip strength for this equation.

Biological age = 45.8 - 1. _____ + 2. _____ + 3. _____

+ 4. _____ + 5. _____ - 6. _____

(Plot on a graph--App. C)   Biological age _____

Radiation Research Foundation Chapter 10

CALCULATION SHEET
JAPANESE TEST BATTERY FOR MEN
RADIATION EFFECTS RESEARCH FOUNDATION
Equation III

Name: _____   Date of Exam : ___/___/___

                                                              Date of Birth: ___/___/___

                                                              Chronological Age: _____

1. *Handgrip strength, dominant hand,
   in kg .... : _____ x 0.327 = _____

2. Audiometry, right ear,
   in dB at 4,000 hz .... : _____ x 0.0949 = _____

3. Vibratory sensitivity, left
   medial malleolus, in volts ...... : _____ x 0.258 = _____

4. Visual acuity (decimal) .... : _____ x 3.06   = _____

*Non-Asian subjects should use the conversion scale in Fig. B. 6-3 to obtain an adjusted handgrip strength for this equation.

Biological age = 60.2 - 1. _____ + 2. _____ + 3. _____ + 4. _____

(Plot on a graph--App. C)   Biological age _____

Chapter 10   **Radiation Research Foundation**

CALCULATION SHEET
JAPANESE TEST BATTERY FOR WOMEN
RADIATION EFFECTS RESEARCH FOUNDATION
Equation IV

Name: _____   Date of Exam : ___/___/___

                                                               Date of Birth: ___/___/___

                                                               Chronological Age: _____

1. *Handgrip strength, dominant hand,
   in kg .... : _____ x 0.485 = _____

2. Audiometry, right ear,
   in dB at 4,000 hz .... : _____ x 0.141 = _____

3. Vibratory sensitivity, left
   medial malleolus, in volts ...... : _____ x 0.329 = _____

4. Visual acuity (decimal) .... : _____ x 2.19   = _____

*Non-Asian subjects should use the conversion scale in
Fig. B. 6-3 to obtain an adjusted handgrip strength for
this equation.

Biological age = 51.9 - 1. _____ + 2. _____ + 3. _____ + 4. _____

(Plot on a graph--App. C)   Biological age _____

REFERENCES

Belsky, J. L., Moriyama, I. M., Fujita, S., Kawamoto, S. Aging studies in atomic bomb survivors. Radiation Effects Research Foundation, *Technical Report RERF TR 11-78*.

Curtis, H. J. *Biological Mechanisms of Aging*. Charles C. Thomas, Springfield, 1966.

Finch, S. C., Beebe, G. W. Review of thirty years study of Hiroshima and Nagasaki atomic bomb survivors. II. Biological effects. F. Aging. *J Radiat Res* (Tokyo) 16 (Suppl): 108-21, 1975.

Hirose, I., Fujisawa, J., Fujino, T., Okamoto, A. Amplitude of visual accommodation in atomic bomb survivors. *ABCC TR 9-67*.

Hollingsworth, J.W. Personal communication, 25 Feb 1985.

Hollingsworth, J.W., Ishii, G. Skin aging and hair graying in Hiroshima. *Geriatrics* 16: 27-36, 1961.

Hollingsworth, J. W., Hashizume, A, Jablon, S. Correlations between tests of aging in Hiroshima subjects--An attempt to define "Physiologic Age". *Yale J Biol Med*, 38: 11-26, Aug 1966.

Hollingsworth, D. R., Hollingsworth, J. W., Bogitch, S., Keehn, R. J. Neuromuscular tests of aging. *ABCC TR 1-69*.

Jablon, S. Personal Communications. 20 September 1983, 26 October 1983, 19 April, 1984.

Jones, M. Personal Communication. 11 October 1983.

Shock, N.W., Greulich, R. C., Costa, P. T., Andres, R., Lakatta, E. G., Arenberg, D., and Tobin, J. D., *Normal Human Aging: The Baltimore Longitudinal Study of Aging*. USDHHS, PHS, NIA, 1984.

Chapter 11

FINNISH TEST BATTERIES
University of Jyvaskyla

Researchers at the University of Jyvaskyla in Finland have conducted aging measurement studies since the early 1970s. It is one of the few research institutions in the world that has tenaciously maintained an interest in this important work, producing a stream of research papers on this subject.

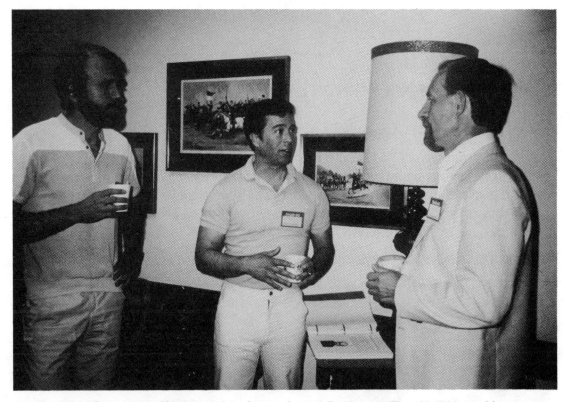

Fig. 11-1. **Dr. Harri Suominen (l), the author (center), and Professor Eino Heikkinen (r)**.

Chapter 11 — University of Jyvaskyla

Professor Eino Heikkinen (*Fig. 11-1*), of the Department of Health Sciences at the University, reported on the first study in the series in 1974 (Heikkinen, 1974). Although he conducted extensive studies using his original test battery--like the researchers from the ABCC (Chapter 10)--he did not disclose the equations in the original article. He recently retrieved the data from his archives and kindly provided the previously unpublished equation for inclusion in this book (Suominen, 1 Apr 1986).

EQUIPMENT FOR HEIKKINEN'S FIRST TEST BATTERY:

1. Spirometer (Appendix A. 2-1).
2. Vibrometer (Appendix A. 5-8).
3. Audiometer (Appendix A. 3-1).

TESTS IN HEIKKINEN'S FIRST TEST BATTERY:

1. Vital capacity (VC) (Appendix B. 2-2), in liters.
2. Vibratory sensitivity (VS) (Appendix B. 5-6) of the lateral malleolus (outside ankle), measured in volts with the vibrometer. Heikkinen used a custom-made vibrometer that registered in an arbitrary unit score. The score can be obtained by determining the vibratory threshold in volts, and then converting to arbitrary units using the conversion table in Fig. B. 5-10 in Appendix B.
3. Auditory acuity (AA) (Appendix B. 3-1), in decibels for each ear at 4,000 Hz. The value for the better ear is used.

HEIKKINEN'S FIRST EQUATION FOR MEN:

Biological age = 29.44 + 0.38 CA - 4.36 (VC) + 1.34 (VS) + 0.147 (AA)

EFFECT OF EXERCISE ON AGING AND AGING RATES

Dr. Harri Suominen (*Fig. 11-1*), an exercise physiologist in Heikkinen's Department, conducted a series of follow-up studies from 1975 to 1978, using a modification of the original test battery. His subjects were 44 men ranging in age from 31 to 72 years. Half were athletes from local running or orienteering clubs, and half were sedentary but otherwise healthy men. Suominen's goal was to determine whether physical training had any effect on the aging process (Suominen, 1978).

It has been hypothesized that since elderly people have many of the characteristics of physically unfit younger subjects, it is easy to assume that improvement of physical fitness in young and middle-aged people will increase their life span and consequently reduce their rate of aging (Shock).

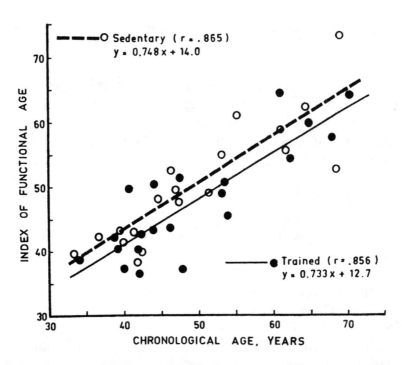

Fig. 11-2. **Comparison of chronological age and "index of functional age" (biological age) in trained and sedentary men.** Although the trained men generally scored younger biologically than their age-matched sedentary counterparts, the aging rates (slopes of regression lines) are identical in both groups (Suominen, 1978).

Dr. Ralph S. Paffenbarger and colleagues (1986) in the Department of Family, Community and Preventive Medicine, Stanford U. School of Medicine, recently confirmed the beneficial effects of exercise in reducing all causes of mortality. Paffenbarger found that all-cause mortality rates *decreased* as physical activity *increased*. Mortality rates became stabilized at minimum levels at an exercise intensity of 3,500 kcal/week or greater.

Some gerontologists continue to quibble about the differences between aging and disease (see Chapter 3 for more on this subject). They claim that it is *disease*--not the aging process--that is detrimental, and that our efforts should be directed at improving the quality (not necessarily the quantity) of life. I pointed out in Chapter 3 that the two goals are not mutually exclusive--that it is possible and preferable to have *both*. Paffenbarger's study indicates that exercise is a means of accomplishing this dual objective of reducing the incidence of the chronic degenerative diseases, as well as extending the life expectancy.

Although Suominen found that the athletes generally scored biologically younger than their age-matched sedentary counterparts, their aging *rates* appeared to be essentially the same (*Fig. 11-2*). These results seem to confirm the findings of an ongoing longitudinal study at San Diego State University alleging that exercise does not affect the aging rate, despite its many beneficial effects on health (Wallace).

Some scientists interpret these findings as an indication that exercise is of little use in an age retardation/health optimization program. I think they suggest the opposite.

Exercise obviously resets the biological age to a more youthful level (see Chapter 13 for another comparison of the effect of exercise appearing to corroborate Suominen's findings). Therefore, there *must* be a period during the transition from a deconditioned to a conditioned state during which the aging rate is temporarily reversed. How else would the conditioned subjects consistently score younger biologically post-conditioning?

Unfortunately, this reversal is limited and cannot be maintained indefinitely. The aging rate soon resumes its inexorable progression. However, if other modalities can be found that exert similar dramatic affects of "re-setting" biological ages to more youthful levels, the cumulative effect will clearly result in significant de facto reductions in the overall aging rate.

The concept of "step-wise" increases in lifespan (due to successive reductions in aging rate) was described and illustrated (*Fig. 11-3*) by Dr. Donald Carpenter (1980), who proposed the hypothetical possiblity of greatly increasing the lifespan by the progressive use of various incremental life-extending modalities (which may be available now or in the near future).

This approach was further supported in a recent article in the *New England Journal of Medicine* by Dr. Ed Schneider, former Deptuty Director of the NIA, and his colleague Dr. J. D. Reed (1985). The authors stated that, "...it is possible that 'segmental' interventions may be developed that will have important impacts on specific aging processes. An example would be the potential for arresting or reversing the decline in immune function that occurs with aging. Rejuvenation of the immune system might successfully delay the increased susceptibility of older people to infectious diseases and thus lead to a marked *increase in the quantity* as well as the quality of life.

"Segmental interventions can be assessed in laboratory animals and in human beings through the measurement of specific *biologic markers of aging* [such as are the subject of this book]. Such markers should be reproducible, noninvasive measures of specific molecular, cellular and organ functions that change over relatively short periods of time."

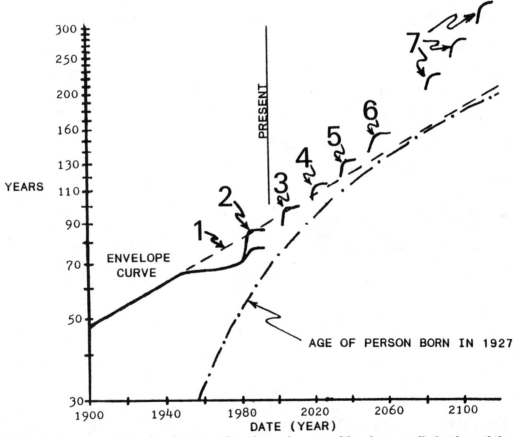

Fig. 11-3. **Effect of segmental aging intervention therapies, resulting in overall slowing of the aging rate and extension of the lifespan (Carpenter).** Hypothetical effect of successive applications of optimal regimens of potentially effective age-retarding agents. 1. Physical conditioning (Wallace); 2. Caloric restriction (Walford); 3. Antioxidant therapy (Harman); 4. Restoration of immune function (Goldstein, et al); 5. "Death Hormone" blocking drugs (Regelson); 6. Chelation therapy (Bjorksten); 7. Other proposed age-retarding agents (Schneider and Reed; Mann; Pearson and Shaw).

Suominen does not recommend the clinical use of his aging measurement system at this time. He thinks the reliability of his equation may be questioned because of the relatively small number of participants in the study and the lack of longitudinal comparative data of the aging rates of all trained and control subjects (Suominen, July 14, 1984). Despite his reservations, our experience with his equation give remarkably accurate results. Furthermore, since all tests included in his battery are integral parts of other systems in this book, its completion will not require a great deal of additional effort.

REQUIREMENTS FOR SUOMINEN'S TEST BATTERY:

1. Equipment for determining maximal oxygen uptake (VO_2max):

    a. Bicycle ergometer (Appendix A. 1-2). or:

    b. Laboratory treadmill (Appendix A. 1-3) with or without a metabolic cart or other instrument capable of computing VO_2max (Appendix A. 1-4).

    or:

    c. Two-step staircase (Appendix A. 1-5).

2. Spirometer (Appendix A. 2-1).

3. Sphygmomanometer and stethoscope (Appendix A. 1-1).

4. Vibrometer (Appendix A. 5-8).

5. Audiometer (Appendix A. 3-1).

6. Wechsler Digit Symbol test kit (Appendix A. 5-14).

TESTS IN SUOMINEN'S TEST BATTERY:

1. Maximal oxygen uptake (VO_2max) in liters/min (Appendix B. 1-5).

2. Vital capacity (VC) (Appendix B. 2-2), in liters.

3. Systolic blood pressure (SBP) (Appendix B. 1-1) (supine), in mm Hg.

4. Vibratory sensitivity (VS) (Appendix B. 5-6) of the lateral malleolus (outside ankle), measured in volts with a vibrometer. Suominen's custom-made vibrometer registered in an arbitrary unit score. After determining the vibratory threshold in volts, convert to units using the conversion table in *Fig. B. 5-10*, Appendix B.

5. Auditory acuity (AA) (Appendix B. 3-1), in decibels for each ear at 4,000 Hz. The value for the better ear is used.

6. Digit Symbol test (DS) (Appendix B. 5-8).

SUOMINEN'S EQUATION FOR MEN:

Biological age = 69.51 - 2.27 (VO$_2$max) - 3.68 (VC) + 0.0092 (SBP) + 0.736 (VS) + 0.128 (AA) - 0.148 (DS)

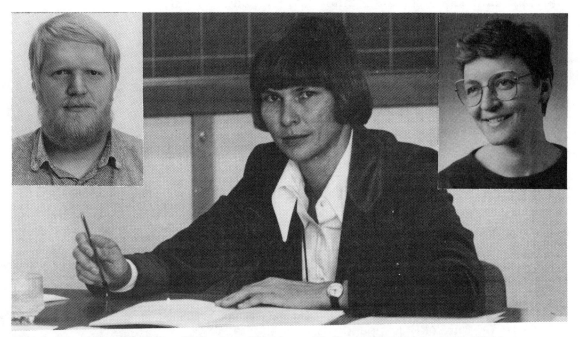

Fig. 11-4. **Left to right: Pertti Era, M.S., Anja Kiiskinen, Ph.D., and Terttu Parkatti, Ph.Lic.**

ADDITIONAL TEST BATTERIES

Further studies were conducted by another group associated with Heikkinen and Suominen. These were conducted by Dr. Anja Kiiskinen and her colleagues, Terttu Parkatti, Ph. Lic., and Pertti Era, M.S., (*Fig. 11-4*) (Kiiskinen, et al). They tried to construct a simple test battery that could: be conducted rapidly; require no complicated instruments or highly trained personnel; measure essential body functions; and be sensitive and reliable. Kiiskinen modified some of the tests of Heikkinnen and Suominen, and included women and younger subjects.

REQUIREMENTS FOR KIISKINEN'S TEST BATTERY:

1. Vibrometer (Appendix A. 5-8).
2. Berens near-point indicator; Krimsky-Prince rule; or yardstick and near-vision cards (Appendix A. 4-1).
3. Spirometer (Appendix A. 2-1).
4. Sphygmomanometer and stethoscope (Appendix A. 1-1).
5. Handgrip dynamometer (Appendix A. 6-1).
6. Three-choice reaction time apparatus (Appendix A. 5-12).
7. Purdue pegboard (Appendix A. 5-2).

TESTS IN KIISKINEN'S TEST BATTERY:

1. Vibratory sensitivity (VS) of the medial malleolus (Appendix B. 5-6), in volts (subsequently converted to arbitrary units as in Suominen's test).
2. Near vision (NV) (Appendix B. 4-1), in diopters.
3. Vital capacity (VC) (Appendix B. 2-2), in liters.
4. Pulse pressure (PP) (Appendix B. 1-4), in mm Hg.

5. Handgrip strength (HGS) (Appendix B. 6-2), in kg.

6. Three-choice reaction time (RT3) (Appendix B. 5-13. a), in milliseconds.

7. Finger dexterity (FD), using a modified Purdue pegboard test (Appendix B. 5-1.b). The standard test is modified in that only the first ten holes (of fifty possible) are filled with a pin, washer and socket. Tape is placed over the remaining holes. The score is the time in seconds to complete the test.

KIISKINEN'S AGING MEASUREMENT EQUATIONS:

I. (Men) Biological age = 69.9 + 1.147 (VS) - 1.920 (NV) - 2.110 (VC) + 0.066 (PP) - 0.024 (HGS) + 0.013 (RT_3) + 0.044 (FD)

II. (Women) Biological Age = 76.8 + 0.503 (VS) - 2.683 (NV) - 2.133 (VC) + 0.079 (PP) - 0.012 (HGS) + 0.001 (RT_3) + 0.105 (FD)

CORRECTION FACTORS FOR KIISKINEN'S EQUATIONS:

Although not in their original paper, the researchers calculated correction factors for inclusion in this book (Parkatti), correcting the artifactual errors inherent in the regression method (see Chapters 7 and 14 for extended discussions of this subject). The correction factors are in Table 11-I. The correction factor should be added to or subtracted from the biological age.

CONTINUING STUDIES AT THE UNIVERSITY OF JYVASKYLA:

Heikkinen continued his research, further refining and improving his test batteries (Heikkinen, et al, 1984). Although he did not describe the exact test batteries and equations in his latest paper, he again kindly sent this information for inclusion in this book (Heikkinen, 1985).

REQUIREMENTS FOR HEIKKINEN'S TEST BATTERIES:

1. Audiometer (Appendix A. 3-1).
2. Handgrip dynamometer (Appendix A. 6-1).
3. Equipment for determining maximal oxygen uptake (VO_2max) (see Suominen's test battery).
4. Choice reaction-time apparatus (Appendix A. 5-13. a).
5. Bio-mechanical force platform (Appendix A. 5-11).
6. Sphygmomanometer and stethoscope (Appendix A. 1-1).
7. Friedmann visual field analyzer (Appendix A. 4-3).
8. Wechsler Block Design test set (Appendix A. 5-15).

TESTS IN HEIKKINEN'S TEST BATTERIES:

1. Auditory accuity (AA) (Appendix B. 3-1) at 4,000 Hz, in dB.
2. Handgrip strength (HGS) (Appendix B. 6-2), in kg.
3. Maximal oxygen uptake (VO_2max) (Appendix B. 1-5) in ml/kg.min. Although Heikkinen used a bicycle ergometer, any of the methods of measuring VO_2max should give valid longitudinal measurements.
4. 4-choice reaction time (RT_4) (Appendix B. 5-13. a) in milliseconds.
5. Static balance (SB) (Appendix B. 5-11. b), in mm.
6. Systolic blood pressure (SBP) (Appendix B. 1-1) in mm Hg in the sitting position.
7. Dark adaptation test (DA) (Appendix B. 4-3), in sec.
8. Block design (BD) (Appendix B. 5-10).

HEIKKINEN'S EQUATIONS FOR MEN:

I. Biological age = 31.24 + .245 (CA) + .227 (AA) - .235 (HGS) - .309 (VO$_2$max) + .013 (RT$_4$) + 0.028 (SB) + .076 (SBP) + .012 (DA)

II. Biological age = 31.0 + .248 (CA) + .239 (AA) - .307 (HGS) + .004 (RT$_4$) + .118 (SBP) + .017 (DA) - .429 (BD)

III. Biological age = 47.6 + .260 (CA) + .270 (AA) - .328 (HGS) + .003 (RT$_4$) + .021 (SB) + .015 (DA) - .463 (BD)

HEIKKINEN'S EQUATIONS REVISED:

Because the dark adaptation and static balance tests require equipment available only in major research institutes, these test batteries are of little use for most clinicians. At my request, Heikkinen and his staff calculated another set of equations especially for inclusion in this book, deleting these tests (Suominen, 29 Nov 1985). These revised equations are:

I. a. Biological age = 33.1 + .279 (CA) + .257 (AA) - .270 (HGS) - .353 (VO$_2$max) + .010 (RT$_4$) + .114 (SBP)

II. a. Biological age = 29.3 + .259 (CA) + .262 (AA) - .307 (HGS) + .004 (RT$_4$) + .148 (SBP) - .522 (BD)

III. a. Biological age = 51.0 + .289 (CA) + .306 (AA) - .336 (HGS) + .003 (RT$_4$) - .579 (BD)

All of these equations have built-in correction factors, and do not require additional manipulations to improve their accuracy. Heikkinen cautions that his measurement systems may not give the requisite accuracy for the uses that I propose, due to their lack of longitudinal and cross-cultural validation. I think that his reservations are overcautious and unnecessary. Our preliminary computer verifications indicate that his test batteries appear to be quite accurate.

Table 11-I. **Biological Age Correction Table--Kiiskinen**

Chronological Age	Men	Women
35	-0.8295	-0.8335
36	-0.6994	-0.7274
37	-0.5693	-0.6213
38	-0.4392	-0.5152
39	-0.3091	-0.4091
40	-0.179	-0.303
41	-0.0489	-0.1969
42	0.0812	-0.0908
43	0.2113	0.0153
44	0.3414	0.1214
45	0.4715	0.2275
46	0.6016	0.3336
47	0.7317	0.4397
48	0.8618	0.5458
49	0.9919	0.6519
50	1.122	0.758
51	1.2521	0.8641
52	1.3822	0.9702
53	1.5123	1.0763
54	1.6424	1.1824
55	1.7725	1.2885
56	1.9026	1.3946
57	2.0327	1.5007
58	2.1628	1.6068
59	2.2929	1.7129
60	2.423	1.819
61	2.5531	1.9251
62	2.6832	2.0312
63	2.8133	2.1373
64	2.9434	2.2434
65	3.0735	2.3495
66	3.2036	2.4556
67	3.3337	2.5617
68	3.4638	2.6678
69	3.5939	2.7739
70	3.724	2.88

Table 11-I. (cont'd)

Chronological Age	Men	Women
71	3.8541	2.9861
72	3.9842	3.0922
73	4.1143	3.1983
74	4.2444	3.3044
75	4.3745	3.4105
76	4.5046	3.5166
77	4.6347	3.6227
78	4.7648	3.7288
79	4.8949	3.8349
80	5.025	3.941
81	5.1551	4.0471
82	5.2852	4.1532
83	5.4153	4.2593
84	5.5454	4.3654
85	5.6755	4.4715

Chapter 11 — University of Jyvaskyla

CALCULATION SHEET
FINNISH TEST BATTERY FOR MEN
UNIVERSITY OF JYVASKYLA
Heikkinen

Name: _____   Date of Exam : ___/___/___

　　　　　　　　　　　　　　　　　　　　Date of Birth: ___/___/___

　　　　　　　　　　　　　　　　　　　　Chronological Age : _____

1. Vital capacity, in liters .... : _____ x 4.36   = _____

2. Vibratory sensitivity,
    lateral malleolus, in volts
    = _____ units
    (use the conversion scale in
    Fig. B. 5-10, Appendix B) ...... : _____ x 1.346 = _____

3. Auditory acuity at 4,000 Hz,
    in decibels .... : _____ x 0.147 = _____

Biological age = 29.44 + 0.38 CA _____ − 1. _____ + 2. _____
+ 3. _____

(Plot on a graph--App. C)   Biological age = _____

University of Jyvaskyla   Chapter 11

CALCULATION SHEET
FINNISH TEST BATTERY FOR MEN
UNIVERSITY OF JYVASKYLA
Suominen

Name: _____   Date of Exam : ___/___/___

                                                                                      Date of Birth: ___/___/___

                                                                                      Chronological Age: _____

1. Maximal oxygen uptake,
   in liters per minute .... : _____ x 2.27   = _____

2. Vital capacity, in liters .... : _____ x 3.68   = _____

3. Systolic blood pressure
   (supine), in mm Hg .... : _____ x 0.0092 = _____

4. Vibratory sensitivity,
   lateral malleolus, in volts
   = _____ units
   (use the conversion scale in
   Fig. B. 5-10 in Appendix B) .... : _____ x 0.736 = _____

5. Auditory perception at
   4,000 Hz, in decibels .... : _____ x 0.128 = _____

6. Digit Symbol test .... : _____ x 0.148 = _____

Biological age = 69.51 - 1. _____ - 2. _____ + 3. _____

+ 4. _____ + 5. _____ - 6. _____

(Plot on a graph--App. C)   Biological age = _____

| Chapter 11 | University of Jyvaskyla |

CALCULATION SHEET
FINNISH TEST BATTERY FOR MEN
UNIVERSITY OF JYVASKYLA
Kliskinen Equation I

Name: _____   Date of Exam : ___/___/___

　　　　　　　　　　　　　　　　　　　　　　Date of Birth: ___/___/___

　　　　　　　　　　　　　　　　　　　　　　Chronological Age: _____

1. Vibratory sensitivity,
   medial malleolus, in volts
   = _____ units
   (use the conversion scale in
   Fig. B 5-10, Appendix B) .... : _____ x 1.147 = _____

2. Near vision, in diopters .... : _____ x 1.920 = _____

3. Vital capacity, in liters .... : _____ x 2.110 = _____

4. Pulse pressure, in mm Hg .... : _____ x 0.066 = _____

5. Handgrip strength, in kg .... : _____ x 0.024 = _____

6. Three-choice reaction time,
   in milliseconds .... : _____ x 0.013 = _____

7. Finger dexterity, in sec
   required to fill 10 holes ...... : _____ x 0.044 = _____

Biological age = 69.9 + 1. _____ - 2. _____ - 3. _____

+ 4. _____ - 5. _____ + 6. _____ + 7. _____

+ _____ correction factor (CF) (From Table 11-I)

(Plot on a graph--App. C) Corrected biological age _____

University of Jyvaskyla   Chapter 11

CALCULATION SHEET
FINNISH TEST BATTERY FOR WOMEN
UNIVERSITY OF JYVASKYLA
Kiiskinen Equation II

Name: _____   Date of Exam : ___/___/___

                                         Date of Birth: ___/___/___

                                         Chronological Age: _____

1. Vibratory sensitivity,
     medial malleolus, in volts
     = _____ units
     (use the conversion scale in
     Fig. B. 5-10, Appendix B). ..... : _____ x 0.503 = _____

2. Near vision, in diopters .... : _____ x 2.683 = _____

3. Vital capacity, in liters .... : _____ x 2.133 = _____

4. Pulse pressure, in mm Hg .... : _____ x 0.079 = _____

5. Handgrip strength, in kg .... : _____ x 0.012 = _____

6. Three-choice reaction time,
     in milliseconds .... : _____ x 0.001 = _____

7. Finger dexterity, in sec
     required to fill 10 holes ...... : _____ x 0.105 = _____

Biological age = 76.8 + 1. _____ - 2. _____ - 3. _____

+ 4. _____ - 5. _____ + 6. _____ + 7. _____

= _____ correction factor (From Table 11-I)

(Plot on a graph--App. C) Corrected biological age _____

CALCULATION SHEET
FINNISH TEST BATTERY FOR MEN
UNIVERSITY OF JYVASKYLA
Heikkinen Equation I

Name: _____   Date of Exam : ___/___/___

Date of Birth: ___/___/___

Chronological Age: _____

1. Auditory accuity, 4,000 Hz, in dB : _____ x 0.227 = _____

2. Handgrip strength, in kg .... : _____ x 0.235 = _____

3. Maximal oxygen uptake, in ml/kg.min: _____ x 0.309 = _____

4. Four-choice reaction time,
   in milliseconds .... : _____ x 0.013 = _____

5. Static balance, in mm .... : _____ x 0.028 = _____

6. Systolic blood pressure, in mm Hg : _____ x 0.076 = _____

7. Dark adaptation, in sec .... : _____ x 0.012 = _____

Biological age = 31.2 + .245 CA _____ + 1. _____ - 2. _____
- 3. _____ + 4. _____ + 5. _____ + 6. _____ + 7. _____

(Plot on a graph--App. C)   Biological age _____

| University of Jyvaskyla | Chapter 11 |

CALCULATION SHEET
FINNISH TEST BATTERY FOR MEN
UNIVERSITY OF JYVASKYLA
Heikkinen Equation 1 a

Name: _____   Date of Exam : ___/___/___

　　　　　　　　　　　　　　　　　　　　Date of Birth: ___/___/___

　　　　　　　　　　　　　　　　　　　　Chronological Age: _____

1. Auditory accuity, 4,000 Hz, in dB : _____ x 0.257 = _____

2. Handgrip strength, in kg .... : _____ x 0.270 = _____

3. Maximal oxygen uptake,
      in ml/kg.min .... : _____ x 0.353 = _____

4. Four-choice reaction time,
      in milliseconds .... : _____ x 0.010 = _____

5. Systolic blood pressure, in mm Hg : _____ x 0.114 = _____

Biological age = 33.1 + .279 CA _____ + 1. _____ − 2. _____

− 3. _____ + 4. _____ + 5. _____

(Plot on a graph--App. C)   Biological age _____

Chapter 11	University of Jyvaskyla

CALCULATION SHEET
FINNISH TEST BATTERY FOR MEN
UNIVERSITY OF JYVASKYLA
Heikkinen Equation II

Name: _____ Date of Exam : ___/___/___

Date of Birth: ___/___/___

Chronological Age: _____

1. Auditory accuity, 4,000 Hz, in dB   : _____ x 0.239 = _____

2. Handgrip strength, in kg .... : _____ x 0.307 = _____

3. Four-choice reaction time,
    in milliseconds .... : _____ x 0.004 = _____

4. Systolic blood pressure, in mm Hg   : _____ x 0.118 = _____

5. Dark adaptation, in sec ....   : _____ x 0.017 = _____

6. Block design ....   : _____ x 0.429 = _____

Biological age = 31.0 + .248 CA _____ + 1. _____ - 2. _____

+ 3. _____ + 4. _____ + 5. _____ - 6. _____

(Plot on a graph--App. C)   Biological age _____

University of Jyvaskyla   Chapter 11

CALCULATION SHEET
FINNISH TEST BATTERY FOR MEN
UNIVERSITY OF JYVASKYLA
Heikkinen Equation II a

Name: _____   Date of Exam : ___/___/___

                                         Date of Birth: ___/___/___

                                         Chronological Age: _____

1. Auditory accuity, 4,000 Hz, in dB   : _____ x 0.262 = _____

2. Handgrip strength, in kg ....   : _____ x 0.307 = _____

3. Four-choice reaction time,
     in milliseconds ....   : _____ x 0.004 = _____

4. Systolic blood pressure, in mm Hg   : _____ x 0.148 = _____

5. Block design   X 0.522 =   = (5)

Biological age = 29.3 + .259 CA _____ + 1. _____ - 2. _____

+ 3. _____ + 4. _____ - 5. _____

(Plot on a graph--App. C)   Biological age _____

123

CALCULATION SHEET
FINNISH TEST BATTERY FOR MEN
UNIVERSITY OF JYVASKYLA
Heikkinen Equation III

Name: _____   Date of Exam : ___/___/___

                                                              Date of Birth: ___/___/___

                                                              Chronological Age: _____

1. Auditory accuity, 4,000 Hz, in dB : _____ x 0.270 = _____

2. Handgrip strength, in kg .... : _____ x 0.328 = _____

3. Four-choice reaction time,
   in milliseconds .... : _____ x 0.003 = _____

4. Static balance, in mm .... : _____ x 0.021 = _____

5. Dark adaptation, in sec .... : _____ x 0.015 = _____

6. Block design .... : _____ x 0.463 = _____

Biological age = 47.6 + .260 CA _____ + 1. _____ - 2. _____

+ 3. _____ + 4. _____ + 5. _____ - 6. _____

(Plot on a graph--App. C)   Biological age _____

University of Jyvaskyla Chapter 11

CALCULATION SHEET
FINNISH TEST BATTERY FOR MEN
UNIVERSITY OF JYVASKYLA
Heikkinen Equation III a

Name: _____ Date of Exam : ___/___/___

 Date of Birth: ___/___/___

 Chronological Age: _____

1. Auditory accuity, 4,000 Hz, in dB : _____ x 0.306 = _____

2. Handgrip strength, in kg .... : _____ x 0.336 = _____

3. Four-choice reaction time,
   in milliseconds .... : _____ x 0.003 = _____

4. Block design .... : _____ x 0.579 = _____

Biological age = 51.0 + .289 CA _____ + 1. _____ − 2. _____

+ 3. _____ − 4. _____

(Plot on a graph--App. C) Biological age _____

REFERENCES

Bjorksten, J. Possibilities and limitations of chelation as a means for life extension. *Rejuvenation*, Vol. VII, No. 3, Sept 1980, pp. 67-72.

Carpenter, D. G. Correction of biological aging. *Rejuvenation*. Vol. VIII, No. 2, Jun 1980, pp. 31-49.

Goldstein, A. L., Low, T. L. K., Hall, N., Naylor, P. H., and Zatz, M. M. Thymosin: Can it retard aging by boosting immune capacity? in: *Modern Aging Research--Intervention in the Aging Process, Part A: Quantitation, Epidemiology, and Clinical Research*, by Regelson, W., and Sinex, F. M. (eds), New York, Alan R. Liss, 1983.

Harman, D. Free radical theory of aging: The "free radical" diseases. *AGE*, Vol. 7, No. 4, October, 1984, pp. 111-131.

Heikkinen, E. Assessment of Functional Ageing, in: *Lectures on Gerontology, Vol. I: On Biology of Ageing, Part B*. A. Vidik (ed). New York, Academic Press, 1982.

Heikkinen, E., Kiiskinen, A., Kayhty, B., Rimpela, M., and Vuori, I. Assessment of Biological Age, *Gerontologia* Vol. 20: 33-43 1974.

Heikkinen, E., Arajarvi, R. L., Era, P., Jylha, M., Kinnunen, V., Liskinen, A.L., Leskinen, E., Masseli, E., Pohjolainen, P., Rahkila, P., Suominen, H., Turpeinen, P., Vaisanen, M., and Osterback, L. Functional capacity of men born in 1906--10, 1926--30, and 1946--50. A Basic Report. *Scand J Soc Med Suppl* 33, 1984.

Heikkinen, E. Personal communications, 8 March 1984, 15 January 1985, 26 June 1985.

Kiiskinen, A., Era, P., and Parkatti, T. Functional age of relatively young and old female and male employees in the machine industry. *IRCS Medical Science: Biochemistry; Clinical Medicine; Environmental Biology and Medicine; Social and Occupational Medicine*, Vol. 9, pp. 6-7 (1981).

Mann, J. *Secrets of Life Extension*. New York. Bantam Books, 1982.

Paffenbarger, R. S., Hyde, R. T., Wing, A. L., Hsieh, C. C. Physical activity, all-cause mortality, and longevity of college alumni. *N Engl J Med*, 1986. 314: 605-613.

Parkatti, T. Personal communication, 7 May, 1985.

Pearson, D, and Shaw, S. *Life Extension*. New York, Warner Books, 1981.

Regelson, W. The evidence for pituitary and thyroid control of aging: Is age reversal a myth or reality? The searach for a "death hormone", in: *Modern Aging Research--Intervention in the Aging Process, Part B: Basic Research and Pre-clinical Screening*, by Regelson, W., and Sinex, F. M. (eds), New York, Alan R. Liss, 1983.

Schneider, E. L., and Reed, J. D. Life Extension, *New England Journal of Medicine*. Vol. 312, No. 18, 1985, pp. 1159-1168.

Shock, N. W. Physical activity and the "rate of ageing". in: *The Longevity of Athletes*, Polednak, A. P. (ed.), 1979, Springfield, Charles C. Thomas, pp. 5-13.

Suominen, H. Effects of Physical Training in Middle-Aged and Elderly People, in: Komi, P.V. (ed.), *Studies in Sport, Physical Education and Health*, 11, University of Jyvaskyla, 1978.

Suominen, H. Personal communications, 14 July, 1984; 5 September, 1984; 29 November, 1985; 1 April 1986.

Wallace, J. P. Physical Conditioning: Intervention in aging cardiovascular function. in: *Modern Aging Research--Intervention in the Aging Process, Part A: Quantitation, Epidemiology, and Clinical Research*, by Regelson, W., and Sinex, F. M. (eds), New York, Alan R. Liss, 1983.

Walford, R. L. *Maximum Life Span*, New York, W. W. Norton and Company, 1983.

Chapter 12

AMERICAN TEST BATTERY
Gerontology Research Center

The Gerontology Research Center (GRC) of The National Institute on Aging (NIA), one of the member institutes of the National Institutes of Health, is conducting a comprehensive long-term study on the effects of aging on a large group of men (between 500 and 600 at any given time). This study has been continuing for over a quarter of a century (Shock, et al). About every year and a half, these men (women have also recently been added to the study) undergo numerous biochemical, physiological and psychological tests.

Three of the major goals of this study are: to describe the psychological and physiological effects of aging; to develop a means to calculate rates of change in specific variables in individual subjects; and to develop indices of physiological age (Shock, et al).

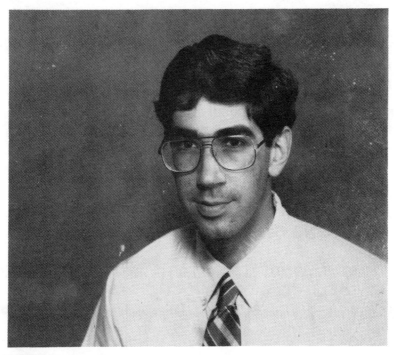

Fig. 12-1. **Dr. Gary Borkan**.

Chapter 12 — Gerontology Research Center

An in-depth, productive analysis of these data was made by Dr. Gary Borkan (*Fig. 12-1*), a resourceful, innovative anthropological researcher for the Veterans Administration Normative Aging Study in Boston. In collaboration with Dr. Arthur Norris, late Chief of the Human Performance Section, Borkan (1982) calculated an aging measurement equation based on his analysis of data from 1,068 men in the NIA's study.

REQUIREMENTS FOR THE GRC TEST BATTERY:

1. Standard clinical laboratory chemistry and hematological tests.
2. Spirometer (Appendix A. 2-1).
3. Handgrip dynamometer (Appendix A. 6-1).
4. Tapping board (Appendix A. 5-10).
5. Stopwatch.

TESTS IN THE GRC EQUATION:

1. Hemoglobin (HB) (Appendix B. 8-2), in mg/100 ml.
2. Forced expiratory volume in 1 second (FEV_1) (Appendix B. 2-1) in liters.
3. Creatinine clearance (CC) (Appendix B. 10-2), in ml per minute.
4. Systolic blood pressure (SBP) (Appendix B. 1-1), in mm Hg, in the supine position. Several measurements are taken, and the average is used.
5. Handgrip strength (HGS) (Appendix B. 6-2), in kg. With the subject seated, three maximum effort repetitions are made with each hand. The value used is the average of the highest score attained with each hand.
6. Tapping test (TT) (Appendix B. 5-13) in min.

BORKAN'S EQUATION FOR MEN:

Biological age = $99.52 - 1.58 (HB) - 6.048 (FEV_1) - .152 (CC) + .197 (SBP) - .361 (HGS) + 6.883 (TT)$

Gerontology Research Center   Chapter 12

CALCULATION SHEET
TEST BATTERY FOR MEN
GERONTOLOGY RESEARCH CENTER

Name: _____ Date of Exam : ___/___/___

                                         Date of Birth: ___/___/___

                                         Chronological Age: _____

1. Hemoglobin in gm/100 ml .... : _____ x 1.58 = _____

2. Forced expiratory volume
   in 1 sec (FEV_1) in liters ...... : _____ x 6.048 = _____

3. Creatinine clearance
   in ml/min .... : _____ x 0.152 = _____

4. Systolic blood pressure
   in mm Hg .... : _____ x 0.197 = _____

5. Handgrip strength in kg .... : _____ x 0.361 = _____

6. Tapping test in min .... : _____ x 6.883 = _____

Biological age = 99.52 - 1. _____ - 2. _____ - 3. _____

+ 4. _____ - 5. _____ + 6. _____

(Plot on a graph--App. C)   Biological age _____

REFERENCES

Borkan, G. A. *The Assessment of Biological Age During Adult-hood*. Doctoral Dissertation. Univ. Michigan. Dissertation Abstracts International, 39/06-A, 3682 (University Microfilms No. 78228-61). 1978.

Borkan, G. A., and Norris, A. H. Assessment of biological age using a profile of physical parameters. *J Gerontol*, 55, 177, 1980.

Borkan, Gary A., and Norris, A. H. Biological age in adult-hood: Comparison of active and inactive U.S. males. *Human Biology*, December 1980, Vol 52, No. 4, pp. 787-802.

Borkan, G. A., Bachman, S. S. Comparison of visually estimated age with physiologically predicted age as indicators of rates of aging. *Social Science in Medicine*, Vol. 16, 197-204, 1982.

Borkan, G. A., Hults, D.E., Gerzof, S. G., Burrows, B. A., and Robbins, A. H. Relationships between computed tomography tissue areas, thickness and total body composition. Annals of *Human Biology*, 1983, Vol. 10, No. 6, 537-546.

Borkan, G. A., Hults, D. E., and Glynn, R. J. Role of longitudinal change and secular trend in age differences in male body dimensions. *Human Biology*, September 1983, Vol. 55, No. 3, pp. 629-641.

Borkan, G. A., Hults, D. E., Gerzof, S. G., Robbins, A. H., and Silbert, C. K. Age changes in body composition revealed by computed tomography. *J Geront* 1983, Vol. 38, No. 6, pp. 673-677.

Borkan, G. A. Factors in clinical aging: Variation in rates of aging. *Intervention in the Aging Process, Part A, Quantitation, Epidemiology, and Clinical Research*, New York, Alan R. Liss, 1983.

Shock, N. W., Greulich, R. C., Andres, R., Arenberg, D., Costa, P. T., Lakatta, E. G., and Tobin, J. *Normal Human Aging: The Baltimore Longitudinal Study of Aging*. U.S. Dept of Health and Human Services, NIH Publication No. 84-2450, November 1984. Wash, D.C. U.S. GPO.

Chapter 13

JAPANESE TEST BATTERIES
University of Kyoto

Dr. Eitaro Nakamura (*Fig. 13-1*), Associate Professor, Department of Physical Education, Kyoto University College of Liberal Arts, in Japan, recently studied the effects of physical conditioning on the rate of aging. His goal and approach were similar to those of Suominen in Finland (Chapter 11).

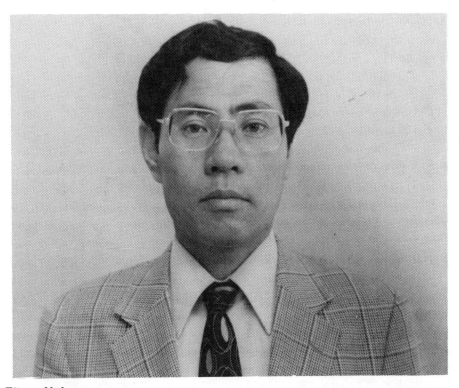

Fig. 13-1. **Dr. Eitaro Nakamura**.

In his first study, Nakamura (1982) reviewed the results of a comprehensive battery of medical examinations given to 390 men during 1979 and 1980. He believed that most of the aging measurement systems developed by other scientists were inadequate in several respects--primarily because most of them contained non-standard or difficult- to- measure tests. He attempted to correct this deficiency by basing his first test battery on 9 standard laboratory tests.

In testing his equation, he found--as did Dirken in Holland (Chapter 7)--that the curve of the regression line was skewed clockwise, causing subjects at the older end of the population to score younger than they should, and those at the younger end to appear older (*Fig. 13-2*).

Although he did not include them in the original article, he subsequently calculated correction factors by which uncorrected biological ages should be adjusted to compensate for this artifactual error (Nakamura, personal communication, 11 Dec 1984). He recalculated the regression line, and found the corrected equation predicted the biological ages of nearly 70% of the subjects within 1.0 standard deviation of their chronological ages (*Fig. 13-3*).

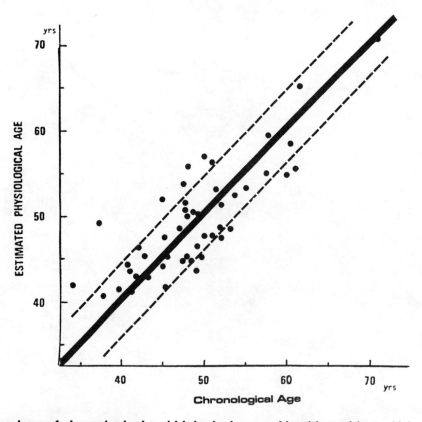

Fig. 13-2. **Comparison of chronological and biological ages of healthy subjects**. Using Nakamura's uncorrected first equation, the line generated by the equation is skewed clockwise, causing those at the older end of the population to score younger than they should, and those at the younger end to appear older (Nakamura, *Jap J Hygiene*).

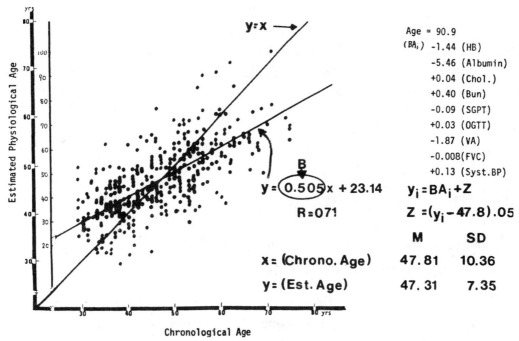

Fig. 13-3. **Comparison of chronological and biological age using Equation I modified by correction factors** (Nakamura, Personal communication, 11 December 1984).

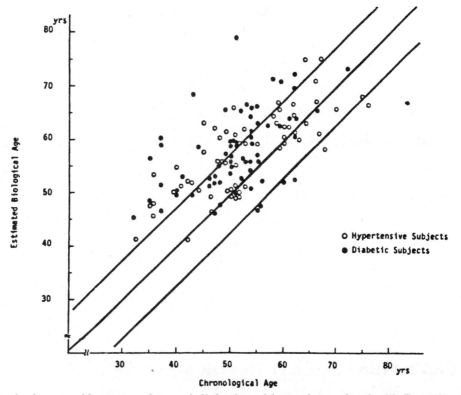

Fig. 13-4. **Biological ages of hypertensive and diabetic subjects determined with Equation I.** As the biological ages were generally older than the chronological ages, this appears to confirm the common belief that these diseases really are correlated with premature aging (Nakamura, *Jap J Hygiene*, 1982).

Next, he used a technique similar to Webster (Chapter 8) and Furukawa (Chapter 9), to test the equation's validity. He calculated the biological ages of 63 hypertensive and 65 diabetic patients, and found that the average biological age for both groups was significantly higher than their average chronological ages (*Fig. 13-4*). This appears to confirm the common belief that diabetes or hypertension are associated with accelerated aging (Anonymous, *Modern Medicine*; Thompson).

REQUIREMENTS FOR NAKAMURA'S FIRST TEST BATTERY:

1. Standard clinical laboratory hematology and chemistry tests.
2. Visual acuity charts (Appendix A. 4-2).
3. Spirometer (Appendix A. 2-1).
4. Sphygmomanometer and stethoscope (Appendix A. 1-1).

TESTS IN NAKAMURA'S FIRST TEST BATTERY:

1. Hemoglobin (HB) (Appendix B. 8-2) in mg/100 ml.
2. Albumin (AL) (Appendix B. 9-7) in mg/100 ml.
3. Cholesterol (CHOL) (Appendix B. 9-1) in mg/100 ml.
4. Urea nitrogen (BUN) (Appendix B. 9-5) in mg/100 ml.
5. Glutamic pyruvic transaminase (SGPT) (Appendix B. 9-8) in international units.
6. Glucose at one hour during an oral glucose tolerance test (OGTT) (Appendix B. 11-1) in mg/100 ml.
7. Visual acuity, left eye (VA) (Appendix B. 4-2) as a decimal.
8. Forced vital capacity (FVC) (Appendix B. 2-2) in ml.
9. Systolic blood pressure (SBP) (supine) (Appendix B. 1-1) in mm Hg.

NAKAMURA'S FIRST EQUATION FOR MEN:

Biological age = 90.9 - 1.44 (HB) - 5.46 (AL) + 0.04 (CHOL) + 0.40 (BUN) -0.09 (SGPT) + 0.03 (OGTT) - 1.87 (VA) - 0.008 (FVC) + 0.13 (SBP)

University of Kyoto   Chapter 13

FOLLOWUP STUDIES:

Nakamura thinks biological age can be assessed most precisely if the tests measure response to a physiological stress. This concept is shared by many other gerontologists and is discussed at greater length in Chapter 23. His second equation is based on the results of examinations conducted on 51 healthy sedentary men between 32 and 72 years of age.

REQUIREMENTS FOR NAKAMURA'S SECOND TEST BATTERY:

1. Equipment for measuring maximal oxygen uptake (VO_2 max). Nakamura uses the treadmill protocol in Appendix B. 1-5. a., and measures VO_2 max directly with a metabolic cart (Appendix A. 1-4). Other methods described in Appendix B. 1-5 may be used also.

    a. Laboratory treadmill (Appendix A. 1-3) and physiological monitoring system (Appendix A. 1-4) (optional).

    or:

    b. Bicycle ergometer (Appendix A. 1-2).

    or:

    c. Two-step staircase (Appendix A. 1-5).

2. Body weight scale, that measures in kg.

3. Heart rate monitor (Appendix A. 1-6).

4. Spirometer (Appendix B. 2-1).

TESTS IN NAKAMURA'S SECOND TEST BATTERY:

1. Maximal oxygen uptake (VO_2 max) (Appendix B. 1-5). Two values for this test are necessary: One is the VO_2 max in ml/kg.min (used directly in the equation); the other is in ml/min, used to calculate the rate of oxygen removal. These values may be easily converted into each other by either multiplying or dividing by the subject's body weight in kg.

2. Maximal voluntary ventilation in one minute (MVV_1) (Appendix B. 2-4), performed immediately after completion of the exercise test.

3. Heart rate (HR). The resting heart rate is recorded. The subject then performs a sub-maximum exercise stress test as described in Appendix B. 1-5 (treadmill, bicycle, or step test), and the maximum heart rate is recorded. The heart rate is again recorded three minutes after termination of exercise. These values are used in the computation of the heart rate recovery ratio.

4. Heart rate recovery ratio (RR), (Appendix B. 1-8. c).

5. Oxygen removal rate (ORR) (Appendix B. 1-8. d), determined by dividing VO_2 max (in ml/min) by MVV_1.

NAKAMURA'S SECOND EQUATION FOR MEN:

Biological age = 91.26 - 0.385 (VO_2 max in ml/kg.min) + 0.149 (ORR) - 0.234 (HR max) + 0.137 (RR)

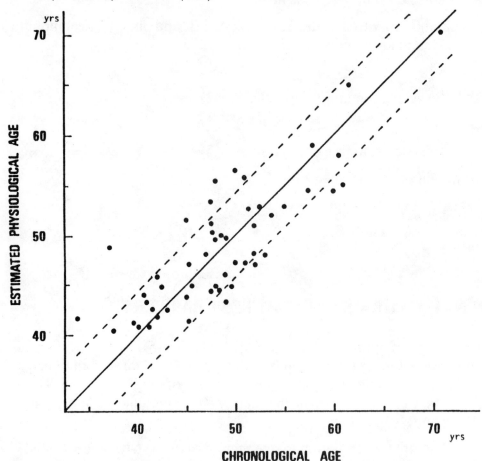

Fig. 13-5. **Comparison of chronological age vs biological age of untrained subjects, using Equation II.** (Nakamura, *Kyoiku Igaku*).

COMPARISONS BETWEEN TRAINED AND UNTRAINED SUBJECTS:

The plot of biological ages from Equation II also requires a correction factor to obtain accurate results (*Table 13-1*). After correction, Nakamura found that over 72% of the untrained subjects had biological ages within plus or minus one standard deviation of their chronological ages (*Fig. 13-5*).

Equation II was applied to men who had been participating in a vigorous tennis conditioning program. The majority of participants in the study scored below the 45° line (representing normal aging), indicating that the trained subjects were biologically younger than their chronological ages. Overall, the mean biological ages of the subjects were 4.33 years younger than their chronological ages (*Fig. 13-6*).

An additional attempt to validate the measurement system was made by evaluating longitudinal data on 10 other subjects who had been participating in a similar program for 5-6 years. Their biological ages showed an average improvement of 7 years (*Fig. 13-7*), thereby apparently confirming the hypothesis that conditioned individuals may be biologically younger than their deconditioned counterparts. See Chapter 11 for additional discussion of this subject.

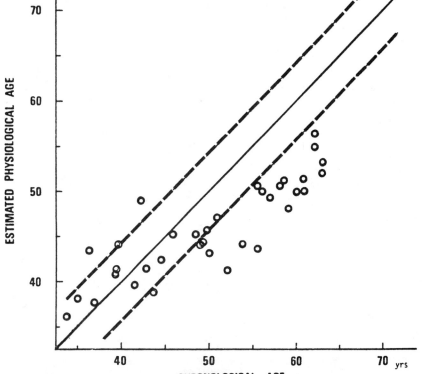

Fig. 13-6. **Biological ages of trained subjects compared to their chronological ages.** Note their relatively youthful biological ages (Nakamura, *Kyoiku Igaku*, 1982).

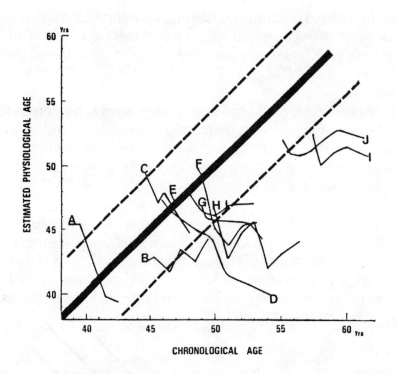

Fig. 13-7. **Changes in biological ages resulting from 5-6 years of tennis training**. This illustrates the reduction in biological age obtainable from physical conditioning (Nakamura, *Kyoiku Igaku*, 1982).

RECENT STUDIES IN KYOTO:

Nakamura is continuing his research, and recently sent details of yet another just-completed study (*J Kyoto Pref U Med*). This equation is unique in that it is based on data from 462 exceptionally healthy men, selected from a pool of 6,000. The men were found to be totally free from disease, and any changes should therefore be solely due to aging. This will eliminate the criticism of many aging measurement studies that changes were due to disease, not age.

Having learned of the artifactual skewing of the regression lines from his earlier studies, Nakamura calculated built-in correction factors for his latest equation.

University of Kyoto	Chapter 13

REQUIREMENTS FOR NAKAMURA'S THIRD TEST BATTERY:

Requirements are the same as for Equation I.

TESTS IN NAKAMURA'S THIRD TEST BATTERY:

The tests are the same as Equation I, except for the deletion of SGPT and addition of:

1. Glutamic oxaloacetic transaminase (SGOT) (Appendix B. 9-11).
2. Albumin/globulin ratio (A/G) (Appendix B. 9-12).
3. Resting heart rate (HRR).

NAKAMURA'S THIRD EQUATION FOR MEN:

$$BA = 12.09\,[2.616 - 0.102\,(HB)] - 0.646\,(AL) + 0.002\,(CHOL) \\ + 0.031\,(BUN) + 0.024\,(SGOT) + 0.005\,(OGTT) - 0.3\,(VA) \\ + 0.026\,(HRR) - 0.0005\,(FVC) + 0.018\,(SBP) + 50.86 \\ - [34.25 - 1.1\,(\text{Chronological age}) + 0.008\,(\text{Chronological age})^2]$$

TABLE 13-I. Correction factors

Chronological Age	Equation I	Equation II
35	-6.4	-4.9469
36	-5.9	-4.5769
37	-5.4	-4.2069
38	-4.9	-3.8369
39	-4.4	-3.4669
40	-3.9	-3.0969
41	-3.4	-2.7269
42	-2.9	-2.3569
43	-2.4	-1.9869
44	-1.9	-1.6169
45	-1.4	-1.2469
46	-0.9	-0.8769

(continued on next page)

TABLE 13-I. Correction factors (continued)

Chronological Age	Equation I	Equation II
47	-0.4	-0.5069
48	0.1	-0.1369
49	0.6	0.2331
50	1.1	0.6031
51	1.6	0.9731
52	2.1	1.3431
53	2.6	1.7131
54	3.1	2.0831
55	3.6	2.4531
56	4.1	2.8231
57	4.6	3.1931
58	5.1	3.5631
59	5.6	3.9331
60	6.1	4.3031
61	6.6	4.6731
62	7.1	5.0431
63	7.6	5.4131
64	8.1	5.7831
65	8.6	6.1531
66	9.1	6.5231
67	9.6	6.8931
68	10.1	7.2631
69	10.6	7.6331
70	11.1	8.0031
71	11.6	8.3731
72	12.1	8.6831
73	12.6	9.0531
74	13.1	9.4231
75	13.6	9.7931
76	14.1	10.1631
77	14.6	10.5331
78	15.1	10.9031
79	15.6	11.2731
80	16.1	11.6431
81	16.6	12.0131
82	17.1	12.3831
83	17.6	12.7531
84	18.1	13.1231
85	18.6	13.4931

University of Kyoto   Chapter 13

CALCULATION SHEET
JAPANESE TEST BATTERY FOR MEN
KYOTO UNIVERSITY
Equation I

Name: _____   Date of Exam : ___/___/___

                                          Date of Birth: ___/___/___

                                          Chronological Age: _____

1. Hemoglobin in mg/100 ml .... : _____ x 1.44 = _____

2. Albumin in gm/100 ml .... : _____ x 5.46 = _____

3. Cholesterol in mg/100 ml .... : _____ x 0.04 = _____

4. Blood urea nitrogen, in mg/100 ml : _____ x 0.40 = _____

5. Serum glutamic pyruvic
     transaminase, in units/ml ...... : _____ x 0.09 = _____

6. Oral glucose tolerance test
     at 1 hour in mg/100 ml .... : _____ x 0.03 = _____

7. Visual acuity as a decimal ...... : _____ x 1.87 = _____

8. Forced vital capacity in ml ..... : _____ x 0.008 = _____

9. Systolic blood pressure, in mm Hg : _____ x 0.13 = _____

Biological age = 90.9 - 1. _____ - 2. _____ + 3. _____

+ 4. _____ - 5. _____ + 6. _____ - 7. _____ - 8. _____

+ 9. _____ + correction factor _____ (Table 13-I)

(Plot on a graph--App. C) Corrected biological age _____

CALCULATION SHEET
JAPANESE TEST BATTERY FOR MEN
KYOTO UNIVERSITY
Equation II

Name: _____ Date of Exam : ___/___/___

Date of Birth: ___/___/___

Chronological Age: _____

1. Maximal oxygen uptake,
   in ml/kg.min .... : _____ x 0.385 = _____

2. Rate of oxygen removal,
   in ml/min .... : _____ x 0.149 = _____

3. Maximum heart rate .... : _____ x 0.234 = _____

4. Recovery ratio .... : _____ x 0.137 = _____

Biological age = 91.26 - 1. _____ + 2. _____ - 3. _____

+ 4. _____ + correction factor _____ (Table 13-II)

(Plot on a graph--App. C) Corrected biological age _____

University of Kyoto   Chapter 13

CALCULATION SHEET
JAPANESE TEST BATTERY FOR MEN
KYOTO UNIVERSITY
Equation III

Name: _____   Date of Exam : ___/___/___

                                         Date of Birth: ___/___/___

                                         Chronological Age: _____

1. Hemoglobin, in mg/100 ml .... : _____ x 0.102 = _____

2. Albumin, in gm/100 ml .... : _____ x 0.646 = _____

3. Albumin/globulin ratio .... : _____ x 1.343 = _____

4. Cholesterol, in mg/100 ml .... : _____ x 0.002 = _____

5. Urea nitrogen, in mg/100 ml ..... : _____ x 0.031 = _____

6. Glutamic oxaloacetic
     transaminase, in units/ml ...... : _____ x 0.024 = _____

7. Oral glucose tolerance test
     at 1 hour, in mg/100 ml .... : _____ x 0.005 = _____

8. Visual acuity, as a decimal ..... : _____ x 0.3   = _____

9. Resting heart rate .... : _____ x 0.026 = _____

10. Forced vital capacity, in ml .... : _____ x 0.0005 = _____

11. Systolic blood pressure, in mm Hg : _____ x 0.018 = _____

12. Chronological age .... : _____ x 1.1   = _____

13. Chronological age squared .... : _____ x 0.008 = _____

Biological age = 12.09 x [2.616 - 1. _____] - 2. _____

 - 3. _____ + 4. _____ + 5. _____ + 6. _____ + 7. _____

 - 8. _____ + 9. _____ - 10. _____ + 11. _____ + 50.86

 - [34.25 - 12. _____ + 13. _____]

(Plot on a graph--App. C)   Biological age _____

REFERENCES

Anonymous. Hypertensive diabetics a higher death risk, *Modern Medicine*, November 1984, pp. 37-41.

Nakamura, E., Kimura, M., Nagata, H., Miyao, K., and Ozeki, T. Evaluation of the progress of aging based on specific biological age as estimated by various physiological functions. *Nippon Eiseigaku Zasshi (Jap J Hygiene)*, 1982, Feb; 36(6): 853-62.

Nakamura, E. The aged people and its physiological ages in relation to work capacity. *Kyoiku Igaku (Education and Medicine)* (1982) 28: 2-11.

Nakamura, E. The assessment of physiological age based upon a principal component analysis of various physiological variables. *J Kyoto Pref Univ Med*. 1985, 94(8): 757-769.

Nakamura, E. Personal Communications. 22 Jul 1983; 28 Dec 1983; 20 Jun 1984; 11 December 1984; and 19 Feb 1986.

Thompson, M. K. *The Care of the Elderly in General Practice*. Churchill Livingston, Edinburgh, 1984, p. 127.

Chapter 14

SOVIET TEST BATTERY
Minsk Institute of Gerontology

An interesting series of experiments was conducted by scientists from the Academy of Sciences, Byelorussian Soviet Socialist Republic in Minsk, USSR. The first two studies involved the development of a battery of tests for biological age in laboratory rats (Dyundikova, et al; and Dubina, et al, 1983).

Continuing their research, they extended their studies to humans, using longitudinal data from men and women collected over a ten-year period (Dubina, et al, 1984). These data were collected at the Institute of Gerontology in Kiev (Mints, et al) and are also the basis for a slightly different measurement system described in Chapter 16.

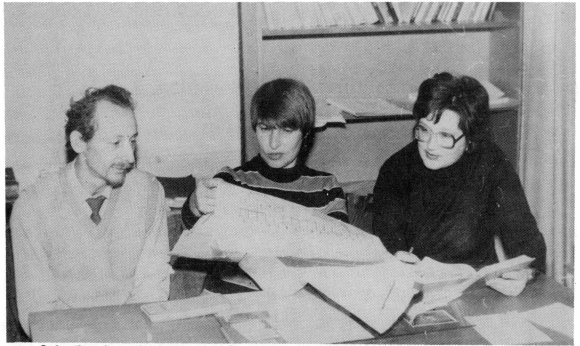

Fig. 14-1. **Scientists from the Institute of Gerontology in Minsk.** From left to right: Drs. E. V. Zhuk, T. L. Dubina, and V. A. Dyundikova.

147

Chapter 14 — Minsk Institute of Gerontology

The research of Dubina and her colleagues (*Fig. 14-1*) is unique in several ways. First, their test group ranged in age from 60 to 100 years. No other study to date has examined this upper end of the aging scale so extensively. Second, the equations were calculated from longitudinal data. This contrasts with the generally isolated, cross-sectional measurements most often used by others.

REQUIREMENTS FOR THE MINSK TEST BATTERY:

1. Handgrip dynamometer (Appendix A. 6-1).
2. Vibrometer (Appendix A. 5-7).

TESTS IN THE MINSK EQUATIONS:

1. Handgrip strength (HGS) (Appendix B. 6-2), in kg.
2. Short term memory (STM) (Appendix B. 5-9).
3. Vibratory sensitivity (VS), right index finger (Appendix B. 5-8), in decibels. Due to limited availability of vibrometers that record in decibels, it is recommended that the sensitivity be recorded in volts and converted to decibels using the conversion scale in *Fig. B. 5-9*.

THE MINSK AGING MEASUREMENT EQUATIONS:

I. Men: Biological age = 93.02 - 0.561 (HGS) - 0.096 (STM) + 0.435 (VS)

II. Women: Biological age = 84.30 - 0.639 (HGS) - 0.086 (STM) + 0.641 (VS)

CORRECTION FACTORS FOR EQUATION-DERIVED BIOLOGICAL AGES

Dubina was unaware of Dirken's earlier work in Holland (Chapter 7), showing that the slope through the means of biological ages tends to be skewed clockwise, causing younger members of populations to appear older and older members to score younger (*Fig. 14-2*). She arrived at her conclusions independently. Like Dirken, she solved this artifactual distortion by calculating correction factors to be added to or subtracted from the uncorrected biological ages.

Dubina thinks correction factors are necessary and must be calculated separately for each population studied (Dubina, 23 Sept 1984). I agree that they may sometimes be required. But I don't think it is necessary to recalculate them for each population. This is based on my assumption that the equations are derived from large representative populations whose age-related values and rates of change are similar for all humans.

Despite Dubina's doubts regarding the inter-population validity of equations and correction factors, she kindly provided her correction factors (not published in her article) for inclusion in this book (*Table 14-I*) (Dubina, 7 May, 1985).

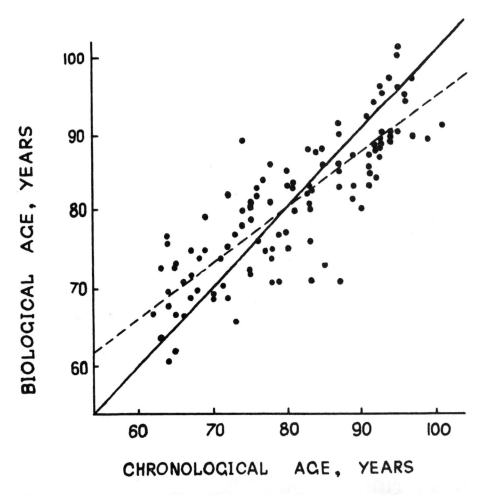

Fig. 14-2. **Individual biological ages for women 60 to 100 years old, using Equation I.** The dashed line shows the clock-wise skewed linear relation between biological and chronological age. This gives a false impression of younger subjects appearing older, and older subjects appearing younger (Dubina, et al, 1984).

ABILITY TO DISCERN DIFFERENCES IN AGING RATES:

One of the most important aspects of Dubina's studies is her graphic evidence that sequential aging measurements reveal differences in aging rates of individuals within a group (*Fig. 14-3*). This confirms the thesis of this book that aging rates can be assessed accurately and can be used to evaluate age-retarding regimens and protocols.

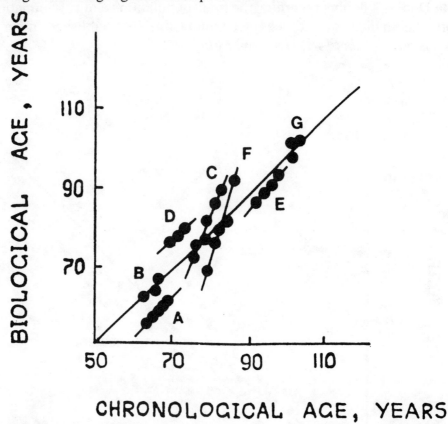

Fig. 14-3. **Longitudinal assessment of biological age in six subjects, showing differences in aging rates** (Dubina, et al, 1984). Four subjects appear to be aging at a normal rate while two subjects are apparently aging significantly faster than normal. If similar results can be demonstrated for larger numbers of subjects, this will confirm that aging rates can be longitudinally assessed using techniques discussed in this book.

USE OF CORRECTION FACTORS:

Using *Table 14-I*, find the appropriate correction factor for the subject's chronological age, and add it to the biological age to determine the corrected biological age.

Table 14-I. Correction factors

Chronological Age	Men	Women
35	−14.7264	−13.7858
36	−14.3724	−13.4848
37	−14.0184	−13.1838
38	−13.6644	−12.8828
39	−13.3104	−12.5818
40	−12.9564	−12.2808
41	−12.6024	−11.9798
42	−12.2484	−11.6788
43	−11.8944	−11.3778
44	−11.5404	−11.0768
45	−11.1864	−10.7758
46	−10.8324	−10.4748
47	−10.4784	−10.1738
48	−10.1244	−9.8728
49	−9.7704	−9.5718
50	−9.4164	−9.2708
51	−9.0624	−8.9698
52	−8.7084	−8.6688
53	−8.3544	−8.3678
54	−8.0004	−8.0668
55	−7.6464	−7.7658
56	−7.2924	−7.4648
57	−6.9384	−7.1638
58	−6.5844	−6.8628
59	−6.2304	−6.5618
60	−5.8764	−6.2608
61	−5.5224	−5.9598
62	−5.1684	−5.6588
63	−4.8144	−5.3578
64	−4.4604	−5.0568
65	−4.1064	−4.7558
66	−3.7524	−4.4548
67	−3.3984	−4.1538
68	−3.0444	−3.8528
69	−2.6904	−3.5518
70	−2.3364	−3.2508
71	−1.9824	−2.9498
72	−1.6284	−2.6488
73	−1.2744	−2.3478
74	−0.9204	−2.0468
75	−0.5664	−1.7458
76	−0.2124	−1.4448
77	0.1416	−1.1438
78	0.4956	−0.8428
79	0.8496	−0.5418
80	1.2036	−0.2408
81	1.5576	0.0602
82	1.9116	0.3612
83	2.2656	0.6622
84	2.6196	0.9632
85	2.9736	1.2642

Chapter 14 — Minsk Institute of Gerontology

Table 14-II. Word lists for Short Term Memory Test*

List A	List B	List C	List D
Drum	Desk	Book	Nose
Curtain	Ranger	Flower	Turkey
Bell	Bird	Train	Color
Coffee	Shoe	Rug	House
School	Stove	Meadow	River
Parent	Mountain	Harp	Lamb
Moon	Glasses	Salt	Gun
Garden	Towel	Finger	Pencil
Hat	Cloud	Apple	Church
Farmer	Boat	Chimney	Fish

*Adapted from Taylor, E. M.

Minsk Institute of Gerontology Chapter 14

CALCULATION SHEET
SOVIET TEST BATTERY FOR MEN
MINSK INSTITUTE OF GERONTOLOGY

Name: _____ Date of Exam : ___/___/___

                                                                                              Date of Birth: ___/___/___

                                                                                              Chronological Age: _____

1. Handgrip strength,
   dominant hand, in kg .... : _____ x 0.561 = _____

2. Short term memory,
   verbal memory score .... : _____ x 0.096 = _____

3. Vibratory sensitivity,
   index finger, dominant hand,
   in volts _____ = decibels .... : _____ x 0.435 = _____

Biological age = 93.02 - 1. _____ - 2. _____ + 3. _____

+ correction factor _____ (Table 14-I)

(Plot on a graph--App. C) Corrected biological age _____

| Chapter 14 | Minsk Institute of Gerontology |

**CALCULATION SHEET
SOVIET TEST BATTERY FOR WOMEN
MINSK INSTITUTE OF GERONTOLOGY**

Name: _____ Date of Exam : ___/___/___

Date of Birth: ___/___/___

Chronological Age: _____

1. Handgrip strength,
     dominant hand, in kg .... : _____ x 0.639 = _____

2. Short term memory,
     verbal memory score .... : _____ x 0.086 = _____

3. Vibratory sensitivity,
     index finger, dominant hand,
     in volts _____ = decibels .... : _____ x 0.641 = _____

Biological age = 84.30 − 1. _____ − 2. _____ + 3. _____

+ correction factor _____ (Table 14-I)

(Plot on a graph--App. C) Corrected biological age _____

REFERENCES:

Dubina, T. L., Dyundikova, V. A., and Zhuk, E. V. Biological age and its estimation. II. Assessment of biological age of albino rats by multiple regression analysis. *Experimental Gerontology*, 1983 (18)1: 5-18.

Dubina, T.L., Mints, A. Ya., and Zhuk, E.V. Biological age and its estimation. III. Introduction of a correction to the multiple regression model of biological age and assessment of biological age in cross-sectional and longitudinal studies. *Experimental Gerontology*, 1984 (19)4: 133-143.

Dubina, T.L. Personal communications, 23 Sept 1984, and 7 May, 1985.

Dyundikova, V. A., Silvon, Z. K., and Dubina, T. L. Biological age and its estimation. I. Studies of some physiological parameters in albino rats and their validity as biological age tests. *Experimental Gerontology*, 1981 (16)1: 13-24.

Mints, A. Ya., Dubina, T. L., Lysenyk, V. P., and Zhuk, E. V. Defining the biological age of an individual and an appraisal of the degree of aging. *Physiologichiski Zhurnal*, 1984, Vol 30, No. 1, pp. 39-45.

Taylor, E. M. *Psychological Appraisal of Children With Cerebral Defects*. Boston, Harvard University Press, 1959.

Chapter 15

SOVIET TEST BATTERIES
Kiev Institute of Gerontology--I

Scientists at the Institute of Gerontology, Academy of Medical Sciences, in Kiev, USSR, are conducting long-term aging measurement studies with men and women. One aspect of the studies is to determine if there is a difference in aging rates between the sexes. Professor Anatoli V. Tokar, Scientific Director of the Institute, and Dr. Vladimir P. Voitenko, Head of the Genetics Laboratory (*Fig. 15-1*) evaluated data from 197 men and women between the ages of 19 and 73 at the Department of Longitudinal Clinical Observations of the Institute. They found that during youth, women tend to age faster, demonstrated by their more rapid sexual maturation (This is not really aging, however. Aging is, by definition, *deleterious* [Strehler], and does not begin until after maturity). Conversely, they found that males tend to age faster in old age, confirmed by the generally longer life expectancies of females.

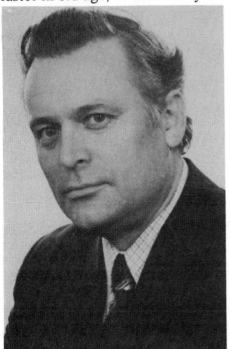
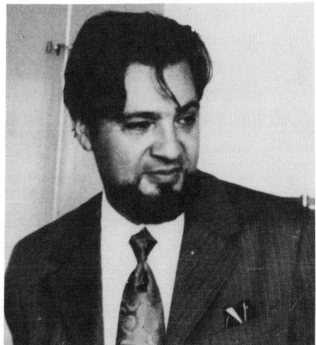

Fig. 15-1. **Professor Anatoli V. Tokar (left), and Dr. Vladimir P. Voitenko (right).**

157

Chapter 15 — Kiev Institute of Gerontology--I

REQUIREMENTS FOR THE KIEV TEST BATTERIES:

1. Sphygmomanometer and stethoscope, (Appendix A. 1-1).
2. Arterial pulse-wave velocity measuring instrument (Appendix A. 1-8).
3. Spirometer (Appendix A. 2-1).
4. Berens near-point indicator or Krimsky-Prince rule, (Appendix A. 4-1).
5. Audiometer (Appendix A. 3-1).
6. Body weight scale (in kg).
7. Wechsler Digit Symbol test kit (Appendix A. 5-14).
8. Sophisticated immunological tests (lymphocyte blast transformation test).

TESTS IN THE KIEV TEST BATTERIES:

1. Systolic blood pressure (SBP) (Appendix B. 1-1), in mm Hg.
2. Arterial pulse-wave velocity from the carotid to the radial artery (APWVc-r) (Appendix B. 1-8), in meters/second.
3. Vital capacity (VC) (Appendix B. 2-1) in ml.
4. Near vision (NV) (Appendix B. 4-1), in diopters.
5. Auditory acuity (AA) at 4,000 Hz (Appendix B. 3-1), in decibels.
6. Static balance (SB) (Appendix B. 5-11. a), in sec.
7. Weight (WT) (Appendix B. 6-14), in kilograms.
8. Wechsler Digit Symbol test (DS) (Appendix B. 5-8), in number of correct answers within 90 seconds.
9. Lymphocyte blast transformation test (LBT) (Appendix B. 12-2).

KIEV AGING MEASUREMENT EQUATIONS FOR MEN AND WOMEN:

MEN:

I. Biological age = 56.244 + 0.064 (SBP) + 0.769 (APWVc-r) - 0.002 (VC) - 2.186 (NV) + 0.211 (AA) - 0.040 (SB) - 0.072 (WT) - 0.259 (DS) - 0.117 (LBT)

II. Biological age = 50.660 + 0.065 (SBP) + 0.718 (APWVc-r) - 0.001 (VC) - 2.129 (NV) + 0.206 (AA) - 0.033 (SB) - 0.227 (DS)

III. Biological age = 58.918 + 0.929 (APWVc-r) - 0.002 (VC) - 2.275 (NV) + 0.222 (AA) - 0.250 (DS)

IV. Biological age = 61.904 - 2.414 (NV) + 0.266 (AA) - 0.318 (DS)

V. Biological age = 68.899 - 5.058 (NV)

WOMEN:

VI. Biological age = 22.396 + 0.141 (SBP) + 0.958 (APWVc-r) - 0.004 (VC) - 0.643 (NV) + 0.297 (AA) - 0.064 (SB) - 0.174 (WT) - 0.151 (DS) - 0.020 (LBT)

VII. Biological age = 25.350 + 0.154 (SBP) + 1.318 (APWVc-r) - 0.004 (VC) - 0.888 (NV) + 0.362 (AA) - 0.066 (SB) - 0.112 (DS)

VIII. Biological age = 40.608 + 1.726 (APWVc-r) - 0.004 (VC) - 0.888 (NV) + 0.495 (AA) - 0.178 (DS)

IX. Biological age = 50.542 - 0.869 (NV) + 0.568 (AA) - 0.340 (DS)

Chapter 15   Kiev Institute of Gerontology--I

CALCULATION SHEET
SOVIET TEST BATTERY FOR MEN
KIEV INSTITUTE OF GERONTOLOGY
Equation I

Name: _____   Date of Exam : ___/___/___

                                                                      Date of Birth: ___/___/___

                                                                      Chronological Age: _____

1. Systolic blood pressure, in mm Hg : _____ x 0.064 = _____

2. Arterial pulse-wave velocity
   (carotid to radial artery),
   in m/sec .... : _____ x 0.769 = _____

3. Vital capacity, in ml .... : _____ x 0.002 = _____

4. Near vision, in diopters .... : _____ x 2.186 = _____

5. Auditory acuity at 4,000 Hz,
   in decibels .... : _____ x 0.211 = _____

6. Static balance, in sec .... : _____ x 0.040 = _____

7. Weight, in kg .... : _____ x 0.072 = _____

8. Digit Symbol test .... : _____ x 0.259 = _____

9. Lymphocyte blast transformation
   test, in counts per min .... : _____ x 0.117 = _____

Biological age = 56.244 + 1. _____ + 2. _____ − 3. _____

− 4. _____ + 5. _____ − 6. _____ − 7. _____ − 8. _____

− 9. _____

(Plot on a graph--App. C)   Biological age _____

Kiev Institute of Gerontology--I Chapter 15

CALCULATION SHEET
SOVIET TEST BATTERY FOR MEN
KIEV INSTITUTE OF GERONTOLOGY
Equation II

Name: _____ Date of Exam : ___/___/___

Date of Birth: ___/___/___

Chronological Age: _____

1. Systolic blood pressure, in mm Hg : _____ x 0.065 = _____

2. Arterial pulse-wave velocity
   (carotid to radial artery)
   in m/sec .... : _____ x 0.718 = _____

3. Vital capacity, in ml .... : _____ x 0.001 = _____

4. Near vision, in diopters .... : _____ x 2.129 = _____

5. Auditory acuity
   at 4,000 Hz, in decibels .... : _____ x 0.206 = _____

6. Static balance, in sec .... : _____ x 0.033 = _____

7. Digit Symbol test .... : _____ x 0.227 = _____

Biological age = 50.660 + 1. _____ + 2. _____ − 3. _____
− 4. _____ + 5. _____ − 6. _____ − 7. _____

(Plot on a graph--App. C)   Biological age _____

Chapter 15 Kiev Institute of Gerontology--I

CALCULATION SHEET
SOVIET TEST BATTERY FOR MEN
KIEV INSTITUTE OF GERONTOLOGY
Equation III

Name: _____ Date of Exam : ___/___/___

Date of Birth: ___/___/___

Chronological Age: _____

1. Arterial pulse-wave velocity
   (carotid to radial artery),
   in m/sec .... : _____ x 0.929 = _____

2. Vital capacity, in ml .... : _____ x 0.002 = _____

3. Near vision, in diopters .... : _____ x 2.275 = _____

4. Auditory acuity
   at 4,000 Hz, in decibels .... : _____ x 0.222 = _____

5. Digit Symbol test .... : _____ x 0.250 = _____

Biological age = 58.918 + 1. _____ − 2. _____ − 3. _____

+ 4. _____ − 5. _____

(Plot on a graph--App. C)   Biological age _____

Kiev Institute of Gerontology--I Chapter 15

**CALCULATION SHEET
SOVIET TEST BATTERY FOR MEN
KIEV INSTITUTE OF GERONTOLOGY
Equation IV**

Name: _____ Date of Exam : ___/___/___

Date of Birth: ___/___/___

Chronological Age: _____

1. Near vision, in diopters .... : _____ x 2.414 = _____

2. Auditory acuity
   at 4,000 Hz, in decibels .... : _____ x 0.266 = _____

3. Digit Symbol test .... : _____ x 0.318 = _____

Biological age = 61.904 - 1. _____ + 2. _____ - 3. _____

(Plot on a graph--App. C)   Biological age _____

Chapter 15 — Kiev Institute of Gerontology--I

CALCULATION SHEET
SOVIET TEST BATTERY FOR MEN
KIEV INSTITUTE OF GERONTOLOGY
Equation V

Name: _____ Date of Exam : ___/___/___

Date of Birth: ___/___/___

Chronological Age: _____

1. Near vision, in diopters .... : _____ x 5.058 = _____

Biological age = 66.899 - 1. _____

(Plot on a graph--App. C)   Biological age _____

Kiev Institute of Gerontology--I Chapter 15

CALCULATION SHEET
SOVIET TEST BATTERY FOR WOMEN
KIEV INSTITUTE OF GERONTOLOGY
Equation VI

Name: _____ Date of Exam : ___/___/___

Date of Birth: ___/___/___

Chronological Age: _____

1. Systolic blood pressure,
   in mm Hg .... : _____ x 0.141 = _____

2. Arterial pulse-wave velocity
   (carotid to radial artery),
   in m/sec .... : _____ x 0.958 = _____

3. Vital capacity, in ml .... : _____ x 0.004 = _____

4. Near vision, in diopters .... : _____ x 0.643 = _____

5. Auditory acuity
   at 4,000 Hz, in decibels .... : _____ x 0.297 = _____

6. Static balance, in sec .... : _____ x 0.064 = _____

7. Weight, in kg .... : _____ x 0.174 = _____

8. Digit Symbol test .... : _____ x 0.151 = _____

9. Lymphocyte blast transformation
   test, in counts per min .... : _____ x 0.020 = _____

Biological age = 22.396 + 1. _____ + 2. _____ − 3. _____

− 4. _____ + 5. _____ − 6. _____ − 7. _____ − 8. _____

− 9. _____

(Plot on a graph--App. C)   Biological age _____

Chapter 15   Kiev Institute of Gerontology--I

CALCULATION SHEET
SOVIET TEST BATTERY FOR WOMEN
KIEV INSTITUTE OF GERONTOLOGY
Equation VII

Name: _____   Date of Exam : ___/___/___

                                        Date of Birth: ___/___/___

                                        Chronological Age: _____

1. Systolic blood pressure,
   in mm Hg .... : _____ x 0.154 = _____

2. Arterial pulse-wave velocity
   (carotid to radial artery),
   in m/sec .... : _____ x 1.318 = _____

3. Vital capacity, in ml .... : _____ x 0.004 = _____

4. Near vision, in diopters .... : _____ x 0.888 = _____

5. Auditory acuity
   at 4,000 Hz, in decibels .... : _____ x 0.362 = _____

6. Static balance, in sec .... : _____ x 0.066 = _____

7. Digit Symbol test .... : _____ x 0.112 = _____

Biological age = 25.350 + 1. _____ + 2. _____ - 3. _____

- 4. _____ + 5. _____ - 6. _____ - 7. _____

(Plot on a graph--App. C)   Biological age _____

Kiev Institute of Gerontology--I Chapter 15

CALCULATION SHEET
SOVIET TEST BATTERY FOR WOMEN
KIEV INSTITUTE OF GERONTOLOGY
Equation VIII

Name: _____ Date of Exam : ___/___/___

   Date of Birth: ___/___/___

   Chronological Age: _____

1. Arterial pulse-wave velocity
   (carotid to radial artery),
   in m/sec .... : _____ x 1.726 = _____

2. Vital capacity, in ml .... : _____ x 0.004 = _____

3. Near vision, in diopters .... : _____ x 0.888 = _____

4. Auditory acuity
   at 4,000 Hz, in decibels .... : _____ x 0.495 = _____

5. Digit Symbol test .... : _____ x 0.178 = _____

Biological age = 40.608 + 1. _____ - 2. _____ - 3. _____

+ 4. _____ - 5. _____

(Plot on a graph--App. C)   Biological age _____

Chapter 15   Kiev Institute of Gerontology--I

CALCULATION SHEET
SOVIET TEST BATTERY FOR WOMEN
KIEV INSTITUTE OF GERONTOLOGY
Equation IX

Name: _____   Date of Exam : ___/___/___

                                                                                       Date of Birth: ___/___/___

                                                                                       Chronological Age: _____

1. Near vision, in diopters .... : _____ x 0.869 = _____

2. Auditory acuity
    at 4,000 Hz, in decibels .... : _____ x 0.568 = _____

3. Digit Symbol test .... : _____ x 0.340 = _____

Biological age = 50.542 − 1. _____ + 2. _____ − 3. _____

(Plot on a graph--App. C)   Biological age _____

REFERENCES

Cheberotev, D. F., Tokar, A. V., and Voitenko, V. P. (eds), *Gerontology and Geriatrics Yearbook*, 1984, Kiev, AMS, USSR.

Strehler, B. L. *Time, Cells and Aging*, 2d edition. New York, Academic Press, 1977, p. 14.

Tokar, A.V., and Voitenko, V. P. Personal communication, 15 February 1985.

Voitenko, V.P., and Tokar, A.V. The Assessment of Biological Age and Sex Differences of Human Aging. *Experimental Aging Research*, Volume 9, Number 4, 1983, pp. 239-244.

Voitenko, V. P. Personal communications, 22 August 1984; and 18 April 1986.

Chapter 16

SOVIET TEST BATTERY
Kiev Institute of Gerontology--II

Dr. Abram Ya. Mints (*Fig. 16-1*) is the Senior Scientific Worker and Chief, Department of Age Changes of the Nervous System, Gerontology Research Institute, Academy of Medical Sciences, in Kiev, USSR. In conjunction with scientists from the Section on Gerontology, AMS, USSR, in Minsk, he conducted a series of studies on women ranging in age from 60 to 101 years (Mints, et al). Mints and his colleagues calculated an age-predicting equation based on the same data used by Dubina, et al, whose work is described in Chapter 14.

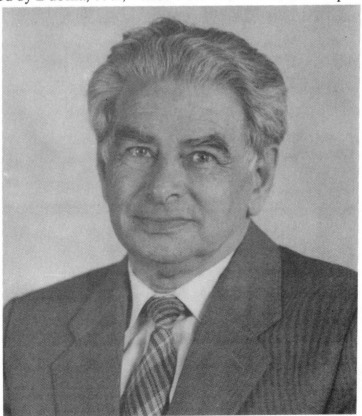

Fig. 16-1. **Dr. Abram Ya. Mints.**

REQUIREMENTS FOR MINTS' TEST BATTERY:

1. Handgrip dynamometer (Appendix A. 6-1).
2. Vibrometer (Appendix A. 5-8).
3. 12-lead electrocardiograph (Appendix A. 1-7).
4. Arterial pulse-wave velocity measuring apparatus (Appendix A. 1-8).
5. Clinical laboratory chemistry tests.

TESTS IN MINTS' TEST BATTERY:

1. Handgrip strength (HGS), in kg (Appendix B. 6-2).
2. Vibratory sensitivity of the index finger (VS), in decibels (Appendix B. 5-6).
3. Short term memory (STM), in number of words recalled (Appendix B. 5-9).
4. Amplitude of T-wave deflection in lead V5 (T_{V5}) on a 12-lead ECG, in mm (Appendix B. 1-9).
5. Arterial pulse-wave velocity from the femoral to the posterior tibial arteries ($APWV_{f-pt}$), in meters/second (Appendix B. 1-10).
6. Serum lecithin to cholesterol ratio (L/C) (Appendix B. 9-10).

MINTS' EQUATION FOR WOMEN:

Biological age = 87.13 + 0.653 (VS) - 0.087 (STM) - 0.622 (HGS) + 0.062 (T_{V5}) - 0.376 ($APWV_{f-pt}$) - 0.478 (L/C)

Kiev Institute of Gerontology--II   Chapter 16

CALCULATION SHEET
SOVIET TEST BATTERY FOR WOMEN
KIEV INSTITUTE OF GERONTOLOGY--II

Name: _____   Date of Exam : ___/___/___

                                                            Date of Birth: ___/___/___

                                                            Chronological Age: _____

1. Vibratory sensitivity,
   index finger, in decibels .... : _____ x 0.653 = _____

2. Short term memory,
   in number of words recalled ..... : _____ x 0.087 = _____

3. Handgrip strength, in kg .... : _____ x 0.622 = _____

4. Amplitude of T-wave deflection
   in lead V5, in mm .... : _____ x 0.062 = _____

5. Arterial pulse wave velocity
   (femoral to posterior tibial
   arteries), in meters/second ..... : _____ x 0.376 = _____

6. Serum lecithin/cholesterol ratio : _____ x 0.478 = _____

Biological age = 87.13 + 1. _____ - 2. _____ - 3. _____

+ 4. _____ - 5. _____ - 6. _____

(Plot on a chart--App. C)   Biological age _____

REFERENCES

Dubina, T. L., Mints, A. Ya., and Zhuk, E. V. Biological age and its estimation. III. Introduction of a correction to the multiple regression mode of biological age and assessment of biological age in cross-sectional and longitudinal studies. *Exp Ger*, Vol 19, pp. 133-143, 1984.

Mints, A. Ya., Dubina, T. L., Lysenyk, V. P., Zhuk, E. V. Determination of individual biological age and evaluation of aging degree. *Physiologichiski Zhurnal*, 1984, Vol. 30, No. 1., pp. 39-45.

Mints, A. Ya. Personal communications: 27 March, 1985; and 25 Sep, 1985.

Chapter 17

GERMAN TEST BATTERY
Karl Marx University
Leipzig (GDR)

Few scientists involved with aging measurement--except perhaps Heikkinen in Finland (Chapter 11)--have pursued the subject as persistently as Werner Ries, M.D. (*Fig. 17-1*), Professor, Department of Medicine, Karl Marx University in Leipzig, GDR, and his colleagues Drs. Dagmar Poethig, Ilse Sauer, and Mrs. Erika Schmidt. Ries and his group have conducted aging measurement studies since 1972, continually refining and improving their systems.

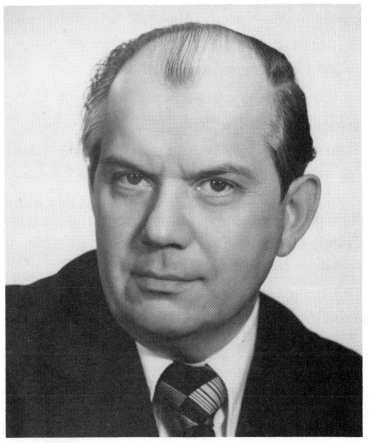

Fig. 17-1. **Professor Werner Ries.**

175

Much of Ries' work has been published only in German, and the complete test batteries and equations in his aging measurement systems have never previously been published in any language. However, he kindly provided the details of his most recent and most accurate version for inclusion in this book. It is a comprehensive test battery incorporating 37 separate tests.

EQUIPMENT REQUIRED FOR THE LEIPZIG TEST BATTERY:

1. Sphygmomanometer and stethoscope (Appendix A. 1-1).
2. Spirometer (Appendix A. 2-1).
3. a. Equipment for drawing arterial blood and blood gas analyzer (Appendix A. 1-9).
   or:
   b. Transcutaneous oxygen monitor (Appendix A. 1-10).
4. Heart rate monitor (Appendix A. 1-6).
5. Charts for measuring visual acuity (Appendix A. 4-2).
6. Audiometer (Appendix A. 3-1).
7. Stroop color-word test set. (Appendix A. 5-16).
8. Finger goniometer (Appendix A. 6-8).
9. Handgrip dynamometer (Appendix A. 6-1).
10. Landolt test sheets for the concentration test (Appendix A. 5-6).
11. Dental exam.
12. Geromat™ (Fig. 17-2). This instrument was designed by Ries and his colleague, Dr. Dagmar Poethig, and assembled by the medical equipment lab of the Halberstadt District Hospital. It was conceived along the lines of Hochschild's H-SCAN (Chapter 21), in that several functions (tapping rate, hand-eye coordination, visual and auditory reaction times) are evaluated using a single instrument. Unlike the H-SCAN, however, the Geromat™ scores do not in themselves give a biological age, but must be incorporated with the results of the other tests in Ries' test battery. At the present time, there are only two of these instruments in existence--one in Ries' lab in Leipzig, and the other in Halberstadt.

Ries and his colleagues are in the process of technically improving the Geromat, to include several other tests. They are investigating the possibility of producing a commercial version.

Karl Marx University — Chapter 17

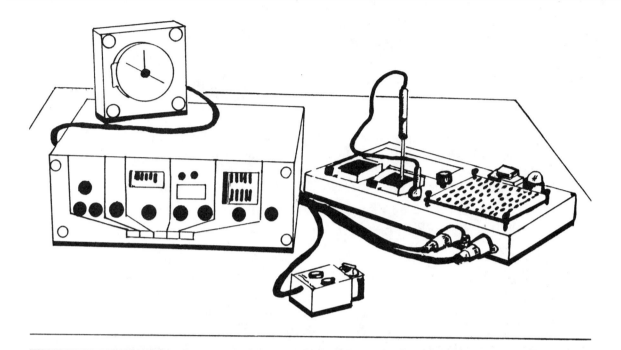

Fig. 17-2. **The Geromat™.**

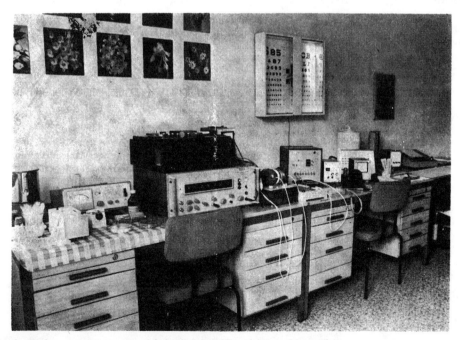

Fig. 17-3. **Leipzig aging measurement laboratory** (Poethig and Israel).

Chapter 17 Karl Marx University

TESTS IN THE LEIPZIG TEST BATTERY:

1. Systolic blood pressure (SBP) (Appendix B. 1-1), in mm Hg.

2. Diastolic blood pressure (DBP) (Appendix B. 1-3), in mm Hg.

3. Vital capacity (VC) (Appendix B. 2-1), as a per cent of normal. This value is automatically calculated by most spirometers.

4. Arterial oxygen tension (pO_2) (Appendix B. 1-11), in mm Hg.

5. Visual acuity of each eye (VA_L, VA_R) (Appendix B. 4-2), as a per cent (i.e., 20/20 = 100%, 20/40 = 50%, 20/200 = 10%, etc).

6. Auditory acuity (AA) (Appendix B. 3-1). Values for hearing loss in decibels at 500, 1,000, 2,000, and 4,000 Hz are determined in both ears, and then converted to percentage hearing loss at each frequency, using *Table B. 2-I*. Values used in the equation are the percentage hearing loss in each ear ("L" = left, "R" = right) at 2,000 and 4,000 Hz ($AA_{L2,000}$, $AA_{L4,000}$, $AA_{R2,000}$ and $AA_{R4,000}$) and the sum (S) of the percentage hearing loss in each ear at all frequencies tested (AA_{LS}, AA_{RS}).

7. Color Word Test (Appendix B. 5-12), in time in seconds needed for the first row (CW_1), second row (CW_2), and third row (CW_3).

8. Landolt Concentration time (Appendix B. 5-4. b.), using the Landolt test sheets (Appendix A. 5-6). The score is the time in seconds to complete the test (C_T) and number of errors (C_E).

9. Handgrip strength (HGS) (Appendix B. 6-2), in kg.

10. Tendon extensibility of the left and right fifth fingers (TE_L, TE_R) (Appendix B. 6-15), in degrees.

11. Caries index (CI) (Appendix B. 7-1).

12. Heart rate after exercise (Appendix B. 1-8. a.). Values are the resting heart rate (HRr), after 20 deep knee bends (HRmax), change in heart rate (HRmax - HRr = ΔHR), and the time needed to execute the 20 knee bends (Tkb).

The following tests use the Geromat™:

13. Tapping rate (TR) (Appendix B. 5-14. f).

14. Hand-eye coordination (H-EC) (Appendix B. 5-14. d).

15. Stepping-stone maze (Maz) (Appendix B. 5-14. e).

16. Reaction time (RT).
    a. Light reaction time (RT_L) (Appendix B. 5-14. a).
    b. Clock reaction time (RT_C) (Appendix B. 5-14. b).
    c. Auditory reaction time (RT_A) (Appendix B. 5-14. b).

LEIPZIG AGING MEASUREMENT EQUATIONS:

MEN:

Biological age = 48.7 ln (0.0067 SBP + 0.01 DBP - 0.0134 HRr
 - 0.00909 HRmax - 0.0101 ΔHR + 0.0222 T_{kb} - 0.01 VC
 - 0.0256 pO_2 - 0.125 TR_1 - 0.125 TR_2 - 0.143 TR_6 - 0.143 TR_7
 + 0.02 Ve + 0.00769 Vt - 0.00625 HGS - 0.00667 (TE_L + TE_R)
 - 0.01 VA_R - 0.01 VA_L + 0.025 $AA_{R2,000}$ + 0.0667 $AA_{R4,000}$
 + 0.01 AA_{RS} + 0.025 $AA_{L2,000}$ + 0.0667 $AA_{L4,000}$ + 0.01 AA_{LS}
 + 0.03125 CI + 0.0833 CW_1 + 0.0476 CW_2 + 0.01515 CW_3
 + 0.0027 Ct + 0.0667 Ce + 0.00192 Maz_{t1} + 0.00667 Maz_A
 + 0.00833 Maz_B + 0.286 Maz_{t2} + 0.0025 RT_V + 0.00769 RT_C
 + 0.00167 RT_A + 12.828) - 70.27

WOMEN:

Biological age = 55.55 ln (0.0067 SBP + 0.01 DBP - 0.0134 HRr
 - 0.00909 HRmax - 0.0101 ΔHR + 0.0222 T_{kb} - 0.01 VC
 - 0.0256 pO_2 - 0.125 TR_1 - 0.125 TR_2 - 0.143 TR_6 - 0.143 TR_7
 + 0.02 Ve + 0.00769 Vt - 0.00625 HGS - 0.00667 (TE_L + TE_R)
 - 0.01 VA_R - 0.01 VA_L + 0.025 $AA_{R2,000}$ + 0.0667 $AA_{R4,000}$
 + 0.01 AA_{RS} + 0.025 $AA_{L2,000}$ + 0.0667 $AA_{L4,000}$ + 0.01 AA_{LS}
 + 0.03125 CI + 0.0833 CW_1 + 0.0476 CW_2 + 0.01515 CW_3
 + 0.0027 Ct + 0.0667 Ce + 0.00192 Maz_{t1} + 0.00667 Maz_A
 + 0.00833 Maz_B + 0.286 Maz_{t2} + 0.0025 RT_V + 0.00769 RT_C
 + 0.00167 RT_A + 12.828) - 90.64

CALCULATION SHEET
GERMAN TEST BATTERY FOR MEN
KARL MARX UNIVERSITY IN LEIPZIG, GDR

Name: _____   Date of Exam : ___/___/___

   Date of Birth: ___/___/___

   Chronological Age: _____

1. Systolic blood pressure, in mm Hg : _____ x 0.0067   = _____

2. Diastolic blood pressure, in mm Hg: _____ x 0.01   = _____

3. Resting heart rate .... : _____ x 0.0134   = _____

4. Post-exercise pulse rate .... : _____ x 0.00909 = _____

5. Change in pulse rate .... : _____ x 0.0101   = _____

6. Time for exercise completion,
   in sec .... : _____ x 0.0222   = _____

7. Vital capacity as a % of normal   : _____ x 0.01   = _____

8. Arterial oxygen tension, in mm Hg : _____ x 0.0256   = _____

9. Tapping rate, 1st period,
   in taps per sec .... : _____ x 0.125   = _____

10. Tapping rate, 2nd period,
    in taps per sec .... : _____ x 0.125   = _____

11. Tapping rate, 6th period,
    in taps per sec .... : _____ x 0.143   = _____

12. Tapping rate, 7th period,
    in taps per sec .... : _____ x 0.143   = _____

13. Hand-eye coordination,
    number of errors .... : _____ x 0.02   = _____

14. Hand-eye coordination,
    in sec .... : _____ x 0.00769 = _____

15. Handgrip strength--sum of
    left _____ and right _____
    hands, in kg .... : _____ x 0.00625 = _____

Karl Marx University   **Chapter 17**

16. Tendon extensibility, sum of
    left _____ and right _____
    fifth fingers, in degrees ...... : _____ x 0.00667 = _____

17. Visual acuity, right eye, as a % : _____ x 0.01 = _____

18. Visual acuity, left eye, as a % : _____ x 0.01 = _____

19. Auditory acuity, right ear
    at 2,000 Hz, as a % .... : _____ x 0.025 = _____

20. Auditory acuity, right ear
    at 4,000 Hz, as a % .... : _____ x 0.0667 = _____

21. Auditory acuity, right ear, sum
    of 500 _____, 1,000 _____,
    2,000 _____ and 4,000 _____ Hz,
    as a % .... : _____ x 0.01 = _____

22. Auditory acuity, left ear
    at 2,000 Hz, as a % .... : _____ x 0.025 = _____

23. Auditory acuity, left ear
    at 4,000 Hz, as a % .... : _____ x 0.0667 = _____

24. Auditory acuity, left ear, sum
    of 500 _____, 1,000 _____,
    2,000 _____ and 4,000 _____ Hz,
    as a % .... : _____ x 0.01 = _____

25. Caries index-# of teeth
    decayed, missing, or filled (DMF): _____ x 0.03125 = _____

26. Color word test, 1st row, in sec : _____ x 0.0833 = _____

27. Color word test, 2nd row, in sec : _____ x 0.0476 = _____

28. Color word test, 3rd row, in sec : _____ x 0.01515 = _____

29. Landolt Concentration, in sec ... : _____ x 0.0027 = _____

30. Landolt Concentration-# of errors : _____ x 0.0667 = _____

31. Maze--completion time, in sec ... : _____ x 0.00192 = _____

32. Maze-# of buttons required ...... : _____ x 0.00667 = _____

33. Maze—# of errors .... : _____ x 0.00833 = _____

34. Maze—time required for
    one step, in sec .... : _____ x 0.286   = _____

35. Visual reaction time
    (light), in msec .... : _____ x 0.0025 = _____

36. Visual reaction time
    (clock), in msec .... : _____ x 0.00769 = _____

37. Auditory reaction time, in sec   : _____ x 0.00167 = _____

Biological age (men) = 48.7 ln [1. _____ + 2. _____

− 3. _____ − 4. _____ − 5. _____ + 6. _____ − 7. _____

− 8. _____ − 9. _____ − 10. _____ − 11. _____ − 12. _____

+ 13. _____ + 14. _____ − 15. _____ − 16. _____ − 17. _____

− 18. _____ + 19. _____ + 20. _____ + 21. _____ + 22. _____

+ 23. _____ + 24. _____ + 25. _____ + 26. _____ + 27. _____

+ 28. _____ + 29. _____ + 30. _____ + 31. _____ + 32. _____

+ 33. _____ + 34. _____ + 35. _____ + 36. _____ + 37. _____

+ 12.828] − 70.27

(Plot on a graph--App. C) Biological age _____

Karl Marx University   Chapter 17

CALCULATION SHEET
GERMAN TEST BATTERY FOR WOMEN
KARL MARX UNIVERSITY IN LEIPZIG, GDR

Name: _____ Date of Exam : ___/___/___

                                                                        Date of Birth: ___/___/___

                                                                         Chronological Age: _____

1. Systolic blood pressure, in mm Hg : _____ x 0.0067 = _____

2. Diastolic blood pressure, in mm Hg: _____ x 0.01 = _____

3. Resting heart rate .... : _____ x 0.0134 = _____

4. Post-exercise pulse rate .... : _____ x 0.00909 = _____

5. Change in pulse rate .... : _____ x 0.0101 = _____

6. Time for exercise completion,
    in sec .... : _____ x 0.0222 = _____

7. Vital capacity as a % of normal : _____ x 0.01 = _____

8. Arterial oxygen tension, in mm Hg : _____ x 0.0256 = _____

9. Tapping rate, 1st period,
    in taps per sec .... : _____ x 0.125 = _____

10. Tapping rate, 2nd period,
     in taps per sec .... : _____ x 0.125 = _____

11. Tapping rate, 6th period,
     in taps per sec .... : _____ x 0.143 = _____

12. Tapping rate, 7th period,
     in taps per sec .... : _____ x 0.143 = _____

13. Hand-eye coordination,
     number of errors .... : _____ x 0.02 = _____

14. Hand-eye coordination,
     in sec .... : _____ x 0.00769 = _____

15. Handgrip strength--sum of
     left _____ and right _____
     hands, in kg .... : _____ x 0.00625 = _____

16. Tendon extensibility, sum of
    left ____ and right ____
    fifth fingers, in degrees ...... : ____ x 0.00667 = ____

17. Visual acuity, right eye, as a % : ____ x 0.01   = ____

18. Visual acuity, left eye, as a % : ____ x 0.01   = ____

19. Auditory acuity, right ear
    at 2,000 Hz, as a % .... : ____ x 0.025   = ____

20. Auditory acuity, right ear
    at 4,000 Hz, as a % .... : ____ x 0.0667 = ____

21. Auditory acuity, right ear, sum
    of 500 ____,   1,000 ____,
    2,000 ____ and 4,000 ____ Hz,
    as a % .... : ____ x 0.01   = ____

22. Auditory acuity, left ear
    at 2,000 Hz, as a % .... : ____ x 0.025   = ____

23. Auditory acuity, left ear
    at 4,000 Hz, as a % .... : ____ x 0.0667 = ____

24. Auditory acuity, left ear, sum
    of 500 ____,   1,000 ____,
    2,000 ____ and 4,000 ____ Hz,
    as a % .... : ____ x 0.01   = ____

25. Caries index-# of teeth
    decayed, missing, or filled (DMF): ____ x 0.03125 = ____

26. Color word test, 1st row, in sec : ____ x 0.0833 = ____

27. Color word test, 2nd row, in sec : ____ x 0.0476 = ____

28. Color word test, 3rd row, in sec : ____ x 0.01515 = ____

29. Landolt Concentration, in sec ... : ____ x 0.0027 = ____

30. Landolt Concentration-# of errors : ____ x 0.0667 = ____

31. Maze--completion time, in sec ... : ____ x 0.00192 = ____

32. Maze-# of buttons required ...... : ____ x 0.00667 = ____

33. Maze-# of errors .... : _____ x 0.00833 = _____

34. Maze--time required for
    one step, in sec .... : _____ x 0.286   = _____

35. Visual reaction time
    (light), in msec .... : _____ x 0.0025 = _____

36. Visual reaction time
    (clock), in msec .... : _____ x 0.00769 = _____

37. Auditory reaction time, in sec   : _____ x 0.00167 = _____

Biological age (women) = 55.55 ln [1. _____ + 2. _____

− 3. _____ − 4. _____ − 5. _____ + 6. _____ − 7. _____

− 8. _____ − 9. _____ − 10. _____ − 11. _____ − 12. _____

+ 13. _____ + 14. _____ − 15. _____ − 16. _____ − 17. _____

− 18. _____ + 19. _____ + 20. _____ + 21. _____ + 22. _____

+ 23. _____ + 24. _____ + 25. _____ + 26. _____ + 27. _____

+ 28. _____ + 29. _____ + 30. _____ + 31. _____ + 32. _____

+ 33. _____ + 34. _____ + 35. _____ + 36. _____ + 37. _____

+ 12.828] − 90.64

(Plot on a graph--App. C) Biological age _____

REFERENCES

Kuhne, K. D., Paul, W., Kockeritz, C. Mikulas, J., Schiemann, S., and Weidinger, V. Zur Bestimmung des biologischen Alters im Rahmen der Halberstadter gerontologischen Studie — 3. Mitteilung: Teilindex III. *Z Alternsforsch*. 40: 6 (1985), 351-356.

Kuhne, K. D., Paul, W., Kockeritz, C., Mikulas, J., Schiemann, S., and Weidinger, V. Zur Bestimmung des biologischen Alters im Rahmen der Halberstadter gerontologischen Studie 2. Mitteilung: Teilindex II. *Z Alternsforsch*. 40:6 (1985) 349-351.

Kuhne, K. D., Paul, W., Kockeritz, C., MIkulas, J. Schiemann, S., and Weidinger, V. Zur Bestimmung des biologischen Alters im Rahmen der Halberstadter gerontologischen Studie 1. Mitteilung: Teilindex I. *Z Alternsforsch*. 40:6 (1985), 339-343.

Poethig, D. *Experimentelle Entwicklung eines klinischen Diagnostikmodelles zur Objektivierung des biologischen Alters des Menschen*, Med. Dissertation B., Leipzig, 1984.

Poethig, D., and Ries, W. Umweltaspekte in der gerontologischen Forschung, *Wiss. Z. Karl Marx Univ. Math Naturwiss*. Vol. 33 (1984), 2, pp. 197-207.

Poethig, D., Hochauf, R., and Michalak, U. Untersuchungen mit dem Gieben-Test zur Alternsdynamik sozialen Verhaltens. *Z Alternsforsch*. 40: 2 (1985), 245-252.

Poethig, D., and Israel, S. Zur bedeutung der bestimmung des biologischen alterns fur die gerontologie. *Z Alternsforsch*. 40: 5 (1985), 313-321.

Ries, W. Personal communications, 18 Feb 1985; 11 April, 1985; 17 Jan 1986; and 18 September 1986.

Ries, W. Problems associated with biological age, in: *Proceedings, IX International Congress of Gerontology and Geriatrics*, Kiev, 1972, 323-326.

Ries, W. Problems associated with biological age. *Exp Ger*, Vol. 9 (1974), pp. 145-149.

Ries, W. *Studien Zum Biologischen Alter*. 1982. Akademie-Verlag, Berlin.

Ries, W. Terminologische und methodische probleme bei der bestimmung des biologischen alters. *Dt Gesundh-Wesen, Zeitschrift fur klinische Medizin*, 38: Heft 11, 401-404.

Ries, W., Sauer, I., Junker, B, Poethig, D., and Schwerdtner, U. Methodische Probleme bei der Ermittlung des biologischen Alters, *Zschr inn Med*, Jahrg. 31 (1976) Heft 4, pp. 109-113.

Ries, W., and Poethig, D. Chronological and Biological Age. *Exp Ger*, Vol. 19, pp. 211-216, 1984.

Roth, N. *Psychophysiologische Analyse von Aktivitatszustand und motorischer Testleistung bei der Ausbildung adaptiver Verhaltensakte des Menschen*, Med. Dissertation B, Leipzig 1976.

Chapter 18

JAPANESE TEST BATTERIES
University of Nagoya

Scientists from the Department of Geriatrics, Nagoya University School of Medicine recently developed another Japanese measurement system. Drs. Hiroshi Shimokata, Fumio Kuzuya and Kazuaki Shibata (*Fig. 18-1*) presented details of their test batteries at the 13th International Congress of Gerontology and Geriatrics in New York City in July, 1985.

In addition to developing a composite equation for *general biological aging status*, they also developed separate equations for external appearance, physiological functions, and physical *condition*. This allowed them to determine the cause of any aberration in biological age and where efforts should be directed to reduce it. This concept is discussed at greater length in Chapter 23.

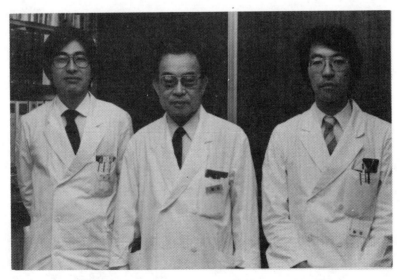

Fig. 18-1. L to R, **Drs. Hiroshi Shimokata, Fumio Kuzuya, and Kazuaki Shibata.**

The Nagoya scientists are unique in being first to actually use results of individual measurements from patients as tools to evaluate physiological and biochemical aspects that contribute to accelerated aging. They used this information to advise the subjects about interventions that could be used to retain their youth and reduce their biological age.

Shimokata is now in the United States, working with the NIA and its Baltimore Longitudinal Study of Aging.

REQUIREMENTS FOR THE NAGOYA BATTERIES:

1. Routine hematological and biochemical tests.
2. Spirometer (Appendix A, 2-1).
3. Vision screening test instrument for near vision test (Appendix A, 4-4).
4. Handgrip dynamometer (Appendix A, 6-1).
5. Tape measure.
6. Stop watch.
7. Master's staircase (Appendix A, 1-5).
8. Scale.
9. Dental exam.
10. Flexibility tester (Appendix A. 6-8. c).

TESTS IN THE NAGOYA EQUATIONS:

1. Anthropometric:
    a. Height (HT), in cm (Appendix B. 6-13).
    b. Weight (WT), in kg (Appendix B. 6-14).
    c. Baldness (B) (Appendix B. 6-10. b).
    d. Grayness (G) (Appendix B. 6-1. b).
    e. Caries index (DMF) (Appendix B. 7-2).

2. Physiological and biochemical:
    a. Near vision (NV), as a decimal (Appendix B. 4-4).
    b. Systolic blood pressure (SBP), in mm Hg (Appendix B. 1-1).
    c. Vital capacity (VC), in ml (Appendix B. 2-2).
    d. Red blood cell count (RBC) (Appendix B. 8-3).
    e. Blood urea nitrogen (BUN), in mg/100 cc (Appendix B. 9-5).
    f. Total protein (TP), in gm/100 cc (Appendix B. 9-13).
    g. Fibrinogen (F), in mg/100 cc (Appendix B. 9-14).
    h. Triglycerides (TRIG), in mg/100 cc (Appendix B. 9-3).
    i. Phospholipids (P), in mg/100 cc (Appendix B. 9-15).
    j. Cholesterol (CHOL), in mg/100 cc (Appendix B. 9-1).
    k. HDL cholesterol (HDL), in mg/100 cc (Appendix B. 9-2).
    l. Alkaline phosphatase (AP) (Appendix B. 9-6) in international units.
    m. Uric acid (UA) (Appendix B. 9-16) in mg/100 cc.

3. Physical condition:
    a. Handgrip strength (HGS), in kg (Appendix B. 6-2).
    b. Static balance (SB), in sec (Appendix B. 5-11 a).
    c. Anteflexion (AF), in cm (Appendix B. 6-11. b).
    d. Heart rate/30 sec (HR), taken 30 sec after completion of 5-minute Master's two-step test, conducted at rate of 90 steps/minute (Appendix B. 1-5. c).

THE NAGOYA EQUATIONS:

I. Appearance

BA = 88.34061 - 0.57600 (HT) + 0.32839 (WT) + 7.09190 (B) + 8.55721 (G)
    + 0.68741 (DMF)

II. Physiological and biochemical functions

BA = 18.89527 - 10.18836 (NV) + 0.18328 (SBP) - 0.00352 (VC) - 0.03719 (RBC)
    + 0.99659 (BUN) - 1.33354 (TP) + 0.05476 (F) + 0.03964 (TRIG) - 0.05075 (P)
    + 0.16270 (HDL)

III. Physical condition

BA = 52.37258 - 0.66986 (HGS) - 0.21602 (SB) + 0.58380 (AF) + 1 0.66389 (2-STEP)

IV. General biological

a. BA = 23.12722 - 0.07215 (SB) - 0.21138 (AF) + 0.30067 (2-STEP)
    + 0.18797 (DBP) + 0.45202 (BUN) + 6.00019 (CR) + 0.02739 (F)
    - 0.06234 (P) + 0.05254 (CHOL) + 0.07278 (HDL) - 3.73141 (NV)
    - 0.24592 (HT) + 4.77109 (B) + 3.84193 (G) + 0.47781 (DMF)

b. BA = 34.72343 - 0.07329 (SB) - 0.24060 (AF) + 0.30132 (2-STEP)
    - 0.00581 (HGS) + 0.00237 (SBP) + 0.18622 (DBP) + 0.00124 (VC)
    - 0.00271 (RBC) + 0.48010 (BUN) + 6.35360 (CR) - 0.82098 (TP)
    - 0.01542 (AP) + 0.02546 (F) + 0.02257 (TRIG) - 0.10261 (P)
    + 0.06172 (CHOL) + 0.12290 (HDL) - 3.65227 (NV) - 0.29118 (HT)
    + 0.00111 (WT) + 4.74923 (B) + 3.67015 (G) + 0.49417 (DMF)

c. BA = 40.4983 - 0.0775652 (SB) - 0.207501 (AF) + 0.19649 (2-STEP)
    - 0.102889 (HGS) + 0.196568 (DBP) + 1.43953E-03 (VC)
    - 1.95778 (UA) + 0.473258 (BUN) + 7.73798 (CR)
    + 0.0260108 (F) + 0.0308529 (CHOL) - 3.41224 (NV)
    - 0.297929 (HT) + 4.83776 (B) + 4.09948 (G) + 0.477932 (DMF)

University of Nagoya   Chapter 18

CALCULATION SHEET
JAPANESE TEST BATTERY FOR MEN
NAGOYA UNIVERSITY
I. Appearance

Name: _____   Date of Exam : ___/___/___

                                                          Date of Birth: ___/___/___

                                                          Chronological Age: _____

1. Height, in cm (non-Asians:
   multiply 0.94 first) .... : _____ x 0.57600 = _____

2. Weight, in kg (non-Asians:
   multiply by 0.72 first) .... : _____ x 0.32839 = _____

3. Baldness score .... : _____ x 7.09190 = _____

4. Grayness score .... : _____ x 8.55721 = _____

5. Caries index (DMF) .... : _____ x 0.68741 = _____

Biological age = 88.34061 − 1. _____ + 2. _____ + 3. _____

+ 4. _____ + 5. _____

(Plot on a graph--App. C)   Biologial age _____

Chapter 18 — University of Nagoya

CALCULATION SHEET
JAPANESE TEST BATTERY FOR MEN
NAGOYA UNIVERSITY
II. Physiological and Biochemical Functions

Name: _____   Date of Exam : ___/___/___

Date of Birth: ___/___/___

Chronological Age: _____

1. Near vision, as a decimal .... : _____ x 10.18836 = _____
2. Systolic blood pressure, in mm Hg : _____ x 0.18328 = _____
3. Vital capacity, in ml .... : _____ x 0.00352 = _____
4. Red blood cell count .... : _____ x 0.03719 = _____
5. Blood urea nitrogen, in mg/100cc : _____ x 0.99659 = _____
6. Total protein, in mg/100 cc ..... : _____ x 1.33354 = _____
7. Fibrinogen, in mg/100 cc .... : _____ x 0.05476 = _____
8. Triglycerides, in mg/100 cc ..... : _____ x 0.03964 = _____
9. Phospholipids, in mg/100 cc ..... : _____ x 0.05075 = _____
10. Cholesterol, in mg/100 cc .... : _____ x 0.08307 = _____
11. HDL cholesterol, in mg/100 cc ... : _____ x 0.16270 = _____

Biological age = 18.89527 - 1. _____ + 2. _____ - 3. _____
- 4. _____ + 5. _____ - 6. _____ + 7. _____ + 8. _____
- 9. _____ + 10. _____ + 11. _____

(Plot on a graph--App. C)   Biological age = _____

University of Nagoya   Chapter 18

CALCULATION SHEET
JAPANESE TEST BATTERY FOR MEN
NAGOYA UNIVERSITY
III. Physical Condition

Name: _____   Date of Exam : ___/___/___

                                                                             Date of Birth: ___/___/___

                                                                             Chronological Age: _____

1. *Handgrip strength in kg .... : _____ x 0.66986 = _____

2. Static balance, in sec .... : _____ x 0.03343 = _____

3. Anteflexion, in cm .... : _____ x 0.01966 = _____

4. Heart rate/ 30 sec after
   two-step exercise test .... : _____ x 0.34042 = _____

*Non-Asian subjects should use the conversion scale in
Fig. B. 6-3 to obtain adjusted handgrip strength values for
this equation.

Biological age = 52.37258 - 1. _____ - 2. _____ + 3. _____

+ 4. _____

(Plot on a graph--App. C)   Biological age = _____

Chapter 18   University of Nagoya

CALCULATION SHEET
JAPANESE TEST BATTERY FOR MEN
NAGOYA UNIVERSITY
General Biological Status IV. a.

Name: _____ Date of Exam : ___/___/___

                                                                        Date of Birth: ___/___/___

                                                                       Chronological Age: _____

1. Static balance, in sec .... : _____ x 0.07215 = _____

2. Anteflexion, in cm .... : _____ x 0.21138 = _____

3. Heart rate 30 sec after
   two-step exercise test .... : _____ x 0.30067 = _____

4. Diastolic blood pressure in mm Hg : _____ x 0.187976 = _____

5. Blood urea nitrogen, in mg/100 ml : _____ x 0.45202 = _____

6. Creatinine, in mg/100 ml .... : _____ x 6.00019 = _____

7. Fibrinogen, in mg/100 ml .... : _____ x 0.02739 = _____

8. Phospholipids, in mg/100 ml .... : _____ x 0.06234 = _____

9. Cholesterol, in mg/100 ml ...... : _____ x 0.05254 = _____

10. HDL, in mg/100 cc .... : _____ x 0.07278 = _____

11. Near vision, as a decimal ...... : _____ x 3.73141 = _____

12. Height, in cm (non-Asians
    multiply by 0.94 first) .... : _____ x 0.24592 = _____

13. Baldness .... : _____ x 4.77109 = _____

14. Grayness .... : _____ x 3.84193 = _____

15. Caries index (DMF) .... : _____ x 0.47781 = _____

Biological Age = 23.12722 − 1. _____ − 2. _____ + 3. _____
+ 4. _____ + 5. _____ + 6. _____ + 7. _____ − 8. _____
+ 9. _____ + 10. _____ − 11. _____ − 12. _____ + 13. _____
+ 14. _____ + 15. _____

(Plot on a graph--App. C)   Biological Age _____

CALCULATION SHEET
JAPANESE TEST BATTERY FOR MEN
NAGOYA UNIVERSITY
General Biological Status IV. b.

Name: _____   Date of Exam : ___/___/___

                                                                     Date of Birth: ___/___/___

                                                                     Chronological Age: _____

1. Static balance, in sec .... : _____ x 0.07329 = _____
2. Anteflexion, in cm .... : _____ x 0.24060 = _____
3. Heart rate 30 sec after
    two-step exercise test .... : _____ x 0.30132 = _____
4. *Handgrip strength in kg .... : _____ x 0.00581 = _____
5. Systolic blood pressure, in mm Hg : _____ x 0.00237 = _____
6. Diastolic blood pressure, in mm Hg: _____ x 0.18622 = _____
7. Vital Capacity, in ml .... : _____ x 0.00124 = _____
8. Red Blood Cell count .... : _____ x 0.00271 = _____
9. Blood urea nitrogen, in mg/100 ml : _____ x 0.48010 = _____
10. Creatinine, in mg/100 ml .... : _____ x 6.35360 = _____
11. Total protein, in gm/100 cc ..... : _____ x 0.82098 = _____
12. Alkaline phosphatase, int'l units : _____ x 0.01542 = _____
13. Fibrinogen, in mg/100 ml .... : _____ x 0.02546 = _____
14. Triglycerides, in mg/100 cc ..... : _____ x 0.02257 = _____
15. Phospholipids, in mg/100 ml ..... : _____ x 0.10261 = _____
16. Cholesterol, in mg/100 ml .... : _____ x 0.06172 = _____
17. HDL, in mg/100 cc .... : _____ x 0.12290 = _____

18. Near vision, as a decimal .... : _____ x 3.65227 = _____

19. Height, in cm (non-Asians
    multiply by 0.94 first) .... : _____ x 0.29118 = _____

20. Weight, in kg (non-Asians
    multiply by 0.72 first) .... : _____ x 0.00111 = _____

21. Baldness .... : _____ x 4.741224 = _____

22. Grayness .... : _____ x 3.67015 = _____

23. Caries index, DMF .... : _____ x 0.49417 = _____

Biological Age = 34.72343 - 1. _____ - 2. _____ + 3. _____

- 4. _____ + 5. _____ + 6. _____ + 7. _____ - 8. _____ + 9. _____

+ 10. _____ - 11. _____ - 12. _____ + 13. _____ + 14. _____

- 15. _____ + 16. _____ + 17. _____ - 18. _____ - 19. _____

+ 20. _____ + 21. _____ + 22. _____ + 23. _____

(Plot on a graph--App. C)   Biological Age _____

*Non-Asian subjects should use the conversion scale in Fig. B. 6-3 to obtain an adjusted handgrip strength for this equation.

| Chapter 18 | University of Nagoya |

CALCULATION SHEET
JAPANESE TEST BATTERY FOR MEN
NAGOYA UNIVERSITY
General Biological Status IV. c.

Name: _____ Date of Exam : ___/___/___

Date of Birth: ___/___/___

Chronological Age: _____

1. Static balance, in sec .... : _____ x 0.0775652 = _____

2. Anteflexion, in cm .... : _____ x 0.207501 = _____

3. Heart rate 30 sec after
   two-step exercise test .... : _____ x 0.19649   = _____

4. *Handgrip strength in kg .... : _____ x 0.102889 = _____

5. Diastolic blood pressure in mm Hg : _____ x 0.196568 = _____

6. Vital capacity, in ml .... : _____ x 1.43953^{-03} = _____

7. Uric acid, in mg/100 ml .... : _____ x 1.95778   = _____

8. Blood urea nitrogen, in mg/100 ml : _____ x 0.473258 = _____

9. Creatinine, in mg/100 ml .... : _____ x 7.73798   = _____

10. Fibrinogen, in mg/100 ml .... : _____ x 0.0260108 = _____

11. Cholesterol, in mg/100 ml ...... : _____ x 0.0308529 = _____

12. Near vision, as a decimal ...... : _____ x 3.41224   = _____

13. Height, in cm (non-Asians
    multiply by 0.94 first) .... : _____ x 0.297929 = _____

14. Baldness .... : _____ x 4.83776   = _____

15. Grayness .... : _____ x 4.09948   = _____

16. Caries Index, DMF .... : _____ x 0.477932 = _____

University of Nagoya   **Chapter 18**

Biological Age = 40.4983 − 1. _____ − 2. _____ + 3. _____
− 4. _____ + 5. _____ + 6. _____ − 7. _____ + 8. _____ + 9. _____
+ 10. _____ + 11. _____ + 12. _____ − 13. _____ − 14. _____
+ 15. _____ + 16. _____

(Plot on a graph--App. C)   Biological Age _____

*Non-Asian subjects should use the conversion scale in Fig. B. 6-3 to obtain an adjusted handgrip strength for this equation.

REFERENCES

Shimokata, H., Shibata, K., Kuzuya, F. Assessment of biological aging status. *J Jap Soc Int Med*, 74: 1344-1347, 1985.

Shimokata, H. Personal communications, 1 Aug, 1985; 26 Aug 1985; 18 October, 1986.

Part III

Miscellaneous Systems

and

Future Prospects

Chapter 19

WHOLE-BODY CALORIMETRY

Dr. Daniel Hershey (*Fig. 19-1*) is Professor of Chemical Engineering, College of Engineering, Department of Chemical and Nuclear Engineering, at the University of Cincinnati in Cincinnati, Ohio, and Vice President for Research and Development of Basal-Tech, Inc., Cincinnati, Ohio. For over a decade, he has devoted an increasing percentage of his time to gerontology, and the development of a unique theory of aging. He approaches gerontological research from a background of chemical engineering and thermodynamics, as well as from the traditional biological and physiological points of view.

Hershey and his students developed the *Entropic Theory of Aging*--an off-shoot of the *Wear and Tear* theory of aging, although much more complex (Dean, 1982; Hershey, 1963, 1974, 1980, 1984a and b). Entropy is a thermodynamic concept that quantifies the increasing disorder occurring in living or non-living systems over time.

Living systems become more disordered with time and hence accumulate entropy. Hershey views death as the ultimate disorder--the state of highest entropy content where all driving forces for life diminish to nothing. He defines *vitality* as the entropy difference between the terminal state of maximum entropy and the actual condition at a given age. He calls this difference "excess entropy" (EE), and the rate of its production "excess entropy production" (EEP).

The rate of *entropy production* in mature mammals decreases continuously. Entropy production nevertheless has a finite cumulative potential that tends toward a minimum value in the vicinity of senile death. The entropy production of a living organism can be determined from its *basal metabolic rate* (BMR) by appropriate thermodynamic equations.

Chapter 19

Whole-Body Calorimetry

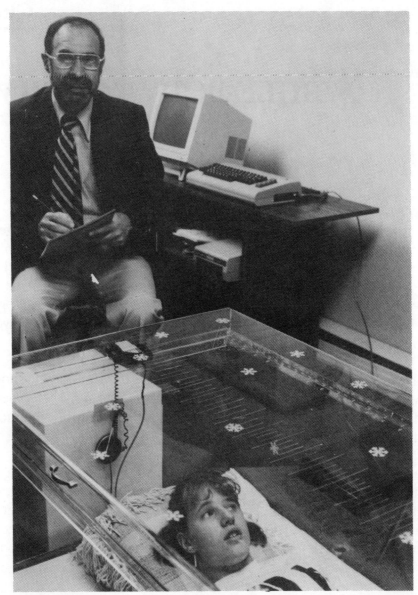

Fig. 19-1. **Daniel Hershey, Ph.D.**

MEASUREMENT OF BASAL METABOLIC RATE

The BMR can be measured directly with a whole-body calorimeter, of which there are several types. Calorimeters, by various methods, measure the total amount of heat liberated by the body. They are generally elaborate, expensive devices, suitable only for large research laboratories. However, Hershey and his colleagues designed, patented, and marketed a computerized, portable (100 pounds), relatively inexpensive calorimeter (*Basal-Tech Personal*

Calorimeter) suitable for use in a physician's office (*Fig. 19-2*). His method requires only about 15 minutes to determine a subject's metabolic rate.

The whole-body calorimeter is a rectangular, transparent box made of 3/8 inch plexiglas, 7 feet long, 3 feet wide, and 2 feet high. As air flows into and out of the calorimeter, the inlet and outlet air temperatures are automatically measured to within 0.1° F by thermocouples whose signals are fed into the computer.

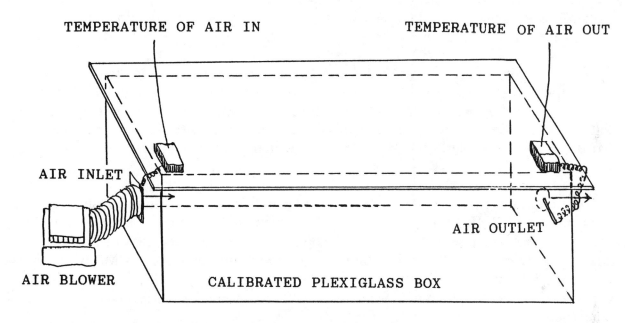

Fig. 19-2. **Whole-body calorimeter**, manufactured by Basal-Tech, Inc.

BMR MEASUREMENTS AND LIFESPAN DETERMINATION

Basal metabolic rate measurements give an indication of "whole body metabolism" (Gump). The BMR is a measure of metabolism as it occurs in the body at rest, and is not specific for any body region, organ or subsystem. The basal state measurement represents the energy requirements of the vegetative functions of the body (i.e., maintenance of body temperature, respiration, circulation, cellular metabolism, and other essential bodily functions required to support life) (Young). During the course of a normal day, such activities as digestion, stress, and physical activity will produce temporary rises in the metabolic rate. The basal rate is a reproducible minimum for a given subject over finite time periods. Presently, BMR measurements are the physician's only readily available tool in the general area of total body energy production (Becker).

BMR values appear to decrease with age. Over short periods of time--say, a few months-- the BMR can be considered to be reasonably constant. This is especially true in later life. Thus, any condition that causes a steady rise in BMR over time is not the normal response of a healthy subject. A variety of physiological and pathological conditions cause such abnormal increases in BMR. The classic causes involve the effect of thyroid hormones on BMR. For example, severe hyperthyroidism can increase the BMR by as much as 100% (Robbins, et al).

BMR measurements have traditionally been used as a diagnostic tool for thyroid-related metabolic abnormalities. However, because of the cumbersome nature of conventional methods of measuring BMR, other diagnostic methods for thyroid abnormalities (such as protein-bound iodine determination and assays of thyroid and thyroid-stimulating hormone levels) have generally become the accepted standard.

With the exceptions of occasional use in the investigation of thyroid status and obesity management, BMR measurement techniques are rarely utilized for other diagnostic possibilities. Hershey thinks that his BMR measurement techniques might be useful in the early diagnosis of a variety of conditions, including cancer, endocrine disorders, and cardiovascular disease, as they drive the BMR off the lifespan track the individual has generated (Hershey and Lee).

To support his hypothesis, Hershey compiled data from many longitudinal and cross-sectional studies of BMR changes with age in both men and women into a series of entropy production tables. These tables reflect the apparent progressive decrease of BMR with increasing age (Hershey, 1980). Some studies conclude that the decrease in BMR with aging is only apparent, and is due to the decreased muscle mass which also occurs with aging. Whichever is the case, it does not invalidate Hershey's concept. He is still measuring very real aging changes.

Using his BMR data and entropy-conversion equations, Hershey can construct "lifespan tracks" for individuals. He found that when the excess entropy reaches zero, the subject is near his lifespan potential, and death may be near. His research yields several guidelines for predicting the longevity of individuals: (1) when the positive-valued EEP of an individual diminishes to zero on an EEP versus age graph, he has reached his lifespan potential and death is imminent; or (2) when the negative-valued EE rises to zero on an EE versus age graph, death is also imminent.

Using longitudinal data for 39 subjects from the NIA's Baltimore Longitudinal Study of Aging and BMR measurements made with the *Basal-Tech Whole-Body Personal Calorimeter*, he found that the calculated lifespan projection agreed with the actual lifespan within 1 year for 16% of the subjects, within 4 years for 48%, and within 7 years for 74%.

Whole-Body Calorimetry — Chapter 19

APPLICATIONS AND AVAILABILITY OF HERSHEY'S CALORIMETERS

Using the whole-body calorimeter-derived basal metabolic rates and entropy production rates, *relative biological ages* (*metabolic-entropy age*) and expected remaining life spans may be determined. Specific details are provided with the calorimeters, and are also contained in Hershey's book, *A New Age Scale for Humans* (Lexington books, 1980), and in a Ph.D. thesis by one of his students, *Analysis to Understand the Thermodynamics of Living Aging Systems*, by William Lee (University of Cincinnati, 1985).

The calorimeter and BMR data are also useful for bariatric physicians (physicians specializing in weight control) who use these data to determine a patient's *daily caloric needs* (DCN) for diet planning and for calculating rates of weight loss. Although this use by bariatric physicians is probably the most common commercial application of the calorimeter, its most important potential use is as a means of measuring biological age. Most bariatric physicians who use the calorimeter will also be able to calculate biological ages, utilizing a computer program Hershey is developing.

Additional information and names and addresses of physicians and exercise physiologists who use Hershey's whole-body personal calorimeter can be obtained from:

Basal-Tech, Inc.
726 Lafayette Avenue
Cincinnati, OH 45220
(513) 751-2723.

Names of physicians specializing in bariatric medicine can be obtained from:

The American Society of Bariatric Physicians
7430 Caley Avenue Suite 210
Englewood, CO 80111, or

The International Academy of Bariatric Medicine
P.O. Box 2888
Littleton, CO 80161.

REFERENCES

Becker, D. V. Metabolic indices, in: *The Thyroid*, Werner, S. D., and Ingbar, S. H. (eds.) New York, Harper and Row, 1971, p. 269.

Dean, W. A New Age Scale for Humans (Review), *J Am Geriatr Soc*, 30(8): 547-548, 1982.

Gump. F. E. Whole body metabolism, in: *Handbook of Shock and Trauma, Vol. I: Basic Science*, Altura, S. M., et al (eds.). in Press, 1983, p. 241.

Hershey, D., Wang, H. *A New Age Scale for Humans*, Lexington Books, Lexington, 1980.

Hershey, D. *Must We Grow Old?* Basal Books, Cincinnati, 1984.

Hershey, D. Entropy, Basal Metabolism and Life Expectancy, *Gerontologia* 7:245-250 (1963).

Hershey, D. *Lifespan and Factors Affecting It*. Charles C. Thomas, Springfield, 1974.

Hershey, D., and Lee, W. Life span potential from excess entropy (EE) and excess entropy production (EEP). *AGE*, 7(4): 149 (#67), Oct 1984.

Lee, W. *Analysis to Understand the Thermodynamics of Living Systems*. Ph.D. Thesis, U. of Cincinnati, 1985.

Lee, W. E., and Hershey, D. The utilization of BMR measurements as a routine diagnostic procedure in normal health maintenance. *Medical Hypotheses*, 16: 147-154, 1985.

Robbins, J., Rall, J. E., and Gorden, P. The thyroid and iodine metabolism, in: *Duncan's Diseases of Metabolism. Endocrinology*, Bondy, P. K., and Rosenberg, L. E. (eds.), Philadelphia, W. B. Saunders, 1974, p. 1009.

Chapter 20

NEUROENDOCRINE TEST BATTERIES
Petrov Research Institute, Lenningrad

Professor Vladimir Dilman (*Fig. 20-1*), a noted Soviet clinical gerontologist, is Chief, Laboratory of Endocrinology, Petrov Research Institute of Oncology, Lenningrad, USSR. Dilman believes that aging is manifested by a progressive inability of the endocrine system to maintain homeostatic conditions within the body (Dilman, 1982, 1984; Dean, June 1983 and August 1983).

NEUROENDOCRINE HOMEOSTATIC DECLINE TEST BATTERIES

The pituitary and the hypothalamus normally maintain hormonal and other metabolic conditions within a narrow "normal" range by a complex system of "negative feedback loops" (*Fig. 20-2*). With age, these feedback systems seem to lose their sensitivity to feedback inhibition, and wider and wider endocrine and metabolic swings occur before the controlling mechanisms are activated to bring the levels back within the normal ranges.

An example is the decline in the body's ability to handle a carbohydrate load, as evidenced by the change in the response of older people to an oral glucose tolerance test (Appendix B. 11-1). Usually the "normal" range for an elderly person would indicate diabetes in a younger person (Thompson).

Dilman believes the concept of "age-adjusted normals" is erroneous. He thinks that *any* deviation from that of a healthy 25-year old should be considered *abnormal*, and should be an indication for gerontotherapeutic intervention.

He designed test batteries (1981) to measure the ability of the hypothalamus and pituitary to control the body's neuroendocrine homeostatic state, and to differentiate between *secondary* failure due to deterioration of the *end organs* (i.e., thyroid, testes, ovaries, or adrenals) or a *primary* failure due to hypothalamic or pituitary dysfunction. He therefore refers to these

Chapter 20

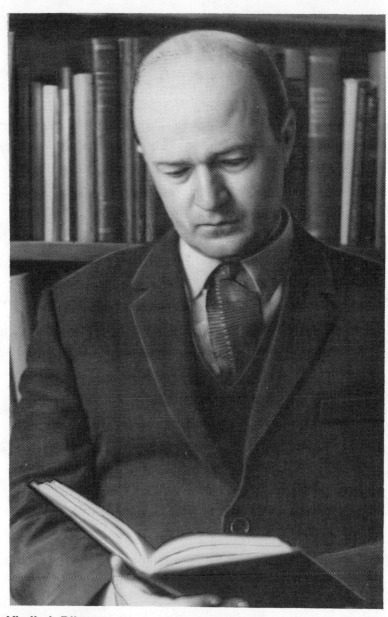

Fig. 20-1. **Professor Vladimir Dilman.**

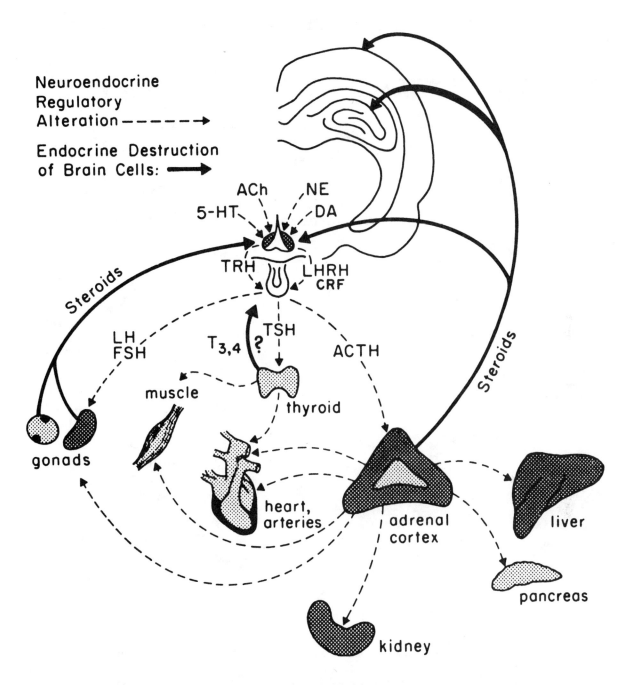

Fig. 20-2. **Control of the hypothalamo-pituitary-adrenal-reproductive axis.** Releasing hormones are evolved by the hypothalamus to control the function of the pituitary. Corticotrophin releasing factor (CRF) and luteinizing hormone releasing hormone (LHRH) stimulate the production of adrenocorticotrophic hormone (ACTH) and follicle stimulating hormone (FSH) and luteinizing hormone (LH) respectively. ACTH stimulates the adrenal cortex to produce adrenal steroids. LH stimulates testosterone secretion by the gonads. Feedback control of hypothalamic activity originates in the gonads, the adrenal cortex and the pituitary (Landfield).

TABLE 20-1. **TESTS FOR EVALUATION OF THE MAIN HOMEOSTATIC SYSTEMS**

Homeostatic System	Primary Test	Secondary Test
Energy System	Insulin stress test	Oral glucose tolerance test (two hour)
	Growth hormone after fat loading	Serum cholesterol
		HDL
		Triglycerides
		Weight
		Basal metabolic rate
Reproductive System	LHRH test	Serum FSH
	Clomiphene test	Serum LH
		Urinary excretion of total gonadotropins and total phenolsteroids
Adaptive System	Dexamethasone suppression test	17 ketosteroid to 17 hydroxycorticosteroid excretion ratio
	Insulin stress test	
	Diurnal cortisol levels	Tests of cell-mediated immunity
"Thyrostat"	T3 suppression test	TSH, T3, and T4 levels
Regulation of MSH and prolactin secretion	L-dopa test	Serum prolactin
	Chlorpromazine test	Serum MSH

batteries as *Secondary* (hypothalamo-pituitary dependent) and Primary (end-organ dependent) batteries (Table 20-I), respectively. His preliminary Secondary battery uses relatively standardized laboratory tests (available from most clinical laboratories), and is used as a screening test battery to identify the presence of neuroendocrine dysfunctions.

The more complex *Primary* battery consists of a number of sophisticated tests (and in some cases experimental protocols) used to identify the specific site of the dysfunction if the *Secondary* tests are consistently abnormal.

SECONDARY BATTERY:

1. Two hour oral glucose tolerance test (OGTT), with simultaneous insulin levels (Appendix B., 11-1). Although the OGTT is a standard test, insulin levels are not routinely determined during screening exams. Dilman has modified the standard test by including insulin levels.
2. Cholesterol (Appendix B. 9-1).
3. HDL cholesterol (Appendix B. 9-2).
4. Triglycerides (Appendix B. 9-3).
5. Body weight (Appendix B. 6-14).
6. Basal metabolic rate (BMR) (Appendix B. 11-2).
7. Follicle stimulating hormone (FSH) (Appendix B. 11-4).
8. Luteinizing hormone (LH) (Appendix B. 11-3).
9. Urinary excretion of total gonadotropins (FSH and LH) and total phenolsteroids (Appendix B. 11-7).
10. 17-ketosteroid /17-hydroxycorticosteroid excretion ratio (Appendix B. 11-12).
11. Tests to evaluate cell-mediated immunity. Immune function is known to decline with age. This results in a reduced resistance to infection, and an increase in auto-immune diseases and cancer (*Fig. 20-3*). Dilman recommends one or more of the following standard immunological tests to evaluate immune function:

    a. Assay of T and B lymphocyte levels in peripheral blood. (Appendix B. 12-1).

    b. Lymphocyte response to phytohemaglutinin (PHA) (Appendix B. 12-2).

    c. Dinitrochlorobenzene (DNCB), tuberculin, or candida contact sensitization skin tests (Appendix B. 12-3).

12. TSH, T₃, and T₄ (Appendix B. 11-8).

13. Prolactin (Appendix B. 11-9).

14. Melanocyte stimulating hormone (MSH) (Appendix B. 11-10).

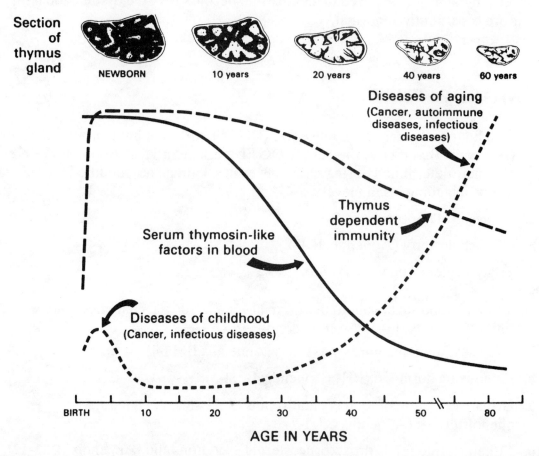

Fig. 20-3. **Decline of thymic-dependent immunity with age**. As serum thymosin-like factors in the blood decrease due to progressive involution of the thymus gland with age, there is an increase in the diseases of aging (Goldstein, et al).

I suggested to Dilman that he include testosterone and estrogen levels, (Appendix B. 11-12, and 11-13), and the LHRH and clomiphene tests. Estrogen and testosterone levels are important because they change markedly with age, have profound effects on the body, and may be easily modulated pharmacotherapeutically. The LHRH and clomiphene tests help to determine whether the cause of hypogonadism is gonadal or pituitary in origin. Dilman (18 Nov 1984) agreed that they should be incorporated.

Petrov Research Institute Chapter 20

Dilman (3 July 1984) thinks the Secondary tests are sufficient for routine periodic evaluations. The more complex Primary tests are required only if there are persistent abnormalities in the Secondary tests, and are used to locate the site of the dysfunction (*hypothalamo-pituitary* vs *end-organ*) indicated by the Secondary test.

PRIMARY BATTERY:

1. **Insulin stress test**. Although this test is a standard endocrinological diagnostic test, it has been modified so much by Dilman that it is described fully below. It assesses the response of the hypothalamo-pituitary-adrenal axis by determining cortisol and growth hormone levels after hypoglycemia has been induced by insulin. The test is potentially dangerous, and the patient must be carefully monitored.

The following are prerequisites:

1. Resting ECG. Ischemic changes or a history of angina are contraindications for the test.
2. Body weight.
3. Fasting blood sugar should be less than 150 mg/100 ml. Diabetics require special monitoring.
4. Fast from midnight preceding the day of the test, and rest in bed until the test.

The test is conducted as follows:

1. Administer 0.1 units/kg of insulin intravenously at time "0" as indicated on the table below. Although the standard insulin stress test utilizes 0.15 units/kg (Wills, 1983), Dilman is concerned that the profound hypoglycemia which may ensue with this dosage may be dangerous for middle-aged and older subjects, and thus recommends the reduced dosage (Dilman, July 1984).
2. The following blood samples are taken at the intervals indicated in the table that follows: Glucose (1 ml in a fluoride tube), cortisol and growth hormone (two 10 ml plain tubes), and thyroid stimulating hormone (TSH) (2 ml in a plain tube). For a normal response, the maximum plasma cortisol value should reach 550 nmol/l, and the increase over basal levels should exceed 190 nmol/l. The growth hormone value should exceed 20 mU/l.

Time (min)	-2	0	+20	+30	+60	+90	+120
Glucose	+		+	+	+	+	+
Cortisol	+			+	+	+	+
GH	+			+	+	+	+
TSH	+		+		+		

2. Thyrotropin Releasing Hormone (TRH) test. This can be conducted simultaneously with the Insulin Stress Test. 200 μg TRH are administered simultaneously with the insulin. Five ml of blood in a plain tube are then collected at the times shown for TSH. In a normal response, the TSH concentration will increase to a peak response between 5 and 20 mU/l at 30 minutes, and then fall by at least one-third of the peak response at 120 minutes (*Fig. 20-4*).

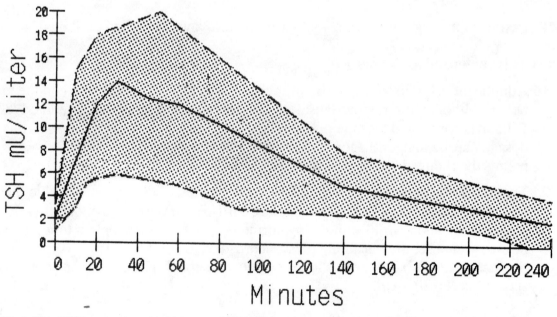

Fig. 20-4. **The TSH response to 500 μg of TRH given intravenously--mean +/- SEM** (Hershman).

3. **Growth hormone level after fat loading.** This is an experimental protocol being developed by Dilman (1 June, 1984). The test is conducted as follows: Five hundred mg of nicotinic acid in 500 ml of saline are administered intravenously over 1-2 hours. From 220 to 250 ml of Intralipid™ (a fat emulsion) are simultaneously injected intravenously at a rate of 1.5-2.0 ml/min. Five thousand units of heparin are given intravenously 15 minutes after the beginning of the Intralipid infusion. Growth hormone levels are drawn at the following times: -30, 0, 30, 60, 90, 120, 180 and 240 minutes.

Growth hormone levels usually rise as a result of the nicotinic acid load because nicotinic acid inhibits lipolysis (*Fig. 20-5*) (Quabbe, et al, 1981; and Quabbe, et al, 1983). Intralipid inhibits the rise of growth hormone, however, and the inhibition becomes even more pronounced with age. Dilman (1 Jun 1984) has not yet established normal values for this test, and does not recommend its accomplishment until further data are obtained. It is included here because it is a potentially valuable test, worthy of further investigation.

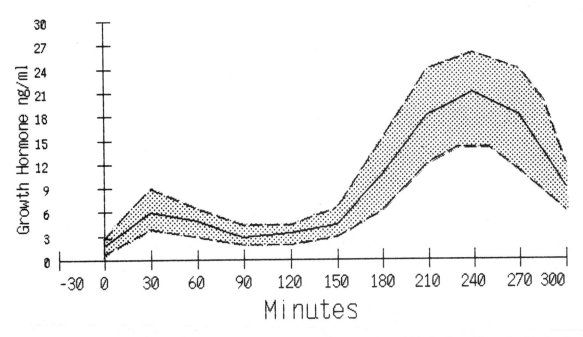

Fig. 20-5. **Serum growth hormone concentrations during nicotinic acid infusion.** Note the bi-phasic growth hormone response. Ingestion of fats (as simulated by the Intralipid infusion) greatly blunts the growth hormone release (Quabbe, et al, 1983).

4. **LHRH test.** 100 μgm of LHRH are injected intravenously, and blood samples are taken before and at 20 and 60 minutes after the injection for determination of LH and FSH (Besser et al). A normal response shows a 4- to 8-fold increase in plasma LH and a 1- to 2-fold increase in plasma FSH (Hodkinson).

5. **Clomiphene test.** Clomiphene blocks the feedback of gonadal steroids on the hypothalamus in both men and women, allowing the release of LH and FSH. A daily dose of 100 mg of clomiphene citrate is given orally for 10 days. Because gonadotropin (FSH and LH) secretion is pulsatile, it is recommended that *before* and *after* the 10 days of treatment the average LH and FSH values of three or four blood samples taken over 20 minutes apart, be compared (Bardin and Paulsen). A rise of over the normal range or a doubling of the basal value is usually observed. A smaller increase occurs in FSH. Lack of normal response suggests pituitary or hypothalamic disease (Hodkinson).

6. **Dexamethasone suppression test** (Appendix B. 11-10).

7. **Diurnal blood cortisol levels** (Appendix B. 11-11).

8. **L-dopa test.** L-dopa, a drug used in the treatment of Parkinson's Disease, inhibits the secretion of prolactin by the pituitary gland (*Fig. 20-6*). This test consists of orally administering 500 mg L-dopa, and measuring blood prolactin levels before, and 1 hour after treatment (Dilman, 15 May 1984; and Frantz).

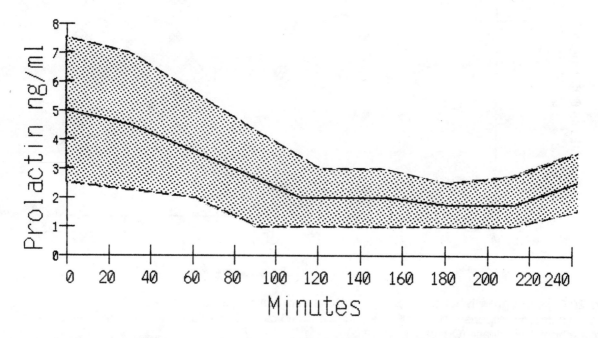

Fig. 20-6. **Prolactin concentrations after the oral administration of 500 mg of L-dopa (Bansal, et al).**

9. Chlorpromazine test. Chlorpromazine (Thorazine) is a drug used in many psychiatric illnesses. In contrast to the inhibition of prolactin secretion by the pituitary caused by L-dopa, chlorpromazine stimulates prolactin secretion. In this test, prolactin levels are measured before, and 1 hour after the oral administration of 25 mg chlorpromazine (*Fig. 20-7*). The effects of chlorpromazine on young healthy subjects should result in a marked increase in prolactin levels (more than 50%). The stimulatory effect in elderly subjects is greatly reduced (Dilman, 15 May, 1984; and Frantz).

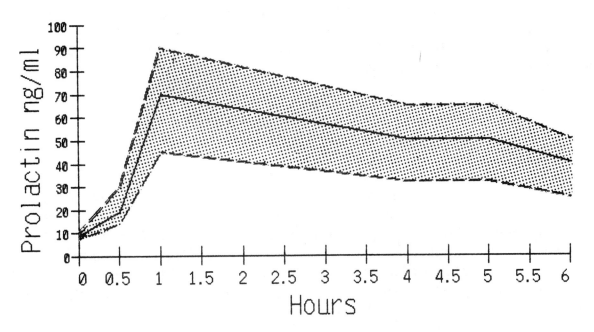

Fig. 20-7. **Chlorpromazine test.** Plasma prolactin levels in normal subjects who received 25 mg chlorpromazine intramuscularly at time zero (Frantz, et al).

Because the L-dopa and chlorpromazine tests (like the growth hormone after fat loading test) are still in the developmental stages, Dilman (3 Jul, 1984; and 17 Jul, 1984) discourages their use until further data are obtained.

10. **TSH blood levels after T3 suppression test (Werner; Dilman, 1 June 1984).** This test is conducted as follows: Baseline thyroid stimulating hormone (TSH) and thyroxin (T4) levels are measured. Fifty µg of triiodothyronine (T3) are given orally each day for 6 days. T4 and TSH levels are again drawn, and compared with the initial levels. Dilman finds that the TSH level normally declines about 34% in young adults, and the T4 level drops about 38%. However, in older subjects (about 50 years old), the TSH declines about 20%, and the T4 level is reduced by about 11%.

CLINICAL USE OF DILMAN'S TEST BATTERIES:

While these test batteries do not give specific biological ages like most of the other aging measurement systems discussed in this book, they clearly do provide an objective assessment of the state of the neuroendocrine homeostatic system. Most importantly, they provide the clinical gerontologist with good indications of both when gerontotherapeutic intervention is indicated, and specifically where the intervention should be directed.

It should be relatively easy to complete many of the tests in the Secondary battery during a periodic aging measurement evaluation or routine examination. Dilman recommends that the Secondary tests be repeated every two years. If any of the Secondary tests are abnormal, they should be repeated within 6 months.

The more complex Primary tests should only be required if one or more of the Secondary tests are persistently abnormal--and then only those tests which will help to isolate the source of the dysfunction indicated by the abnormal Secondary test. Because of the complexity of some of the challenge tests in the Primary battery, and because of the profound effects which they have on the neuroendocrine system, it is advisable not to conduct more than one test at a time. If indicated, the tests should be conducted several weeks apart, to insure that there are no adverse effects from the interactions between them.

DILMAN'S ANTI-AGING PROGRAM

This book is primarily concerned with biological aging measurement, and the subject of specific gerontotherapeutic protocols is intentionally avoided. However, if Dilman's hypothesis is correct, many aspects of aging would be subject to treatment and may even be reversible (Cutler). Therefore, I feel obliged to briefly mention his innovative but controversial therapeutic approach. Dilman recommends the following drugs to be used in an age-retarding program, based on the results of his two test batteries:

1. Phenformin, an oral anti-diabetic drug of the biguanide class, is no longer available in the U.S. It was ordered withdrawn from the market by the FDA due to a significant number of deaths associated with its use by diabetics. Although it is still available in Europe, its use is generally discouraged there as well (Thompson). Dilman also recognizes the hazards of the drug and does not use it in those with frank diabetes, nor does he use it in an orthodox manner for its hypoglycemic effects. He has found that it is a powerful immune stimulant, and he uses it to restore immune functions to more youthful levels (Dilman, 1977). Methformin, a safer drug of the same class, may gain FDA approval, and may be considered for the same use as phenformin.

2. Phenytoin (Dilantin™).

3. Clofibrate (Atromid-S™).

4. Estrogen, progesterone, and *sigetin* (a drug with low estrogen activity and antigonadotropic action, not available in the U.S.).

5. Thyroid hormone.

Space does not permit a full discussion of the use of these drugs in this short chapter. However, in his book, *The Law of Deviation of Homeostasis and Diseases of Aging*, Dilman describes the indications for their use in an age retarding program, and reviews their metabolic and biologic effects.

REFERENCES

Adler, W.H., Nordin, A.A. *Immunological Techniques Applied to Aging Research*. Boca Raton, CRC Press, 1981.

Bansal, S., Louyse, A. L, and Woolf, P.D. Dopaminergic regulation of growth hormone (GH) secretion in normal man: Correlation of L-dopa and dopamine levels with the GH response. *J Clin Endocrinol Metab* 53:301, 1981.

Bardin, C. W., Paulsen, C. A.. 1981, The Testes. In: Williams, R. H. (ed). *Textbook of Endocrinology*, Saunders, Philadelphia, p. 293.

Besser, G. M., McNeilly, A. S., Anderson, D. C., Marshall, J. C., Harsoulis, P., Hall, R., Ormstron, B. J., Hormone-releasing hormone in man. *British Medical Journal*, 3:267-281.

Cutler, R. The Law of Deviation of Homeostasis and Diseases of Aging (book review), *Archives of Gerontology and Geriatrics*, 1985, 4:2, 187-188.

Dean, W., The Law of Deviation of Homeostasis and Diseases of Aging (book review), J Am Ger Soc, June, 1983, pp. 84-5.

Dean, W., A Soviet scientist's anti-aging book, *Anti-Aging News*, Vol. 3, No. 8, August 1983, pp. 93-95.

Dilman, V. Biological age and its determination in the light of elevation mechanism of aging. *Proceedings, IX International Congress of Gerontology and Geriatrics*. Kiev, 1972, 319-322.

Dilman, V. *The Law of Deviation of Homeostasis and Diseases of Aging*, John Wright, PSG Inc., Boston, 1982.

Dilman, V. Three models of medicine. *Medical Hypotheses*, Vol. 15, No. 2, 1984, pp. 185-208.

Dilman, V. Personal communications, 13 Jan 1983; 14 April 1983; 26 Nov 1983; 1 Jun 1984; 3 July, 1984; and 17 July, 1984.

Dilman, V. M., Ostroumova, M. N., Blagosklonnaya, J. V., et al: Metabolic immunodepression. Normalizing effect of phenformin. *Human Physiology*, 3:579-586, 1977.

Frantz, A.G., et al. Studies on prolactin in man, *Recent Prog Horm Res*, 1972, 28:527-90.

Hall, D.A. *The Biomedical Basis of Gerontology*. Boston, John Wright PSG, 1984, p. 143.
Goldstein, A.L., Thurman, G.B., Low, T.L.K., Trivers, G. E., and Rossio, J.L. Thymosin:

The endocrine thymus and its role in the aging process, in: *Physiology and Cell Biology of Aging*, by Cherkin, A., et al (eds). Raven Press, New York, 1979, 51-60.

Hershman, J. H. Use of thyrotropin-releasing hormone in clinical medicine. *Medical Clinics of North America*, Vol. 62, No. 2, March 1978, pp. 313-325.

Hodkinson, M., (ed). *Clinical Biochemistry of the Elderly*. Churchill Livingstone, 1984, 268.

Landfield, P. W. An endocrine hypothesis of brain aging and studies on brain-endocrine correlations and monosynaptic neurophysiology during aging, In: *Parkinson's Disease, Vol 2: Aging and Neuroendocrine Relationships*, by Finch, C. E. (ed), New York, Plenum, 1978, 179-199.

McClure, J.E., Lameris, N., Wara, D. W., and Goldstein, A., L. Immunochemical studies on thymosin: Radioimmunoassay of Thymosin 1. *The Journal of Immunology*, Vol. 128, No. 1, January 1982, pp. 368-375.

Quabbe, H.J., et al. Growth hormone, glucagon, and insulin response to depression of plasma free fatty acids and the effect of glucose infusion. *J Clin Endocr Metab*, 1977, 44: 383-391.

Quabbe, H.J., et al. Growth hormone, cortisol and glucagon concentration during plasma free fatty acid depression. Different effects of nicotinic acid and an adenosine derivative. *J Clin Endocr Metab*, 1983, 57:410-414.

Thompson, M. K. *The Care of the Elderly in General Practice*. Edinburgh, Churchill Livingstone, 1984, p. 37.

Weindruch, R. H., and Walford, R. L. Aging and functions of the RES, pp. 713-748, in: *The Reticuloendothelial System*, Vol. 3, by Cohen, N., and Sigel, M. M. (eds), Plenum Publishing Co., 1982.

Werner, S.C., and Spooner, M. "A new and simple test for hyperthyroidism employing L-triiodothyronine and the 24 hour I131 uptake method". *Bull NY Acad Med* 1955, 31:137-145.

Wills, Michael R, and Havard, B. *Laboratory Investigation of Endocrine Disorders*, Butterworths, Boston, 1983.

Wills, Michael R. Personal communication. 3 Apr 1984.

Chapter 21

THE H-SCAN COMPUTERIZED SYSTEM

Dr. Richard Hochschild (*Fig. 21-1*) is the President of Hoch Company of Corona Del Mar, California, an instruments and computer manufacturing firm. Hochschild thinks that test batteries (as described in Part II of this book) are the best means of assessing biological age and aging rates. However, these systems have several disadvantages: the time required to conduct them; and the potential for error due to varying test conditions and equipment at different locations.

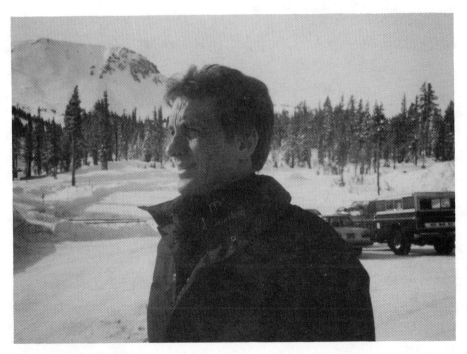

Fig. 21-1. **Dr. Richard Hochschild.**

Chapter 21 — The H-SCAN Computerized System

To overcome these problems, he developed a computerized aging measurement system (H-SCAN) based on concepts and data from other researchers. In developing his system, he surveyed over 250 clinical tests as potential physiological and psychological markers of aging. He selected 14 tests, based on their statistical correlation with chronological age, minimum redundancy of systems tested, adaptability to the computer-driven format, time required to conduct the test, and relevance of the test to mental and physical faculties important in everyday tasks and challenges.

HARDWARE AND SOFTWARE DEVELOPMENT

With the exception of pulmonary functions, none of the tests had previously been automated. The result of Hochschild's efforts was an instrument resembling a video game set, with a screen, six push-buttons, earphones, a breathing tube, an optical viewer, vibrometers, and a printer, in an attractive desk-top unit (*Fig. 21-2*).

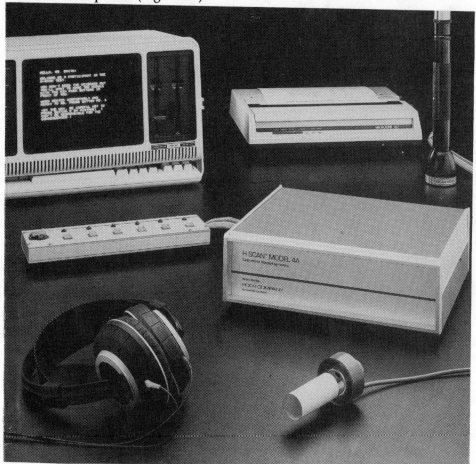

Fig. 21-2. **The H-SCAN.**

The H-SCAN Computerized System — Chapter 21

SUMMARY OF OPERATION

The participant enters his name, height and age into the H-SCAN, and then covers the computer keyboard with a metal cover. The H-SCAN goes to work automatically, giving the participant step-by-step instructions on the screen for performing each test.

If the participant makes an error in technique or tries to cheat, the computer responds—sometimes humorously—explaining what was done wrong and how to do it right. At the end of testing, the H-SCAN prints the results in duplicate (one copy for the participant), giving scores obtained on each test, and the age typical for each score. The computed test ages depend on sex (and for lung function, on height as well), and are based on results of a heterogeneous reference population currently consisting of about 2,100 subjects. The final item on the printout is the net H-SCAN-calculated biological age—a weighted combination of the individual test ages.

INDIVIDUAL H-SCAN TESTS

Following are the fourteen tests comprising the H-SCAN battery, and a brief description of how each test is performed. It is apparent that many of these tests were adapted from the test battery originally developed by Dirken's group in Holland (Chapter 7). Probably the greatest deficiency of the H-SCAN is that it does not test any biochemical or hematological functions.

1. High frequency audiometry (Appendix B. 3-2). A tone randomly starts and stops as it rises and falls in pitch. The tone volume remains at a constant 80 decibels over the entire pitch range from 2,600 Hz to 21,000 Hz. As long as the tone is heard, the participant keeps a button depressed. When the tone is not heard, the button is released. Because the tone turns on and off for random periods, the test is cheat-proof.

2. Auditory reaction time. In this test, the participant presses a button as quickly as possible in response to a tone. Reaction time is displayed on the screen after each trial to motivate the participant to progressively improve. After a practice session of four trials, the test is repeated ten times, and the five fastest response times are averaged for the score.

3. Visual reaction time. This is similar to the preceding test, but uses a visual signal on the screen in place of the audible tone. The participant presses a button, and quickly releases it in response to the signal. After a practice session, the test is repeated 10 times. The score is the average of the 5 best responses.

Chapter 21 — The H-SCAN Computerized System

4. Movement time. This test, measured simultaneously with visual reaction time, is the time required for the finger to jump the 7-inch distance to a predetermined new button after instantly releasing the starting button. It is a measure of muscle movement speed. After several practice trials, the best 5 of 10 trials are averaged. 5. Decision reaction time. In this test, a target signal jumps randomly from button to button. The object is to rapidly follow the target with one finger. After each jump, the destination button becomes the new start button. If a wrong button is hit, that score is discarded and an additional jump is added. After a practice run, the 5 best of 10 "good" jumps are averaged.

6. Decision movement time. This is a continuation of the preceding test, and records the time required for the finger to travel to a new button after releasing the start button. It measures muscle movement speed with a decision step.

7. Forced vital capacity (FVC) (Appendix B. 2-2). The participant blows forcefully and exhaustively as fast as he can through a 1" diameter, 6.5" long plastic tube. The best effort of 3 trials is recorded. As the breath is exhaled through the tube, the curve representing exhaled volume (vertically) vs. time (horizontally) is simultaneously traced on the computer screen to help motivate the participant to maximum effort. Prior curves stay on the screen for comparison during this maneuver.

8. Forced expiratory volume in 1 second (FEV_1) (Appendix B. 2-1). This is determined from the flow data generated for the vital capacity test.

9. Vibratory sensitivity (VS) (Appendix B. 5-7). Vibratory sensitivity is measured at the fingertip using a small round magnet about the size of a 0.25 inch thick dime held between thumb and index finger. The object is to identify which of three target areas is the source of the vibration in the magnet. Following each correct identification, the vibration drops one step in amplitude. The procedure is repeated until the amplitude boundary between a perceptible vibration and an imperceptible one has been crossed several times, and has been carefully defined by the computer.

10. Memory. The H-SCAN memory test is abstract in nature, and involves a target spot that moves on the screen above the six push-buttons. As the target jumps in an irregular sequence from button to button, the participant is asked to watch and memorize the sequence. Upon completing the sequence, he attempts to repeat it by depressing the buttons in the same order. The first sequence is 2 positions long. With each correct repetition one new position is added. If an error is made, no position is added and the sequence is shown again. The test terminates after two successive errors or when the sequence reaches 16 positions. The longest sequence correctly memorized and the location of the error are recorded.

11. Alternate button-tapping. This is a test of muscle speed, control and coordination. The object is to move one finger as rapidly as possible back and forth between two buttons spaced

spaced 7 inches apart. The score is the time required to make 30 round trips. The number of misses is also recorded.

12. Near vision (Appendix B. 4-1). This test was previously unadaptable to computer operation. Hochschild developed a means of accomplishing this test with a novel computer-driven lens system that records the accommodation power of the eye in diopters.

H-SCAN APPLICATIONS

Hochschild (1984) thinks the H-SCAN can detect differences in the rates of aging of individuals receiving effective age-retarding agents in comparison with others receiving a placebo or no therapy at all. Preliminary longitudinal studies appear to be encouraging in this regard.

The H-SCAN has only recently become generally available. Versions of the H-SCAN are now available in both English and German. Further information as to the availability of the H-SCAN can be obtained from: the Hoch Company, 2915 Pebble Drive, Corona Del Mar, California 92625 (714) 759-8066.

REFERENCES

Hochschild, Richard. The H-SCAN--An Instrument for the Automatic Measurement of Physiological Markers of Aging, in: *Intervention in the Aging Process, Part A*, by W. Regelson, and F. M. Sinex, (Eds.), Alan R. Liss, New York, 1983, pp. 113-125.

Hochschild, Richard. Personal communication, 19 July 1984.

Chapter 22

PROSPECTIVE SYSTEMS

The search for aging measurement systems that are more accurate, sensitive, efficient and economical, should have a high priority for clinical gerontologists. This chapter reviews some bio-markers and aging measurement systems currently under development.

PATTERN RECOGNITION ANALYSIS OF URINE METABOLITES

Dr. Bill Vaughan (*Fig. 22-5*), is a Berkeley, California based scientist interested in gerontology and nutrition. He supports the concept of biological aging measurement, but has reservations about the validity of currently available systems. He cites some studies that indicate what he considers an unacceptable lack of precision and reproducibility of laboratory data from one lab to another, and even within the same lab on the same sample. He thinks that errors induced by some laboratory tests vary excessively and invalidate biological age scores. He thinks a more accurate indication of biological age than given by the multiple regression equation methods in Part II are obtainable by *pattern recognition analysis (PRA)*. PRA is a method that correlates the relationships between various biological substances rather than the absolute values of individual substances.

Dr. Arthur B. Robinson (*Fig. 22-1*), former President and Tenured Professor with the Linus Pauling Institute of Science and Medicine, researched the computerized pattern recognition analysis of chemical constituents in blood and urine. Robinson and his associates wanted to discern various patterns that reflected increased susceptibility to various diseases, and even assess biological age (Robinson and Pauling; Robinson et al; Robinson).

In a collaborative study with the late Dr. Arthur Cherkin, formerly of the Veterans Administration Hospital in Sepulveda, California, Robinson analyzed 185 urine vapor substances and urine amines in 235 men ranging in age from 19 to 94 years. He found that 60 of these substances correlated significantly with chronological age.

Chapter 22 — Prospective Systems

In a separate, blind experiment, he classified 70 men according to chronological age. That computerized pattern recognition calculation was accurate to the theoretical limit of their distribution of physiological age.

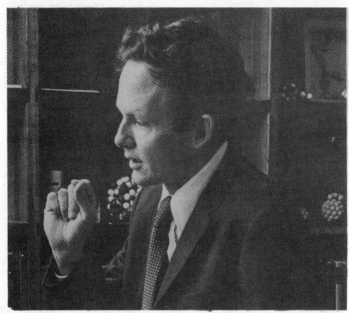

Fig. 22-1. **Dr. Arthur B. Robinson, former President and Director of the Linus Pauling Institute of Science and Medicine.**

Robinson and his associates at the Pauling Institute planned to investigate their pattern recognition analysis-based concept of determining biological age by conducting large-scale longitudinal studies, in cooperation with the Kaiser-Permanente medical group in Northern California. They planned to obtain samples of urine and serum from 50,000 Kaiser members at 6-month intervals over a 5-year period, and planned to perform a computerized pattern recognition analysis part of these samples. Their goals were to develop patterns that indicate predispositions to disease and biological age (Robinson).

Unfortunately, after collecting and analyzing a considerable amount of information, but before completion of the project, Robinson and Pauling had a serious falling out. Robinson left the Pauling Institute--leaving his data behind. The Pauling Institute has apparently discontinued further work on the project.

Robinson is now in Cave Junction Oregon. He has started a small research institute (the Oregon Institute of Science and Medicine) where he hopes to pursue this important line of research.

Dr. Arlen Richardson and his associates in the Department of Chemistry, Illinois State University (Gates, et al, *AGE*; Gates, et al, *Exp Ger*), are conducting similar research. They are still working on a profile for rodents, however, and have not yet extended their work to humans.

DEHYDROEPIANDROSTERONE (DHEA)
as both a bio-marker of aging and a potential anti-aging agent

Dr. Arthur Schwartz (*Fig. 22-2*), of the Fels Research Institute at Temple University, is one of the principal investigators of the clinical applications for the adrenal steroid hormone *dehydroepiandrosterone* (DHEA). With the exception of cholesterol, DHEA is the most common steroid hormone in the body. Despite its relative abundance, the function of DHEA is not fully understood.

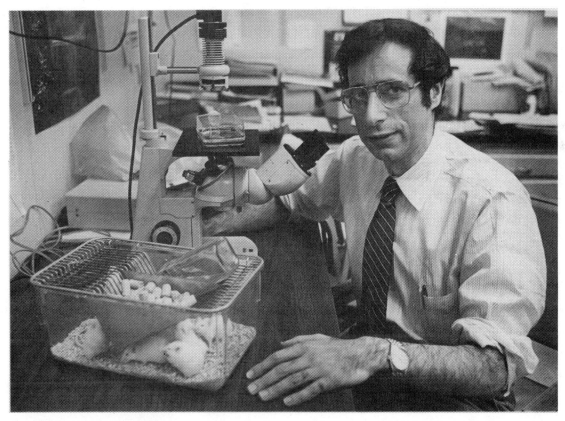

Fig. 22-2. **Dr. Arthur Schwartz.**

Schwartz first became interested in DHEA as a result of a report from British endocrinologist R.D. Bulbrook. In a prospective study of 5,000 apparently healthy women, he monitored urinary breakdown product levels of DHEA for over 10 years. Bulbrook found that 27 of the women developed breast cancer, and *all of them had low levels of DHEA derivatives — some as long as 9 years prior to diagnosis* (Kent, 1982).

DHEA has other roles. It inhibits mammalian glucose-6-phosphate dehydrogenase (G6PDH), the rate-controlling enzyme in the pentose-phosphate shunt, one of the pathways involved in carbohydrate metabolism (*Fig. 22-3*) (Oertel and Benes). This pathway is a major source of extra-mitochondrial nicotinamide-adenine dinucleotide phosphate (NADPH), a necessary co-factor for various bio-chemical processes. They include the synthesis of fatty acids, and ribo- and deoxyribo-nucleotides. DHEA also has anti-cancer, anti-obesity, immuno-enhancing, and possibly anti-aging effects (Schwartz).

It was hypothesized that the beneficial effects of DHEA are due to its inhibition of G6PDH. This was attractive for a number of reasons. For example, the interference with the supply of reduced NADP could explain the effect of DHEA on lipogenesis, while a decreased supply of the product of this reaction (pentose phosphate) could be associated with the antiproliferative properties and the inhibition of tumor development. Furthermore, any nonproductive energy expenditure produced by DHEA would divert calories away from specific metabolic pathways and mimic caloric restriction without actually decreasing food intake (Coleman, et al).

Dr. D. L. Coleman and his associates at The Jackson Laboratory tested this hypothesis with an analog of DHEA (Bromoepiandrosterone-16 α) that inhibits G6PDH 60 times more effectively than DHEA (Pashko, et al). Even at high doses (which dramatically inhibited G6PDH), no improvement in blood glucose or rate of weight gain were noted.

On the other hand, feeding low doses of DHEA had no effect on G6PDH, but had a dramatic effect on the control of diabetes and rate of weight gain (Dr. David Harrison alerted me to this study — Thanks, Dave).

So it appears that other mechanisms are responsible for the beneficial effects of DHEA. Pashko, et al, are pursuing this mechanism by evaluating analogs of DHEA (3 β methyl-androst-5-en-17-one) that do not cause DHEA's adverse (estrogenic) side effects. Coleman (1985) thinks the cause may be due to several metabolites of DHEA (3 α hydroxycholanolone and 3 β hydroxyetiocholanolone).

Prospective Systems Chapter 22

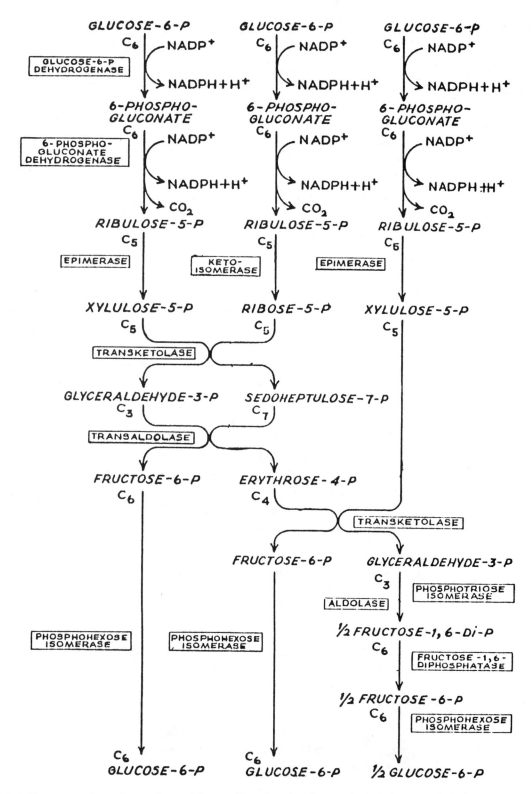

Fig. 22-3. **Pentose-phosphate shunt** (Harper. Reprinted with permission, Lange Medical Publications).

Schwartz worked with tumor-prone mice given DHEA, and found a greatly delayed onset and reduced incidence of both spontaneous and carcinogen-induced tumors. He noted that mice treated with DHEA lost more weight than controls, while consuming the same amount of calories. He is currently studying a strain of mice which characteristically develop *autoimmune hemolytic anemia*. His preliminary data indicate that DHEA may be effective in inhibiting the disease (Schwartz). This apparent immuno-enhancing property of DHEA is highly significant for gerontology, in view of the well-documented adverse effects of aging on immunity.

There is a problem in extrapolating these findings to humans. DHEA has only been effective in large doses. Much of the compound is degraded in the liver before reaching the bloodstream. To overcome this problem, Schwartz and his colleagues at Temple University are trying to synthesize active analogs of DHEA to lower the dose requirements.

Since DHEA undergoes the most marked age-related decline of any steroid hormone (Migeon, et al), scientists see the possibilities of using it as a bio-marker of particular significance.

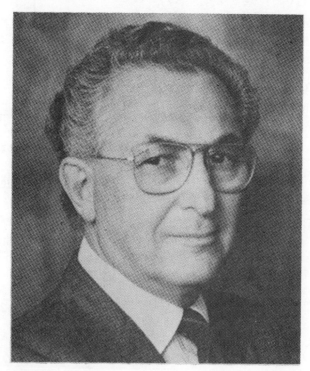

Fig. 22-4. **Dr. Norman Orentreich**.

Dr. Norman Orentreich (*Fig. 22-4*) is Director, Orentreich Foundation for the Advancement of Science (OFAS) in New York City. OFAS, is a research institute that investigates the aging process and diseases of aging. One of their many projects is the potential use of DHEA as a marker of biological age.

Orentreich's laboratory has been analyzing serum samples obtained from 2,500 subjects in the Baltimore Longitudinal Study of Aging of the NIA. The results of this cross-sectional analysis demonstrated a dramatic drop in DHEA levels with age (*Fig. 22-5*). A subsequent study on 15 samples collected longitudinally over 10 years demonstrated a high degree of correlation with the cross-sectional findings (Orentreich).

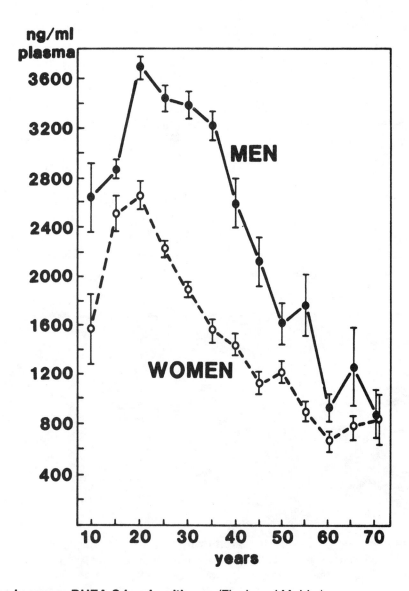

Fig. 22-5. **Changes in serum DHEA-S levels with age** (Finch and Mobbs).

Chapter 22 — Prospective Systems

Exciting conclusions can be drawn from Orentreich's and Schwartz' research. We may have not only a fairly specific bio-marker of biological age, but also a specific means of correcting the biochemical deficiency identified by the bio-marker, with far-reaching potential to delay the rate of development of age-related diseases, and perhaps aging itself.

THE SANAR--a device for evaluating the physiological response to heat stress as a potential bio-marker

Dr. Benjamin Schloss *(Fig. 22-6)* was a nuclear engineer, biophysicist, and maverick gerontologist who died in 1978. He had a varied career, including a secret assignment as Chief, Radiation Monitoring Section for the Manhattan Project, the top-secret group which developed the atomic bomb during World War II. Next he devoted his scientific genius to private industry, and formed the Nucleonics Corporation of America. They designed and manufactured radiation monitoring equipment for government and industry. In the mid-60's, he became interested in aging research, and began attending gerontological scientific meetings. He developed a reputation as a vocal, opinionated, and brilliant but somewhat eccentric scientist.

Because of his many unorthodox ideas and lack of affiliation with any major institution or group, he was not taken more than half seriously by many gerontologists. He became a lone operator, constantly trying to organize international gerontological research programs along the line of the Manhattan Project, and hoped to mass the resources necessary to solve the mystery of the aging process (Rosenfeld).

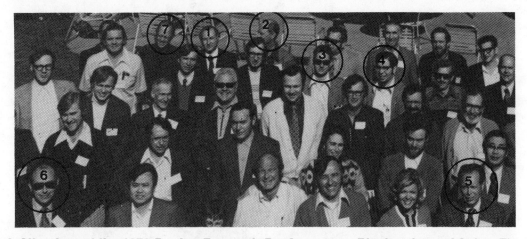

Fig. 22-6. **Attendees at the 1973 Gordon Research Conference on Biochemistry of Aging.** These conferences are restricted to the top research scientists in the world, and attendance is almost "by invitation only". Among those present were Drs. Benjamin Schloss (1), Johan Bjorksten (2), William Vaughan (3), James Florini (4), Denham Harman (5), Jaime Miquel (6), and Mr. Paul Glenn (7).

Prospective Systems Chapter 22

In 1974, he sold his company, moved to Los Angeles, and formed the non-profit Aging Research Institute. Its commercial arm, the Health Improvement Company, concentrated on the development of a biological aging measurement research device, and a similar but less complex unit for home use. Profits from the sales of his home-unit were intended to fund his research.

Schloss called his patented device a *Sanar*, based on the Latin word *sanare* ("to heal")-- deliberately coined to sound like the word *sauna*, which it closely resembled (*Fig. 22-7*). His commercial Sanar (*Fig. 22-8*) was actually a modified home sauna. Several fans mounted at air inlet and outlet ports blew high velocity hot air over the user. The unit contained a thermometer for monitoring cabinet temperatures, an oral thermometer for monitoring temperature of the subject, a digital pulse rate read-out, and a temperature control.

The high velocity hot air caused rapid evaporation of sweat, maximized evaporative cooling, and induced maximum response of the body's thermoregulatory system. This response was manifested by increases in heart rate, cardiac output, respiratory rate, and basal metabolic rate (Dean, 1983). Schloss believed that this would slightly increase caloric consumption, and induce limited cardiovascular training. He felt that the Sanar could be used by people who were either disinclined or unable to exercise. Subsequent studies in Europe indicated that he was probably correct (Dean, 1982; Pribil and Matousek).

However, Schloss had more ambitious plans for his invention than as just another physical fitness "gadget". He knew that the greatest decline of physiological processes and functional capacities with age were those depending upon integrated multi-system coordination. The most significant declines in functional capacities are demonstrated only when the system is stressed (Kohn; Shock, 1977; Thompson). For example, fasting glucose levels (Appendix B. 9-4) may remain relatively unchanged throughout life, while the oral glucose tolerance test (Appendix B. 11-1), which stresses the body with a glucose load, clearly shows age-induced decrements (Andres and Tobin).

Maximal oxygen uptake (VO_2max) (Appendix B. 1-4) is generally considered the best measure of physical fitness and functional capacity. VO_2max decreases significantly and progressively with age (Shock, 1982). It is an integral part of several aging measurement systems (Dirken; Nakamura; Suominen). There are some inherent problems with this test in its current form. Since a near-maximal exercise effort is required, it is obvious that the test is effort-related, and requires a highly motivated subject for accurate results. Someone with a low tolerance for pain may discontinue the test before the levels required for accurate results are achieved. Also, some people may have an underlying physical condition not related to their cardiovascular system (arthritis, for example) that would either prevent their taking the test or produce inaccurate results.

Chapter 22 — Prospective Systems

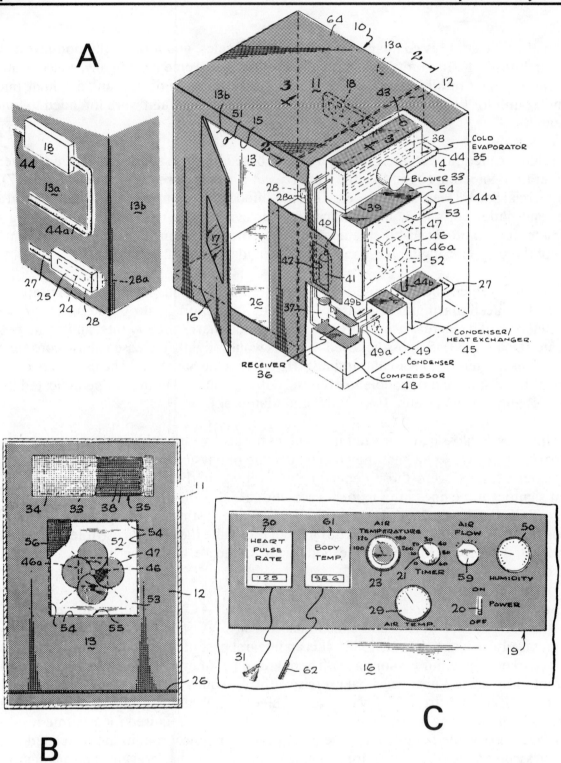

Fig. 22-7. **Schloss' patented therapeutic/diagnostic Sanar.** A. Sanar cabinet. B. Blower assembly. C. Indicator/control panel (Schloss, B.).

242

Prospective Systems | **Chapter 22**

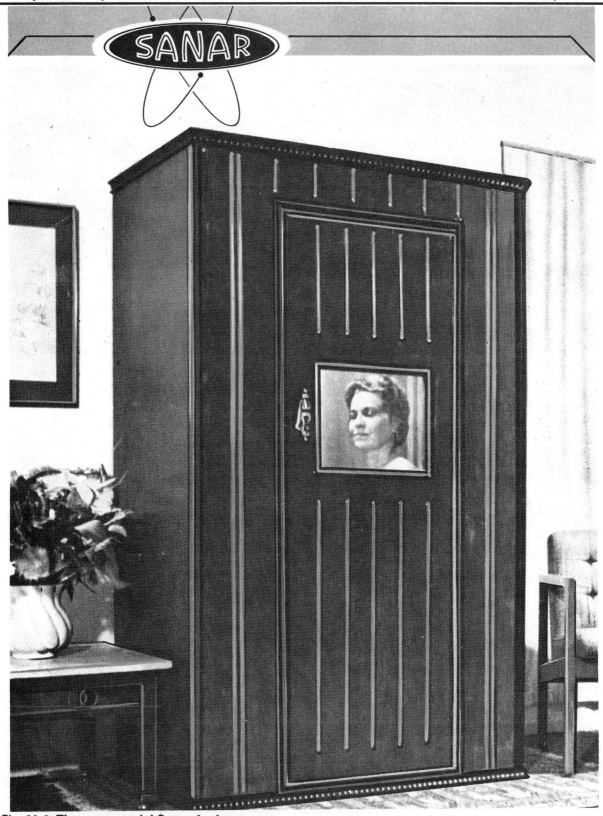

Fig. 22-8. **The commercial Sanar for home use**.

Schloss believed that his research Sanar (or "interaction chamber" as he sometimes called it), would overcome these problems. He knew that the thermoregulatory system of the body is a highly integrated system involving the cardiovascular-pulmonary and neuro-endocrine systems. Core temperature is one of the most tightly regulated physiological variables (Kuhlemeier), and temperature measurements can be made accurately and inexpensively. He also understood that the efficiency of the thermoregulatory system markedly declines with age (Shock, 1977; Kohn; Drinkwater and Horvath).

He planned to evaluate the cardiovascular and thermo-regulatory response to heat stress of supine subjects at rest in a Sanar, under carefully controlled and standardized conditions. He believed that parameters measured in this way (especially oxygen uptake) would provide accurate, reproducible results, due to the lack of influence of motivation, skeletal muscle condition and voluntary effort.

Tables could be constructed to demonstrate the decline of oxygen uptake and other parameters in response to the heat stress like sweat rate, maximum heart rate, and rate of change in core temperature for calculating biological age (Shiffrin; Rosenfeld; Schloss; Kent, 1978).

Unfortunately, just as he was in the final stages of the design and construction of his research Sanar, he contracted acute monocytic leukemia in 1978--most likely a result of his many years of increased radiation exposure. He died several months later. His tragic death robbed the gerontological community of one of its most gifted scientists and enthusiastic supporters, and ended this potentially promising line of research.

Although clinical and experimental applications of the sauna continue to attract the attention of scientists in Scandinavia and Eastern Europe, the physiological effects of saunas remain a surprisingly poorly understood and inadequately researched subject in the US.

ASSESSMENT OF THE EFFICACY OF ANTIOXIDANTS IN LIVING ANIMALS AND HUMANS

One of the more popular and most extensively investigated theories of aging is the Free Radical Theory, conceived by Dr. Denham Harman *(Fig. 22-6)*, Professor of Biochemistry at the University of Nebraska College of Medicine and founder of the American Aging Association. The free radical theory postulates that damage from free radical reactions contribute to aging and age-associated diseases. He has proved that adding various antioxidants to the diet-- both natural (vitamin E, selenium) and synthetic (BHT, BHA, ethoxyquin)--increases the life span of mice, rats, fruit flies and nematodes; inhibits the development of some forms of cancer; enhances humoral and cell-mediated immune responses; and slows the development of autoimmune disorders. Harman (1980) also thinks that free radical reactions may play a significant role in the degradation of the cardiovascular and central nervous systems with age.

Based on the favorable results of the animal studies by Harman and others, many health enthusiasts and life extension experimenters add a variety of antioxidant vitamins, nutrients and chemicals to their diets, hoping to improve their health and live longer lives. A problem with this haphazard method of ingesting various doses of antioxidants is that the optimum combination and dosage has not even been determined for various animal species, let alone for humans. The only available way to determine relative efficacy and appropriate human dosages is to randomly test various antioxidant combinations in trial-and-error life-span studies with different animal species, and then attempt to extrapolate dosages for humans based on the animal dose.

A new technique is being added to the armamentarium of clinical gerontologists that may allow the rapid assessment of the effectiveness and optimal dosages of various antioxidants. Dr. Richard Lippman (*Fig. 22-9*), former Professor of Medical Cell Biology, Uppsala University College of Medicine in Uppsala, Sweden, has developed a new method to measure lipid hydroperoxides and collagen cross-linking in the skin of animals and humans (Lippman, 1984; Lippman, 1985). Using a technique known as *reflective near-infrared spectroscopy*, he utilizes the *Inframatic 8100* reflective, near-infrared spectrometer (*Fig. 22-10*), available from: Basab, Inc., Segetorp, Sweden; and Per Con Prufgerate GmbH, P.O. Box 730-330, D-2000, Hamburg 73, West Germany.

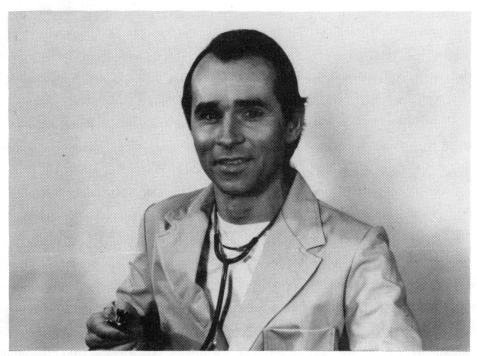

Fig. 22-9. **Dr. Richard Lippman.**

In long-term studies in mice, Lippman has shown progressive increases in normal lipid-hydroperoxide levels and collagen cross-linkages with age. He has demonstrated *reductions* in normal lipid-hydroperoxide levels after oral doses of various antioxidants. Using the spectrometer, he found that each substance tested appears to have an optimum dose-related "window of efficacy". Increases in dosage beyond this optimum level cause a reduction in the effectiveness of the tested antioxidant.

Lippman has only begun preliminary tests with this method. If the "window of efficacy" for various nutrients can be shown to correspond with the dosages which induce maximum increases in life span of various test animals, then this will be of tremendous significance for the quantification of optimum human antioxidant levels.

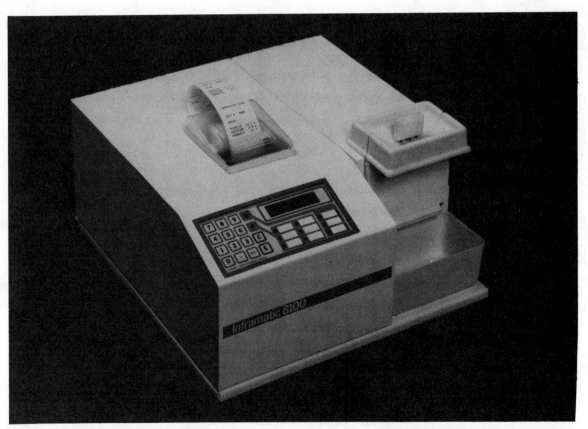

Fig. 22-10. **Inframatic 8100 reflective near infra-red spectrometer**, courtesy Per Con Prufgerate GmbH.

LYMPHOCYTE PEROXIDATION TEST

Dr. Robert Morin, President of the American Longevity Association, has proposed a biological aging measurement based on the rate of peroxidation in lymphocytes (Anonymous, *Longevity Letter*). Morin plans a 2-phase research program to evaluate his ideas. The first phase will study lymphocytes obtained from primate species with different life spans, and from human populations known to have life spans longer or shorter than average (For example, Seventh Day Adventists live about 7 years longer than average. Certain geographical areas in the U.S. differ markedly from others in the life spans of their populations).

These lymphocytes will then be challenged by a source of free radicals to induce damage. Next, the viability of the cells will be observed, and the oxidation products that are formed will be measured. If Morin's hypothesis is correct, cells from longer-lived populations will show greater resistance to oxidative damage. He could then provisionally use such resistance as an index of the rate of aging, and as a marker to identify individuals who are biologically youthful.

If Phase One is successful, he will test the effectiveness of various intervention strategies that protect body tissues against the constant exposure to oxidative damage. Individuals will be tested before and after embarking on dietary and lifestyle modifications designed to reduce this damage.

Unfortunately, this technique does not appear to have imminent clinical applications, and the precision obtainable with the test may be inadequate for short-term evaluation of biological age.

AMES TEST OF DNA DAMAGE

Another potential aging measurement assay is being developed by a group of biochemists headed by Dr. Bruce N. Ames at the UC Berkeley Department of Biochemistry (Ames, B. N.; Ames, B. N., et al; Cathcart, R., et al; Hollstein, M. C., et al). This test measures the amount of thymine glycol and thymidine glycol excreted in urine. Both substances are breakdown products derived from DNA, presumably from repair of oxidized DNA. Despite a great degree of interest which the Ames proposal has generated, the test involves a rather elaborate purification procedure, and the results obtained so far do not qualify it as a measure of the rate of aging in humans.

| Chapter 22 | Prospective Systems |

OTHER POTENTIAL BIO-MARKERS OF BIOLOGICAL AGE

A forthcoming entrant in the growing field of aging measurement is Dr. Fred Abbo, an internist at Scripps Institute in La Jolla, California. Abbo is reluctant to discuss his method due to concern over the possibility of others "beating him to the punch". He reports that he has been working on his system for over a decade, and does not want to lose credit for his efforts. From reports of those who have seen the system, Abbo's approach is similar to that described in Part III, Chapter 23, and Appendix B of this book, in that longitudinal graphic measurements are key factors in his system. He also indicated it would be quite comprehensive, and fully automated, similar to the H-SCAN. He is nearing completion of his project, and hopes to have it commercially available in early 1987. Although it is difficult to evaluate such a system with so few details, Abbo may be on the verge of making a significant contribution to clinical gerontology.

Many other bio-markers are under investigation, and may someday be of practical value for the assessment of human biological age. Some of these include advances in nuclear magnetic resonance imaging technology which can determine tissue energy levels. The future will provide methods in cytogerontology providing biochemical values obtained from biopsy and cell culture techniques that will allow us to probe directly into the nuclear, enzymatic and energy capabilities of cells obtained from our patients in routine screening programs. Additional techniques involving measurement of volatiles in expired air, the supercoiled or oxidized state of DNA will be available. Automated methods for determining age modified changes in protein and peptide patterns in urine and blood are already available awaiting commercial interest (Regelson).

Many of these techniques have been discussed in several books (Bourliere; Reff and Schneider; Regelson and Sinex) two of which I have reviewed elsewhere (Dean, *Rejuvenation*, 1984; Dean, *Archives of Gerontology and Geriatrics*, 1984). These books list many potential bio-markers and may interest gerontologists studying aging measurement systems.

Admittedly, we are at the Wright Brothers or "crystal set" stage of aging measurement. Although some of the earlier tests or systems described in this book may seem somewhat primitive and crude, compared with modern technology, most retain their value.

It is assumed that with increased automation and computerization, data will be rapidly collected and analyzed to rapidly improve the accuracy and cost-effectiveness of aging measurement. I hope this book will be useful in assisting to accomplish these goals.

REFERENCES

Anonymous. News from the American Longevity Association. *Longevity Letter*. January 1985, Vol. 3, No. 1, 2.

Ames, B. N. Mutagens, cancer and aging. Paper presented at the 14th Annual National Meeting, American Aging Association, 18-20 October, 1984.

Ames, B. N., Saul, R. L., Schwiers, E., Adelman, R., and Cathcart, R. Oxidative DNA damage as related to cancer and aging: The assay of thymine glycol, and hydroxymethyluracil in human and rat urine. *Molecular Biology of Aging: Gene Stability and Gene Expression*, Raven (in press).

Andres, R., and Tobin, J. D. Aging, carbohydrate metabolism, and diabetes. *Proc 9th Int Cong Geront*, 1972, 1, 276-80.

Barrett-Connor, E., Khaw, K. T., and Yen, S. S. C. A prospective study of dehydroepiandrosterone sulfate, mortality, and cardiovascular disease. *NEJM*, Vol 315, No 24, 11 Dec 1986, 1519-1524.

Bourliere, F. *The Assessment of Biological Age in Man, Public Health Papers, No. 37*, World Health Organization, Geneva, 1970.

Cathcart, R., Schwiers, E., Saul, R. L., and Ames, B. N. Thymine glycol and thymidine glycol in human and rat urine: A possible assay for oxidative DNA damage. *Proc Nat Acad Sci*, September, 1984, Vol 81, 5633-5637.

Coleman, D. L., Schwizer, R. W., and Leiter, E. H. Effect of genetic background on the therapeutic effects of DHEA in diabetes-obesity mutants and in aged normal mice. *Diabetes*, 1984, 33: 26-32.

Coleman, D. L., Leiter, E. H., and Applezweig, N. Therapeutic effects of DHEA metabolites in diabes mutant mice. *Endocrinology*, 1984, 115: 239-243.

Dean, W. Effects of the sauna. *JAMA*, Jan 1, 1982. Vol 247, No. 1, p. 28.

Dean, W. Proposal for an improved sauna based on thermoregulatory physiology. *Spec Sci Tech*, Vol. 6, No. 1 (1983), pp. 33-36.

Dean, W. Review: *Biological Markers of Aging*, by Reff, M. E, and Schneider, E. L. (eds.) in: *Rejuvenation* September, 1984, Vol. XII, No. 3-4, p. 42.

Dean, W. Review: *Modern Aging Research: Intervention in the Aging Process, Part A: Quantitation, Epidemiology, and Clinical Research*, in: *Archives of Gerontology and Geriatrics* 3 (1984) 351-353.

Dirken, J. M. *Functional Age of Industrial Workers*. Wolers-Noordhoff Publishing Co., Groningen, 1972.

Drinkwater, B. L., and Horvath, S. M. Heat tolerance and aging. *Medicine and Science in Sports*, Vol 11, No. 1, 49-55. 1979.

Gates, S. C., Provancal, S. J., Webb, J. W., and Richardson, A. G. Aging markers detected by metabolic profiling. Paper presented at the 14th Annual Meeting, American Aging Association, 18-20 October, 1984.

Gates, S. C., Provancal, S. J., Webb, J. W., and Richardson, A. Metabolic profiles of rats of different ages. *Exp Ger*, Vol. 19, No. 4, 1984, 272-288.

Harman, D. Free radical theory of aging: Origin of life, evolution, and aging. *AGE*, Vol 3, 100-102, 1980.

Harper, H. A. *Review of Physiological Chemistry*, 14th ed. Lange Medical Publications, Los Altos, 1973, 250.

Hollstein, M.C., Brooks, P., Linn, S., and Ames, B. N. Hydroxymethyluracil DNA glycosylase in mammalian cells. *Proc Nat Acad Sci USA*, Vol. 81, July, 1984, 4003-4007.

Kent, S. DHEA: "Miracle" drug? *Geriatrics*, Vol. 37, No. 9, September, 1982, 157-161.

Kent, S. Measuring human health and aging. *Geriatrics*, Vol. 33, No. 6, June, 1978, 108-111.

Kohn, R. *Principles of Mammalian Aging*. Prentice Hall, Engelwood Cliffs, 1978, 168-169, 183.

Kuhlemeier, K. V. Age related changes in sympathetic function, in: *Experimental and Clinical Interventions in Aging*. Walker, R.F., and Cooper, R. L. (eds). New York, Marcel Dekker, 1983, 355-368.

Lippman, R. D. Measurement of lipid hydroperoxides and collagen elasticity directly in vivo in mice and man, in: *Oxygen Radicals in Chemistry and Biology*, by W. Bors, M. Saran, D. Tait (eds.). Berlin, Walter de Gruyter and Co., 735-739, 1984.

Lippman, R.D. Rapid in vivo quantification and comparison of hydroperoxides and oxidized collagen in aging mice, rabbits and man. *Experimental Gerontology*, Vol 20, 1-5, 1985.

Migeon, C. J., Keller, A. R., Lawrence, B., Shephard, T. H. Dehydroepiandrosterone and androsterone levels in human plasma: Effect of age and sex; day-to-day and diurnal variations. *J Clin Endocrinol Metab*, 17: 1051-1062.

Nakamura, E. The aged people and its physiological ages in relation to work capacity. *Kyoiku Igaku*, 1982, 28: 2-11.

Oertel, G. W., and Benes, P. The effects of steroids on glucose-6-phosphate dehydrogenase. *J Steroid Biochem*, 1972, 3: 493-496.

Orentreich, N. The blood level of DHEA sulfate falls as a person ages. *Annual Report*, Orentreich Foundation for the Advancement of Science, Inc., New York, 1983, 8.

Pashko, L. L., Rovito, R. J., Williams, J. R., Sobel, E. L., and Schwartz, A. G. Dehydroepiandrosterone (DHEA) and 3 ! methylandrost-5-en-17-one. *Carcinogenesis*, 1984, 5: 463-466.

Pashko, L. L., Schwartz, A. G., Abou-Gharbia, M., and Swedrn, D. Inhibition of DNA synthesis in mouse epidermis and breast epithelium by dehydroepiandrosterone and related steroids. *Carcinogenesis*, 1981, 2: 717-721.

Pribil, M., and Matousek, J. The effect of periodical sauna baths on certain signs of the neurovegetative system and physical fitness. *Cas Lek Cesk*, 1978; 117: 1123-1127.

Reff, M. E., and Schneider, E. L. *Biological Markers of Aging*, U.S. D.H.& H.S., N.I.H., P.H.S., N.I.H. Publication No. 82-221, Apr. 1982.

Regelson, W. Personal communication, 18 Feb 1986).

Regelson, W., and Sinex, F. M. (eds.). *Modern Aging Research: Intervention in the Aging Process, Part A: Quantitation, Epidemiology, and Clinical Research*. New York, Alan R. Liss, 1983.

Robinson, A.B., and Pauling, L. Quantitative chromato- graphic analysis in orthomolecular medicine, in: *Orthomolecular Psychiatry*, Hawkins, D., and Pauling, L. (eds.), W. H. Freeman and Co., 1973.

Robinson, A. B., Partridge, D., Turner, M., Teranishi, R. An apparatus for the quantitative analysis of volatile compounds in urine. *J of Chromatography*, 85 (1973) 19-29.

Robinson, A. B. Molecular clocks, molecular profiles, and optimum diets; Three approaches to the problem of aging. *Mechanisms of Aging and Development*, 9, 225-236, 1979.

Rosenfeld, A. *Prolongevity*, Avon Books, New York, 1976, pp. 186-187, 206-207.

Schloss, B. Apparatus for cardiovascular conditioning and other physiological purposes. U.S. Patent No. 4,044,772. Filed Mar 29, 1976, Serial No. 671,592.

Schwartz, A. G., Pashko, L., and Tannen, R.H. Dehydroepiandrosterone: An anti-cancer and possibly anti-aging substance. *Intervention in the Aging Process, Part A: Quantitation, Epidemiology and Clinical Research*, Alan R. Liss, New York, 1983, pp. 267-278.

Shiffrin, N. Is age necessary? *New York*, Nov. 13, 1978, pp. 103-108.

Shock, N. W. Indices of functional age, in: Aging: *A Challenge to Science and Society, Vol. 1, Biology*, by D. Danon, N. W. Shock, and M. Marois (eds.). New York, Oxford U. Press, pp. 270-285.

Shock, N. W. Systems integration, *in: Handbook of the Biology of Aging*, by C. E. Finch and L. Hayflick (eds.), New York, Van Nostrand Reinhold Co., 1977, p. 648.

Suominen, H. Effects of physical training in middle-aged and elderly people, in: Komi, P. V. (ed.), *Studies in Sport, Physical Education and Health*, 11, University of Jyvaskyla, 1978.

Thompson, M. K. *The Care of the Elderly in General Practice*, New York, Churchill Livingstone, 1984.

Part IV

Clinical Application

Chapter 23

SYSTEMS — SELECTION AND USE

When beginning an age-retarding program, a Health Hazard Appraisal (HHA) should be conducted as described in Chapter Two. The HHA will highlight life-style risk factors for diseases or accidents, and compute a risk age and life expectancy based on standard actuarial tables. This value should be entered on a *Risk Age vs. Chronological Age* graph like that in Appendix C.

The HHA should be repeated every 2 years until age 50, and annually thereafter. This is in accordance with guidelines proposed by the Institute of Medicine (1981) of the National Academy of Sciences regarding the recommended frequency for this test for airline pilots. There are several reasons for periodically repeating the HHA: 1) to reinforce avoidance of risks; 2) to find out about newly recognized risk factors identified since the test was last taken (these programs are continually updated); and 3) to determine current risk age.

As previously pointed out, health hazard appraisals do not assess biological age. However, they do provide a measure of increased risks for early demise from non-aging-related causes (i.e., increased chances of dying in accidents if seat belts are not worn). This test clearly identifies the changes necessary to reduce the chances of accidental death or disability.

A periodic health screening exam should be conducted at least annually. A general screening will identify diseases in early stages while they are still treatable, and evaluate biological age. The annual examination should be conducted in accordance with the guidelines proposed by one or more of the major research studies mentioned in Chapter Three and summarized in Table 3-I.

FACTORS TO CONSIDER

Following the preceding recommendations for health screening will evaluate health status in greater depth than during most routine examinations. The next decision is to choose from among the numerous aging measurement systems. Several factors influence this choice. They include expense, population heterogeneity, ethnic variability, gender, test redundancy and test accuracy.

Cost of the tests in the test battery will be a significant consideration for many people. Some of these tests are expensive. Nevertheless, the nutrients, drugs, and chemicals routinely taken by many life extension experimenters are also expensive. **To pursue an age-retarding program without an objective evaluation of whether it is effective or not (or is possibly causing harm) is really a financial (as well as a health) risk.** If some aspect of the program is identified as detrimental to health--and may be *accelerating* the rate of aging--the expense of the measurement tests certainly will be worth their cost.

Another factor to consider is the population from which the equation was derived. There is disagreement among gerontologists regarding the applicability of aging measurement systems for populations geographically, ethnically or occupationally different from the population from which the system was originally developed. Some feel that the test batteries are highly "group specific", and are either not relevant for other populations (Dubina) or that the equation coefficients would at least have to be recalculated (Furukawa).

The problem of ethnic variability has been minimized in this book by the inclusion of numerous *ethnic conversion charts* wherever comparative data are available. Conversion factors have been calculated for parameters such as handgrip strength, height, and weight. These conversion factors correct much of the disparity that would otherwise be present.

Although ethnic/population differences may give somewhat inaccurate *absolute* biological ages, the aging rates should be approximately the same, for two reasons. First, because of the virtually identical maximum life span of all races throughout the world, it is reasonable to assume that the "normal" aging *rate* of all human males and all human females is about the same, regardless of race. Most researchers feel that men and women age at different rates, and that equations calculated for men are inappropriate for women, and vice versa (Voitenko, 1983). This has clearly been demonstrated where separate equations were calculated for both men and women from the same population (Webster; Belsky; Dubina; Voitenko). Furthermore, all variables used in the various measurement systems are highly correlated with age. This correlation appears to be universal, as the same variables seem to demonstrate high correlations with age in all populations (Shock). This has resulted in a large degree of redundancy between measurement systems.

Systems — Selection and Use   Chapter 23

As mentioned in Chapter Five, all systems have been evaluated on a computer model, using the mean age-adjusted data in Appendix B. The results were generally accurate and reproducible. In a few cases, nonsensical results were obtained. Queries to the authors in every case revealed that a misplaced decimal or transposed coefficient had intruded into the equations in the original articles. Appropriate changes were made in the equations in this book, to correct any previously published errors.

The aging measurement systems described in this book are the most scientifically valid ways known to evaluate biological age at the present. No one can yet say for certain which particular system is the most accurate. Table 23-I summarizes these measurement systems, and clearly shows whether they are applicable for men, women, or both.

MEASUREMENT SYSTEM COMPOSITION

Because of the redundancy of sub-tests between systems, only a few additional sub-tests are usually required to complete more than one system. Using more tests and systems makes it easier to identify the most accurate and sensitive system. Also, frequent testing will decrease the chance for gross error, and increase the accuracy of the results. Even more important--if the tests are conducted often, the curve that represents the rate of aging will be smoother and more accurate.

Most physicians will probably prefer to conduct test batteries based primarily on routine laboratory tests, with the addition of several simple tests such as handgrip strength, audiometry, and visual and pulmonary function tests. These tests will also be most acceptable in terms of cost and convenience to the serious experimenter who plans to conduct regular testing every three to six months. Efforts should also be made to conduct test batteries incorporating slightly more expensive or elaborate immunological, metabolic, or endocrine tests on a slightly less frequent basis--every two to three years.

Gerontological psychologists will most likely lean towards measurement systems including tests of neuropsychological functions.

TABLE 23-I.

TEST SYSTEM	MEN	WOMEN
Health Hazard Appraisal (Chapter 2)	x	x
Adult Growth Examination (Chapter 4)	x	x
Anthropometric Test Battery (Chapter 6)	x	
Dutch Test Batteries (Chapter 7)		
Equations I-IV	x	
Australian Test Batteries (Chapter 8)		
Equations I and III		x
Equations II and IV	x	
Japanese Test Batteries--Osaka (Chapter 9)		
Equations I-III	x	
Japanese Test Batteries--RERF (Chapter 10)		
Equations I and III	x	
Equations II and IV		x
Finnish Test Batteries (Chapter 11)		
Heikkinen	x	
Suominen	x	
Kiiskinen		
Equation I	x	
Equation II		x
Heikkinen		
Equations I-III, Ia-IIIa	x	
GRC Test Battery (Chapter 12)	x	
Japanese Test Batteries--Kyoto (Chapter 13)		
Equations I-III	x	
Soviet Test Battery--Minsk (Chapter 14)		
Equation I		x
Equation II		x
Soviet Test Batteries--Kiev-I (Chapter 15)		
Equations I-V	x	
Equations VI-IX		x
Soviet Test Batteries--Kiev-II (Chapter 16)		
Equations I and II		x
German Test Battery--Leipzig (Chapter 17)		
Equation I	x	
Equation II		x
Japanese Test Batteries--Nagoya (Chapter 18)		
Equations I-IV a-c.	x	
Whole-Body Calorimetry (Chapter 19)	x	x
Soviet Neuroendocrine Tests (Chapter 20)	x	x
H-SCAN Computerized Test System (Chapter 21)	x	x

Systems — Selection and Use — Chapter 23

The most accurate test batteries should include tests of cardiovascular functional capacity like *maximal oxygen uptake, heart rate recovery ratio,* and *heart rate recovery rate.* Nathan Shock (1981), Scientific Director, Emeritus, National Institute on Aging, agrees that because of the high correlation of maximal oxygen uptake with age, it should be included in studies where maximum precision in the estimate of biological age is required. The late Robert Kohn (1978) of the Case Western Reserve School of Medicine held that age differences in physiological processes could best be measured when the system was stressed for maximum performance. Robert A. Bruce (1984) of the Department of Medicine, University of Washington School of Medicine, also believes that the measurement of aerobic capacity is the best integrated measure of the functional limits of the whole body which can define the effects of the aging process.

MISCELLANEOUS SYSTEMS

Dilman's *Secondary* and *Primary* test batteries (Chapter 20)--for both men and women--unfortunately do not provide a quantifiable measure of biological age. However, they do provide important information regarding the status of the neuroendocrine and immune systems. They also provide a means to identify the sites of dysfunction where geronto-therapeutic intervention should be applied. The *Secondary* battery should be seriously considered for inclusion in the initial examination, and should be repeated routinely every two years (Dilman, 3 July 1984). If any of the *Secondary* tests become persistently abnormal, the *Primary* battery should be conducted. It is more "site specific" and will help to identify the exact source of the dysfunction.

Hershey's calorimetric method of measuring biological age for both men and women (Chapter 19) is probably one of the simplest, most accurate and best-tested techniques. Unfortunately, it is also one of the more difficult tests to conduct due to the limited geographical distribution of the calorimeters.

The problem with lack of availability may also be encountered in trying to locate an H-SCAN computerized age measuring instrument (Chapter 21). However, high-volume production recently began. It is anticipated that availability of these instruments will improve, and prices will be reduced.

IMPORTANCE OF FREQUENT TESTING

Tests should be done often enough to obtain valid and accurate measurements of functional levels in important systems while the individual is in good health. Testing also must be frequent enough to recognize when a system begins to malfunction before illness develops and the issue is confused with malfunctions in interacting biological systems.

Optimum frequencies have yet to be reliably determined. It is best to conduct frequent measurements during the first year, and whenever making adjustments or changes to an age-retarding program. The more often the measurements are obtained, the more accurately aging rates will be determined.

At this relatively early stage of applied biological aging measurement, it is important to realize that: (1) each individual is his own control; and (2) where one starts on the charts is of much less importance than the slope generated by repeated measurements indicating the rate and direction of aging. Data collected by clinical gerontologists will allow scientists to determine the validity of the various measurement systems, and to revise them as necessary.

Once treatments begin (or after one embarks upon an experimental age-retarding program), frequent testing is still necessary to determine whether the treatments retard or reverse the malfunction. The tests described should help develop a science of preventive medicine by showing when a patient needs treatments and evaluating whether the treatments work.

The most difficult problem is to determine the optimum combination of age-retarding agents. This can only be addressed by further work, in which large numbers of people are repeatedly tested for several years, and the effects of a wide variety of treatments are determined. A few such studies are already in progress, but they probably will fail to produce useful data because they are not coordinated.

Rapid progress will only be possible if standardized sets of tests—as presented in this book—are used so that results can be compared in a central data base. If each physician uses a unique set of tests, as has always been the case, data from different groups cannot be compared. No single group has large enough numbers of people trying enough different treatments over a long enough time to draw meaningful conclusions.

It is vital that all groups agree on an identical standardized set of tests, with results that are summarized in a computerized format in a central data base. Tests in this set should be simple and cheap; their selections should be the highest priority for physicians interested in this area. Of course the standard tests may be supplemented by unique tests in every group, and the best of these should be added to the standard set.

Systems — Selection and Use — Chapter 23

Only a standardized set of tests used on large numbers of people undergoing a wide variety of treatments will make it possible to determine which treatments have been most successful in people similar to each new patient to be treated. As such information expands, it will suggest how treatments should be refined, and selection of treatments will become increasingly more rational and effective.

The immediate value of regular testing is to motivate patients to practice preventive medicine by making lifestyle changes like ceasing smoking, getting regular exercise, altering diets, and using potential age-retarding agents.

Excessive rates of decline in an individual's personal tests will be difficult to ignore, especially since the types of people who participate in testing programs are interested in their health. Even more importantly, the same tests would demonstrate whether the age-retarding program was effective. Thus, patients with regular testing programs would immediately have an opportunity to optimize their programs for their individual health needs (Harrison).

DETERMINING BIOLOGICAL AGING INDEX AND AGING RATES

The *Biological Age vs Chronological Age* (BA vs CA) chart in Appendix C can be used to graphically record biological ages and aging rates for any system. Below are easy-to-follow directions that explain how to perform the calculations and interpret the results. A separate chart should be made for each aging measurement system used.

STEP 1: LABEL THE CHART — Chronological Age axis

1. Enter the subject's current chronological age at the lower left-hand corner of the chart.

2. Label the remainder of the horizontal axis in one-half year intervals greater than the subject's current chronological age. Once labeled, the chart will cover five years. If tests are done more frequently, smaller intervals (less than half a year) can be used.

STEP 2: LABEL THE CHART — Biological Age axis

1. Enter the calculated biological age for each system used along the vertical axis at the 3rd tick mark.

2. Label the vertical axis in about one-half year intervals.

Chapter 23 | Systems – Selection and Use

3. Plot calculated biological ages at corresponding chronological ages each time tests are conducted.

STEP 3: DETERMINE AGING STATUS

Determine aging status by:

A. Calculating the *biological aging index* (BAI) from a single measurement. This will give an index of *relative aging status* that can be compared from one exam to the next.

or:

B. Calculating the *aging rate* by comparing longitudinal measurements. This will probably give more meaningful results. By conducting repetitive measurements over a period of time (6 months to several years) a curve will be generated (c.f. *Fig. 23-1*). The slope of this curve represents the *rate of aging*.

A. CALCULATING BAI FROM SINGLE MEASUREMENTS

1. Divide biological age by chronological age (BA/CA).

2. Interpret the results:

Biological Aging Index	Status
< 1	Retarded aging (biological age is less than chronological age)
1	"Normal" aging (biological age equals chronological age)
> 1	Accelerated aging (biological age is greater than chronological age)

Systems — Selection and Use Chapter 23

B. CALCULATING AGING RATE FROM A SERIES OF MEASUREMENTS

This method determines the *rate of aging* by comparing the change in biological age from one test session to the next.

1. Determine the change in biological age (ΔBA) between test dates: Subtract the first biological age (BA_1) from the most recent test (BA_2):

$$[\ \Delta BA = BA_2 - BA_1]$$

2. Determine the change in chronological age between tests (CA): Subtract the chronological age at the time of the first test (CA_1) from the chronological age at the time of the most recent test (CA_2):

$$[\ \Delta CA = CA_2 - CA_1]$$

3. Calculate the *rate of aging*: Divide the change in biological age (ΔBA) by the change in chronological age (ΔCA) calculated in steps one and two:

$$[\text{Rate of aging} = \Delta BA / \Delta CA]$$

4. Interpret the results:

Rate of Aging	Status
> 1	Accelerated aging rate
1	Normal aging rate
0 to 1	Retarded aging rate
0	Halted aging
< 0	Biological aging reversal

Chapter 23 — Systems – Selection and Use

5. Graphically display the aging rate:

a. Plot the biological age from each test on the corresponding graph at the subject's current chronological age.

b. Interpret the results:

Biological age (BA)	Status
If BA is above the line indicating normal aging:	The subject may be biologically older than average
If BA is below the line indicating normal aging:	The subject may be biologically younger than average

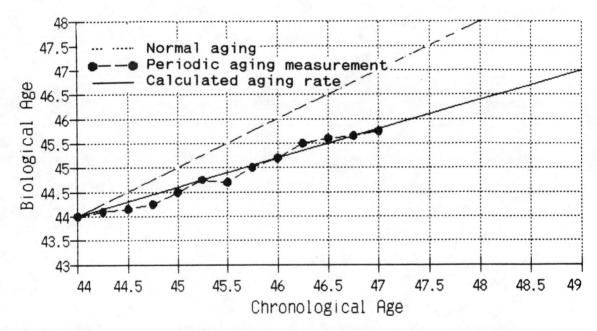

Fig. 23-1. **Sample aging rate measurement chart.** This is a sample chart for a hypothetical 47 year-old male who has been conducting aging measurement tests at three-month intervals for three years. The duration for this particular graph was set at five years. The biological age is somewhat less than the chronological age, and the aging rate is less than one, indicating that he is aging slower than average.

Systems — Selection and Use — Chapter 23

HOW TO REDUCE BIOLOGICAL AGE

Charts representing the rates of decline of most of the tests in the various aging measurement systems are compiled in Appendix B. The curves generally represent mean values for large population samples. Note that there are significant variations of normal ranges for most tests. It is recommended that individual values be plotted on these charts each time they are measured. Ideally, the objective is to maintain values for each test within the ranges of young, healthy adults. Abnormalities may reflect accelerated aging.

By plotting individual values, the *relative biological age* of various organs and organ systems with regard to age-adjusted normals can be compared. This makes it possible for clinical gerontologists to identify specific targets where gerontotherapeutic intervention may be directed in order to bring about a reduction in biological age, and to slow the aging rate. This apparently mechanistic approach of trying to slow/reverse the aging process by attempting to restore various physiological and biochemical parameters to more youthful levels may not be as simplistic as it seems. If these values can be restored to more youthful levels, the more superficial characteristics we associate with age should also appear more youthful.

Even attempts at "cosmetic rejuvenation" such as cosmetic plastic surgery, hair coloring, wearing of toupees, use of hearing aids, or changing from glasses to contact lenses not only impart a more youthful appearance--(although obviously having no effect on the aging process itself)--but may also be of psychological benefit (not an insignificant consideration).

Many techniques directed at the reversal of age-related declines in particular functions may not only restore levels of the primary function to more youthful levels, but may also have secondary beneficial "spin-offs" on other functions. For example, physical exercise causes numerous beneficial changes: reduced systolic and diastolic blood pressure; increased maximal oxygen uptake; improved heart rate recovery; increased glucose tolerance; reduction in cholesterol; increase in HDL cholesterol; increased bone density; and even improved visual acuity (Banta and Monaco; and Monaco and Banta).

Cerebroactive drugs (Spagnoli and Gianni) like Hydergine (ergoloid mesylates), Nootropil (piracetam--not yet available in the U.S.), and other neurotransmitter substances, precursors or enhancers (Schneider and Reed), like L-dopa, Sinimet, choline, DMAE, and centrophenoxine, may improve neuronal functions. This may result in the improvement of a wide variety of psychometric test scores, such as memory, reaction time, and vibratory threshold.

All of the above therapies--although perhaps implemented to improve one or more of the "superficial" test values in Appendix B--have also generally demonstrated improvements in fundamental cellular aging changes. These and other potential therapies are discussed at greater length in the books listed in Appendix D.

AGE RETARDING PROGRAM EVALUATION AND ADJUSTMENT

If repeated measurements show biological age increasing faster than chronological age, the aging rate is apparently faster than average, and an adjustment of the program may be in order. Conversely, if the biological age is increasing at a rate consistently less than the chronological age, the program may be effective, the subject may be aging slower than average, and he will probably outlive his "normally" aging contemporaries.

Once a stable rate of aging on a particular regimen has been obtained, beneficial or detrimental changes in the program should be reflected by corresponding changes in the rate of aging. Major alterations in an age retarding program should be preceded and followed within 3-6 months by repeated measurements. The more effective the program, the less the biological age will change with each additional chronological year. Ideally, on an optimum program, the biological age should actually decrease slightly each year until values in the late 20's are reached, and then stabilize at that youthful level (*Fig. 1-7*).

As the data base grows--from information submitted by clinical gerontologists, age retarding protocols producing favorable as well as detrimental results should be identified. This information will then assist other scientists to refine and improve experimental age retarding protocols.

REFERENCES

Banta, G. R., and Monaco, W. A. The effects of aerobic fitness on visual performance. *J American Aging Association,* 1984, 7(4):147.

Belsky, J. L., Moriyama, I. M., Fujita, S., Kawamoto, S. Aging studies in atomic bomb survivors. Radiation Effects Research Foundation, *Technical Report RERF TR 11-78.*

Bruce, R.A. Exercise, functional aerobic capacity and aging--another viewpoint. *Med Sci Sports Exer*, Vol. 16, No. 1, pp. 8-13, 1984.

Dubina, T. L. Personal communication, 23 September 1984.

Furukawa, Toshiyuki. Personal communication, 21 Jun, 1984. Institute of Medicine: Report of a Study. *Airline Pilot Age, Health, and Performance.* Wash. D.C., National Academy Press, 1981, p. 56.

Harrison, D. E. Personal correspondence, 12 November, 1986.

Kohn, R. R. Principles of Mammalian Aging. Prentice Hall, Inc. Engelwood Cliffs, 1978. p. 183.

Monaco, W., and Banta, G. R. Correlations between aerobic fitness and dynamic visual acuity. *Aviation, Space and Environmental Medicine.* 1985, 56(5):496.

Schneider, E. L., and Reed, J. D. Life Extension, *New England Journal of Medicine.* 312:18, 1985, 1159-1168.

Shock, N.W. *Indices of Functional Age, in: Aging: A Challenge to Science and Society, Vol 1 Biology*, Oxford University Press, New York, 1981. p. 282.

Spagnoli, A., and Tognoni, G. Cerebroactive drugs--clinical pharmacology and therapeutic role in cerebrovascular disorders. *Drugs*, 26:44-69 1983, 44-69.

Voitenko, V. P., and Tokar, A. V. The assessment of biological age and sex differences of human aging. *Experimental Aging Research*, Vol 9, No. 4, 1983.

Walford, R. L. *Maximum Life Span.* New York, W. W. Norton, & Co., 1983.

Webster, I. W., and Logie, A. R. A relationship between functional age and health status in female subjects. *Journal of Gerontology*, 1976, Vol. 31, No. 5, 546-550.

Appendices

Appendix A

Equipment

1. CARDIOVASCULAR

1-1. Sphygmomanometer and stethoscope (*Fig. A. 1-1*), available from most drug stores or surgical supply houses.

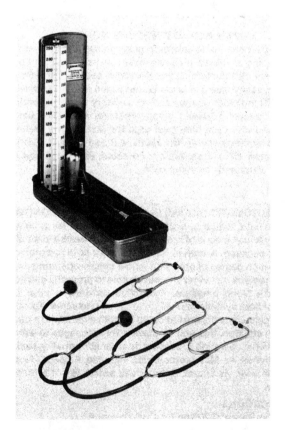

Fig. A. 1-1. **Sphygmomanometer and stethoscope**, courtesy W. A. Baum.

1-2. Bicycle ergometer (*Fig. A. 1-2*). This is not just a fancy exercise bicycle. It is a precision piece of equipment found in many exercise physiology labs and medical offices. The pedal resistance is precisely controlled, and highly reproducible data can be obtained.

There are three major manufacturers of ergometers: Tunturi (Finnish); Monark (Swedish); and Bodyguard (Norwegian). Tunturi ergometers are available from: Amerc, P.O. Box 3825, Bellevue, WA 98009; Monark from: Universal Fitness Products, 20 Terminal Drive South, Plainview, New York 11803; and Bodyguard from: J. Oglaend, Inc., 40 Radio Circle, Mt. Kisco, NY 10549-0096.

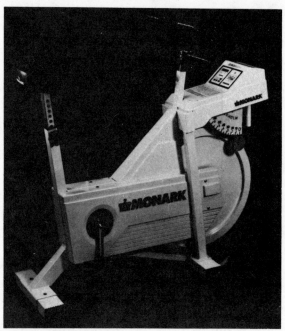

Fig. A. 1-2. **Bicycle ergometer**, courtesy Monark.

1-3. Treadmill (*Fig. A. 1-3*). The most accurate assessment of VO_2max is obtainable with a treadmill. The incline is measured in units of elevation per 100 horizontal units, and is expressed as a percentage. The workload is varied by increasing the speed or incline or both. Treadmills are available from: Quinton Instrument Co., 2121 Terry Ave., Seattle, WA 98121; and Warren E. Collins, Inc., 220 Wood Rd., Braintree, MA 02184 (617) 843-0610.

1-4. Physiological monitoring system (PMS) (*Fig. A. 1-3*). A PMS is an automated mobile system for assessing metabolic, respiratory, and ventilatory variables. It can measure VO_2max directly--the most accurate method. The PMS performs a complete and detailed assessment of a person's metabolic capacities. The data are presented as a summary report, and also as a series of graphic plots. PMS are likely to be available only in well-equipped cardiopulmonary diagnostic centers. They are available from: Sensormedics Corporation, 1630 S. State College Blvd., Anaheim, CA 92806 (714) 385-1905; and Marquette Electronics, Inc., 8200 W. Tower Ave, Milwaukee, WI 53223.

Equipment Appendix A

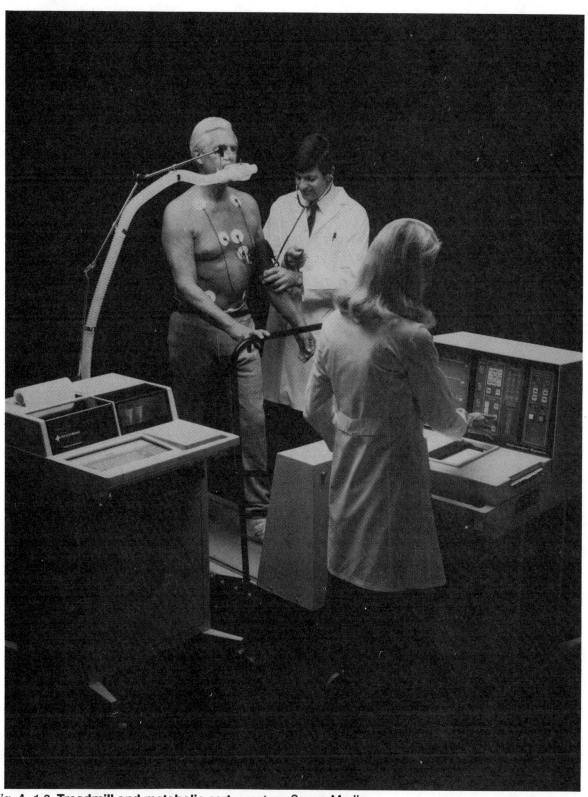

Fig. A. 1-3. **Treadmill and metabolic cart**, courtesy SensorMedics.

1-5. Master's 2-step staircase (*Fig. A. 1-4*). The staircase is a predecessor of the treadmill, but is still used. Staircases are available from: Hausmann Industries, 130 Union Street, Northvale, NJ 07647. Staircases can also be easily built with a minimum of carpentry skill, using step heights of 33 cm for women and 40 cm for men.

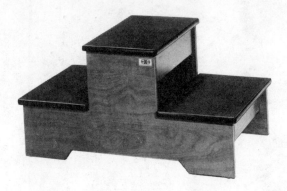

Fig. A. 1-4. **Master's 2-step staircase**, courtesy Hausmann Industries.

1-6. Heart rate monitor (Fig. A. 1-5). Available from: Bio-Sig Instruments, Inc., 5471 Royalmount Ave, Montreal, Quebec H40 1J3, Canada; and Lafayette Instruments.

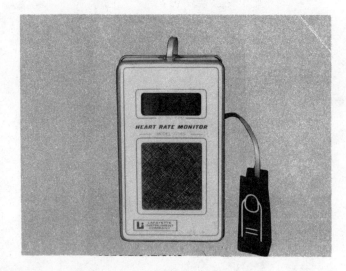

Fig. 1-5. **Heart rate monitor**. Courtesy, Lafayette Instruments.

1-7. Electrocardiograph (*Fig. A. 1-6*). Available from: Brentwood Instruments, Inc., Torrance, CA 90503.

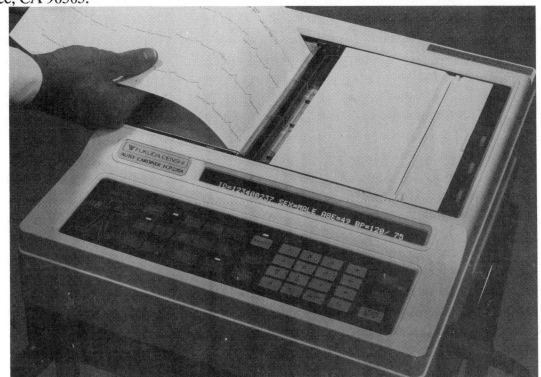

Fig. 1-6. **Electrocardiograph**, courtesy, Brentwood Instruments.

1-8. Instrument for measuring arterial pulse-wave velocity (*Fig. A. 1-7*), available from Lafayette Instrument Co.

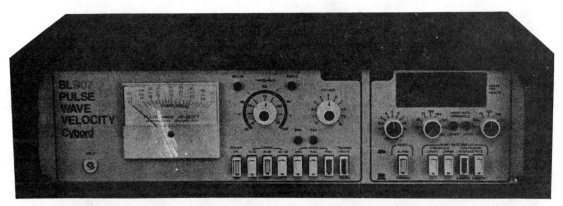

Fig. A. 1-7. **Arterial pulse-wave velocity biofeedback measuring unit, Model BL907**. Courtesy, Autogenic Systems.

1-9. Blood gas analyzer (*Fig. A. 1-8*), for measuring arterial oxygen tension, available from: Radiometer America, Inc., 811 Sharon Dr., Westlake, Ohio 44145; and Sensormedics Corp., 1630 S. State College Blvd., Anaheim, CA 92806.

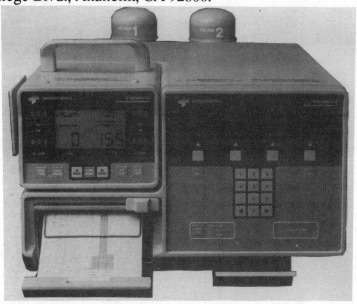

Fig. A. 1-8. **Blood gas analyzer**, courtesy Sensormedics.

1-10. Transcutaneous oxygen monitor (*Fig. A. 1-9*), to measure tissue oxygen tension non-invasively, without an arterial puncture. For routine determinations in normoxic subjects without obvious pulmonary compromise, there is a close correlation between arterial and tissue pO_2. These instruments can be obtained from: Novametrix Medical Systems, Inc., P.O. Box 690, Wallingford, CT 06492; and manufacturers of blood gas analyzers listed above.

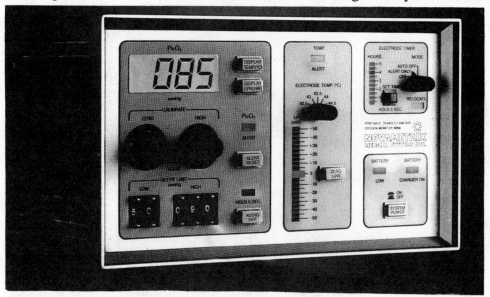

Fig. A. 1-9. **Transcutaneous oxygen monitor**, courtesy, Novametrix.

2. PULMONARY

2-1. Spirometer (*Figs. A. 2-1 and 2-2*), available from: Spirometrics, Inc., 26 Chestnut St., Andover, MA 01810; Medical Equipment Designs, 23521 Ridge Route Drive, Laguna Hills, CA 92653. Accurate pulmonary functions can also be determined using a mini-spirometer like the Pulmometer (*Fig. A. 2-2*). The Pulmometer measures MVV_1, VC, FVC, FEV_1. Available from: Kinetix, 118 Route 17 North, Upper Saddle River, NJ 07458 (201) 934-0505.

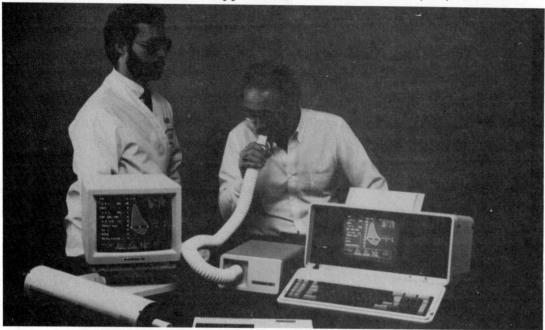

Fig. A. 2-1. **Spirometer**, courtesy Medical Equipment Designs.

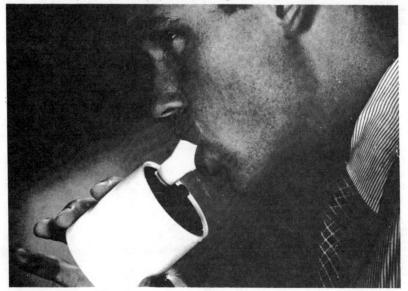

Fig. A. 2-2. **Pulmometer**, courtesy, Kinetix.

3. AUDIOMETRIC

3-1. Audiometer *(Fig. A. 3-1)*, that tests frequencies from 500 through 6,000 Hz. Sources are: Eckstein Bros., Inc., 4807 W. 118th Place, Hawthorne, CA 90250; and Tracor Instruments, Inc., 6500 Tracor Lane, Bldg. 27, Austin, TX 78271.

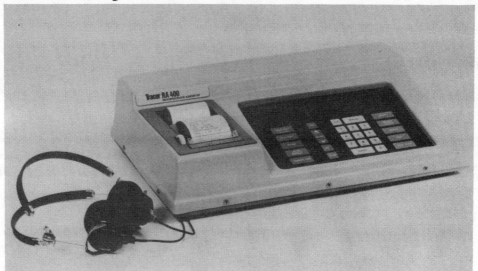

Fig. A. 3-1. **Audiometer**, courtesy Tracor.

3-2. High Frequency Audiometer (*Fig. A. 3-2*). This is a specialized unit that generates signals up to 20,000 Hz at a fixed intensity of 80 decibels. Available from: Demlar Medical, Inc. (Demlar Model 20K Extended High Frequency Audiometer), 121 Estes Dr., Chapel Hill, NC 27514; and Lafayette Instrument Company, (Lafayette Audio Signal Generator, Amplifier, and Speaker), P.O. Box 5729, Lafayette, IN 47903.

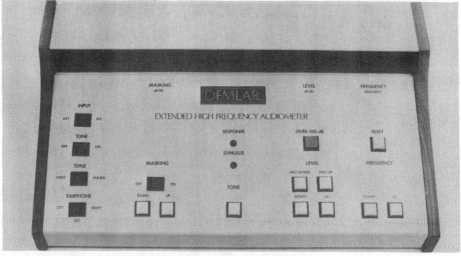

Fig. A. 3-2. **High frequency audiometer**, courtesy Demlar Medical, Inc.

4. VISUAL

4-1. Berens near-point indicator (*Fig. A. 4-1*); Krimsky-Prince Rule (*Fig. A. 4-2*); or yardstick and near-vision cards, for measuring accommodation. Sources are: Richmond Products (Berens near-point indicator), 4089 S. Rogers Circle, Suite 6, Boca Raton, FL 33431; Optical Research Laboratory (Krimsky-Prince Rule) (ORLAB), Brooklyn, NY 11236; or the Age Reduction Corporation, P.O. Box 85152, Dept MB125, San Diego, CA 92138 for a customized instrument designed to be used with subjects older than their mid-40's.

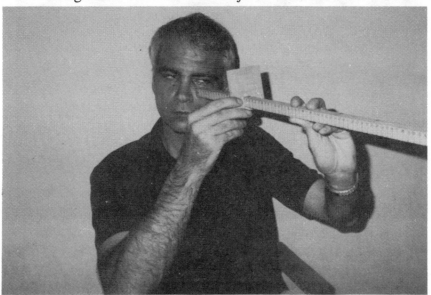

Fig. A. 4-1. **Age Reduction Corporation's improved Beren's near-point indicator**.

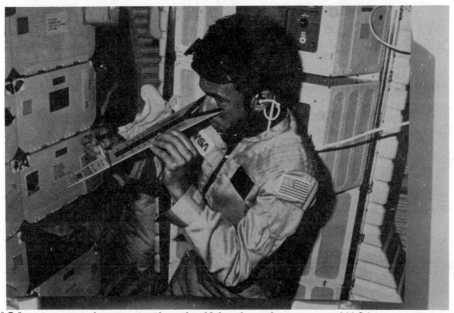

Fig. A. 4-2. **NASA astronaut demonstrating the Krimsky rule**, courtesy NASA.

4-2. Visual acuity charts, available from most medical supply stores, or from: Richmond Products, 4089 S. Rogers Circle, Suite 6, Boca Raton, FL 33431.

4-3. Friedmann visual field analyzer (*Fig. A. 4-3*), for the dark adaptation test (Appendix B. 4-3), manufactured by Clement Clarke International, Ltd., 15 Wigmore Street, London W1H 9LA, England.

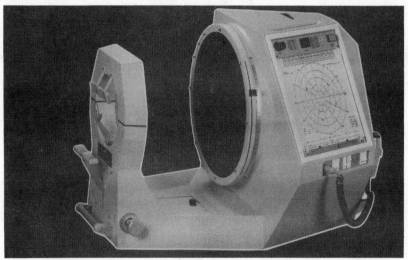

Fig. A. 4-3. **Friedmann Visual Field Analyzer**, courtesy, Clement Clarke, International Ltd.

4-4. FAA Vision Tester (*Fig. A. 4-4*), available from Topcon Instrument Corp, 65 W. Century Rd., Paramus, NJ 07652; Titmus Instruments, P.O. Box 191, Petersburg, VA 23804; and Keystone View, 2212 E. 12th St., Davenport, Iowa 52803.

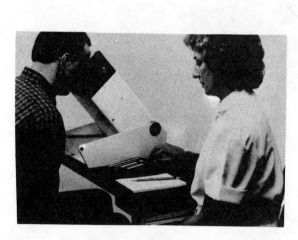
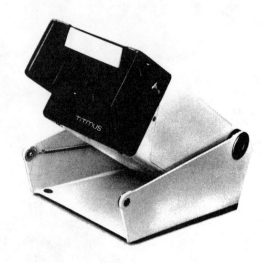

Fig. A. 4-4. **FAA Vision Tester**, courtesy Topcon.

| Equipment | Appendix A |

5. NEUROPSYCHOLOGICAL

5-1. O'Connor Pegboard Test Set (*Fig. A. 5-1*), for the finger dexterity test (Appendix B. 5-1. a). Available from: Lafayette Instrument Co., P.O. Box 5729, Lafayette, IN 47903; J. A. Preston Corp., 60 Page Road, Clifton, N.J. 07012.

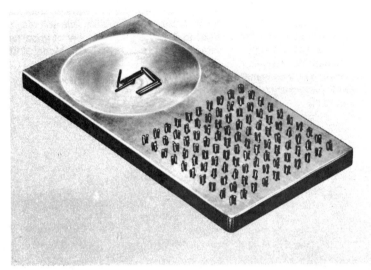

Fig. A. 5-1. **O'Connor Pegboard Test Set**, courtesy Lafayette Instrument Co.

5-2. Purdue Pegboard Set (*Fig. A. 5-2*), for another test of finger dexterity (Appendix B. 5-1. b). Available from: J. A. Preston Corp., 60 Page Road, Clifton, NJ; and Science Research Associates, Inc., 155 N. Wacker Dr., Chicago, IL 60606 (800) 621-0476.

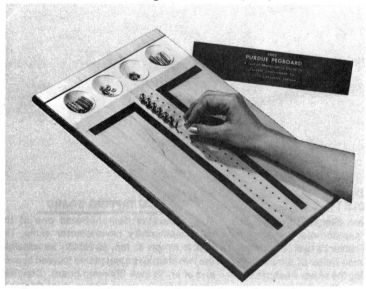

Fig. A. 5-2. **Purdue Pegboard Set**, courtesy, Scientific Research Associates.

5-3. Hand steadiness measuring device (*Fig. A. 5-3*). This is a non-standard item constructed especially for this test. It consists of a brass pin 18 cm long, 3 mm in diameter, weighing 20 gm. The pin is connected to a wire and circuit with a light and a brass plate. 20 holes ranging from 20 to 3.5 mm in diameter are drilled in the plate.

The holes are drilled using a standard set of metric drill bits having the following dimensions:

Hole number	1	2	3	4	5	6	7	8	9	10	...	20
Diameter (mm)	20	18	16	14	12	11	10	9.5	9	8.5	...	3.5

A similar device (Steadiness Tester, Hole Type, Model 32011) is made by Lafayette Instrument Co., Inc., P.O. Box 5729, Lafayette, IN 47903. They need to customize a special plate using the hole dimensions used by the Dutch researchers, and also incorporate their Model 589036 Light Response Unit. Cost for a single unit from Lafayette is estimated to be about $75.

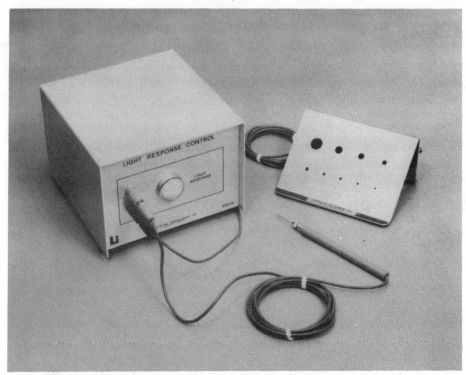

Fig. A. 5-3. **Hand steadiness measuring device**, courtesy Lafayette Instrument Co.

Equipment Appendix A

5-4. Pack of test cards for the Dutch intelligence test (GIT) (*Fig. A. 5-4*). Available from: Swets Publishing Service, Herreweg 347 b, 2161 CA Lisse, The Netherlands; or The Age Reduction Corporation, P.O. Box 85152 Dept MB125, San Diego, CA 92138.

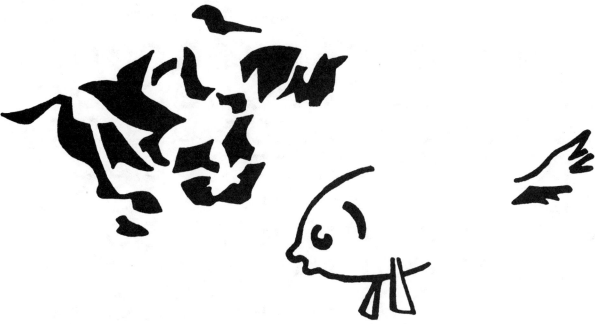

Fig. A. 5-4. **Dutch Intelligence Test cards**, courtesy Swets Publishing Service.

5-5. Bourdon-Wiersma test sheets (*Fig. A. 5-5*). These test sheets have lines consisting of groups of 25 small dots. The groups are formed by 3, 4, or 5 dots in slightly varying configurations. They are also available from the Swets Publishing Service or The Age Reduction Corporation.

Fig. A. 5-5. **Bourdon-Wiersma test sheet**, courtesy Swets Publishing Service.

5-6. Landolt test sheets (*Fig. A. 5-6*) for the Landolt concentration test (App. B. 5-5. b).

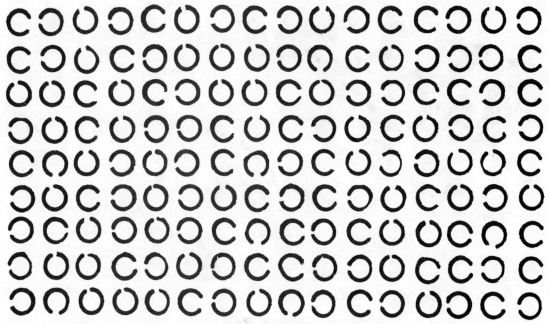

Fig. A. 5-6. **Landolt test sheet**, courtesy Dr. W. Ries.

5-7. Semantic categorization test panel *(Fig. A. 5-7)*. This is another custom-made instrument, consisting of a panel with 4 lights and 4 adjacent switches. The switches are labeled Professions, Animals, Objects, and Towns. Lafayette Instrument Co. again is the source of choice for the device. The words in Table 7-I are pre-recorded on tape.

A tape recorder is used with a programmed switch closure similar to that for advancing slides in a slide projector. The signal is precisely coordinated with the presentation of the words, activating Lafayette's Model 54035 Digital Clock/Counter. There is a 4-switch response panel with 4 indicator lights. Flipping any switch stops the clock. An experimenter's reset button is included in the circuit, allowing the test monitor to clear the light after the correct response and time have been recorded. Cost to fabricate a single unit is approximately $250.

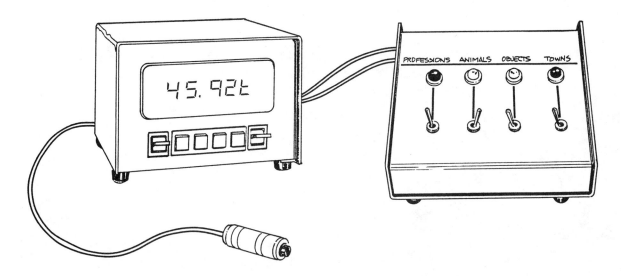

Fig. A. 5-7. **Semantic categorization test panel**, courtesy Lafayette Instrument Co.

5-8. Vibrometer (*Fig. A. 5-8*). This is a research tool and diagnostic instrument used to evaluate peripheral vascular and neurological abnormalities. It is obtainable from: the Bio-Medical Instrument Company, Newbury, Ohio 44065.

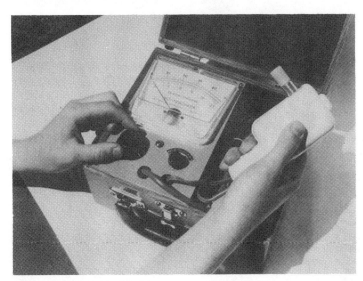

Fig. A. 5-8. **Vibrometer**, courtesy Bio-Medical Instrument Company.

Appendix A — Equipment

A special vibrometer (*Izmeritel Vibratsyonnoi Chuvstvitelnosti* [IVCH-02]) that measures in decibels—for tests by Furukawa (Chapter 9), Dubina (Chapter 14), and Mints (Chapter 16)—is manufactured by Medical Instruments Works, Lvov-19, USSR. Availability of this instrument in the West is unknown. Tests measured in decibels may be performed with Biomedical Instrument's Bio-Thesiometer and the volt-decibel conversion chart in *Fig. A. 5-9*.

5-9. Hand tally counter (*Fig. A. 5-9*), used to measure the tapping rate of the dominant index finger (Appendix B. 5-7. b). Model No. 56016 is available from Lafayette Instrument Co., P.O. Box 5729, Lafayette, IN 47903.

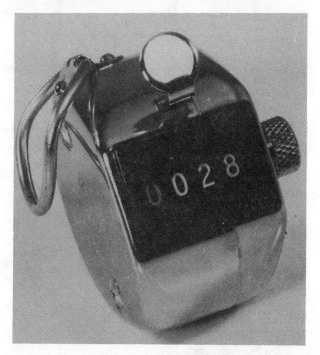
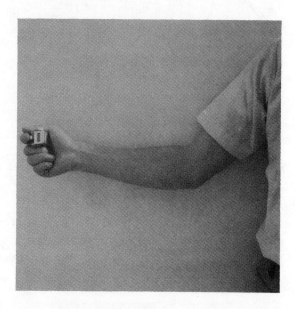

Fig. A. 5-9. **Hand tally counter**, (left), courtesy Lafayette Instrument Co, (right), courtesy Dr. Toshiyuki Furukawa.

5-10. Tapping board (*Fig. A. 5-10*) for use in the GRC tapping test (Appendix B. 5-7. b). The original test described by Borkan (Chapter 12) used a sheet of paper with two 4 mm-wide vertical stripes. The stripes were 142 mm apart, and the test was scored manually. While this method was apparently satisfactory for tax-supported research, it becomes quite tedious in most clinical settings. A more convenient method is to use a customized electronic tapping board available from Lafayette Instrument Co. (specify "Tapping board with 4 mm target/142 mm space on center, Model No. 32012WD" and Single impulse counter, Model No. 58022).

Equipment Appendix A

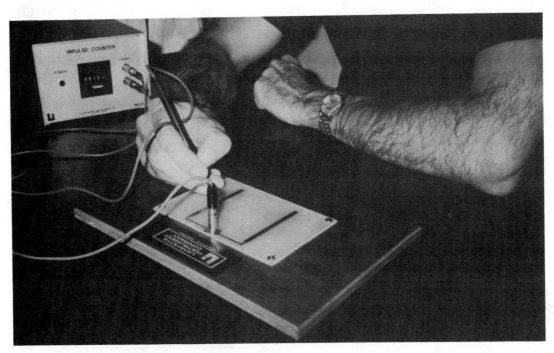

Fig. A. 5-10. GRC Tapping Board.

5-11. Bio-mechanical force platform (*Fig. A. 5-11*), for use in the static balance test. Available from: Kistler Instrument Corporation, 75 John Glenn Drive, Amherst, NY 14120 (716) 691-5100; and Advanced Mechanical Technology, Inc., 141 California Street, Newton, MA 02158 (617) 964-2042.

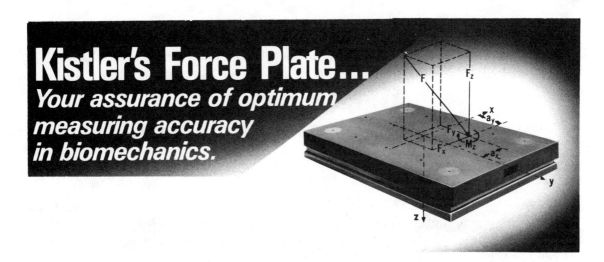

Fig. A. 5-11. **Bio-mechanical force platform**, courtesy, Kistler Instrument Corporation.

5-12. Choice reaction time test device (3 and 4 choice) (*Fig. A. 5-12*), another custom made instrument. It consists of a panel with 4 lights mounted in a horizontal row, 4 cm apart. Below the row of lights is a row of buttons, each corresponding to a light. When the examiner turns on a light, an electric timer starts and runs until the subject presses the button below the light. Lafayette Instruments can make this instrument, using their standard Visual Choice Reaction Time Apparatus, Model 63035, in conjunction with their Model 54035 Digital Stop Clock. Estimated cost is about $400.

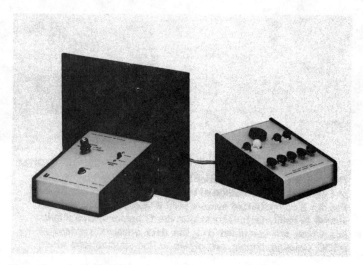

Fig. A. 5-12. **Choice reaction time instrument**, courtesy Lafayette Instrument Co.

5-13. "Bogitch" light extinction device (*Fig. A. 5-13*). This is another custom-made instrument that can be fabricated by Lafayette Instruments. It consists of a row of 10 small lights (similar to flashlight or Christmas tree lights) mounted on a rectangular board. Below each light is a switch that turns the corresponding light off, and simultaneously turns on another randomly located light. The lights are lit in an arbitrary order--3-8-9-5-6-7-2-4-10-1. The subject turns off each light by flipping a corresponding switch. A timer accurate to 1/100 second begins when the first light is turned off, and runs until the last light is turned off. This can be made by Lafayette Instrument Company. Estimated cost is about $200.

Mr. Vern E. Davidson, Vice President, Marketing and Development for Lafayette Instrument Co. can be reached at: (317) 423-1505. Price estimates quoted for all instruments customized by Lafayette are for single units. If numerous inquiries and purchases are made, prices may be reduced.

| Equipment | Appendix A |

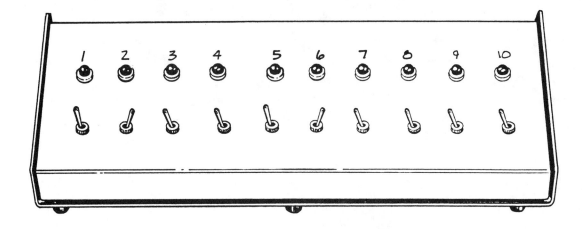

Fig. A. 5-13. **Light extinction device**, courtesy, Lafayette Instrument Co.

5-14. Wechsler Digit Symbol test kit, available from the Psychological Corporation, 7500 Old Oak Boulevard, Cleveland, Ohio 44130.

5-15. Wechsler Block Design test set, available from the Psychological Corporation.

5-16. Stroop color-word test set (*Fig. A. 5-14*). This can be custom-made or obtained from The Age Reduction Corporation, P.O. Box 85152 Dept MB 125, San Diego, CA 92138.

It consists of three test cards. The first card consists of 3 lines of 10 "color words" (red, blue, and green) printed in black ink, repeated in random order. The second card consists of 30 rectangular 3/16" X 1/2" patches (red, blue and green) also in random order. The third card is a list of 30 color words in random order, printed in a color different than designated by the word.

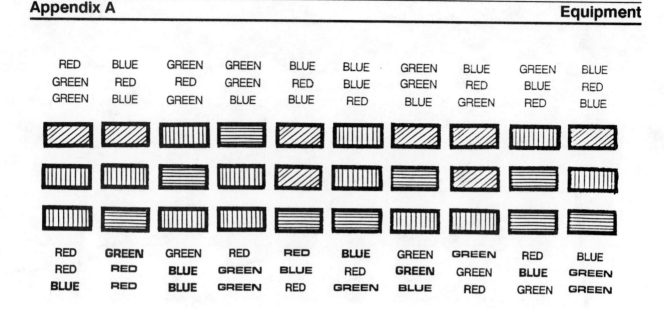

Fig. A. 5-14. Stroop Color Word test set, courtesy Dr. Werner Ries.

6. ANTHROPOMETRIC

6-1. Handgrip dynamometer (*Fig. A. 6-1*), for measuring handgrip strength, available from: Lafayette Instrument Co., P.O. Box 5729, Lafayette, IN 47903; or J. A. Preston Corp., 60 Page Road, Clifton, NJ 07012.

6-2. Anthropometric caliper (*Fig. A. 6-2*), for body measurements. There are several types. One is a professional tool used by anthropologists, consisting of a segmented metal tube with a fixed cross-arm at the top, and a movable sleeve-like cross arm that slides along the entire length of the tube. Professional anthropometric calipers are expensive, costing up to $1500!

Much more reasonably priced instruments give satisfactory results, costing between $8.00 and $85.00, depending on the model selected. They are available from: J. A. Preston Corporation, 60 Page Road, Clifton, NJ 07012, (800) 631-277; Carolina Biological Supply Company, 2700 York Road, Burlington, NC 27215.

Equipment　　　　　　　　　　　　　　　　　　　　　　Appendix A

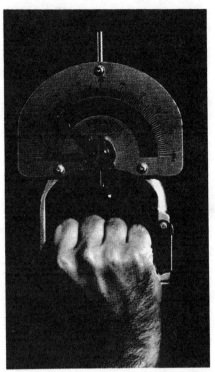

Fig. A. 6-1. **Handgrip dynamometer**, courtesy Lafayette Instrument Co.

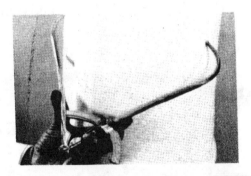

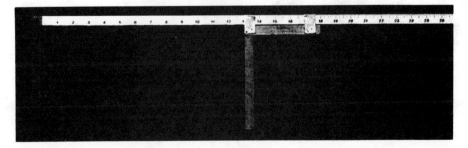

Fig. A. 6-2. **Anthropometric calipers**, courtesy J. A. Preston Corporation.

6-3. Sliding caliper (*Fig. A. 6-3*), for measuring small dimensions, available from: Carolina Biological Supply Company (address above), or from Sears or other suppliers of mechanical or electronic measuring equipment.

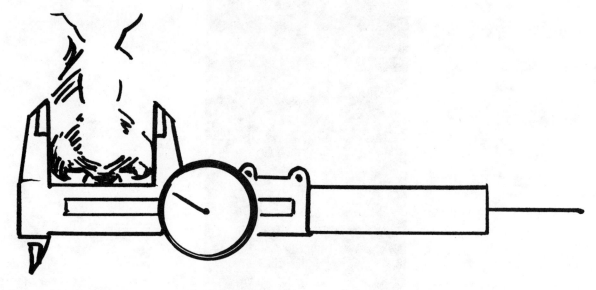

Fig. A. 6-3. **Sliding caliper,** art by Tom Moore.

6-4. Skinfold caliper *(Fig. A. 6-4)*. This is a standard device for measuring skinfold thickness, giving an indication of body fat content. Skinfold calipers are available from: Lafayette Instrument Co., Inc., P.O. Box 5729, Lafayette, IN 47903; and Cambridge Scientific Industries, Cambridge, MD.

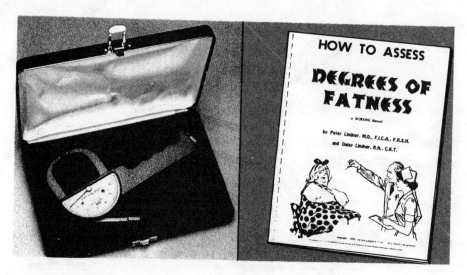

Fig. A. 6-4. **Skinfold caliper,** courtesy Lafayette Instrument Co., Inc.

Equipment Appendix A

6-5. Tape measure.

6-6. Large draftsman's triangle, to measure standing and sitting heights.

6-7. Camera, for recording extent of baldness and grayness, for later comparisons.

6-8. Instruments to measure body flexibility and range of motion.

    a. Goniometer (*Fig. A. 6-5*). This instrument consists of two arms that rotate about a single joint, graduated in degrees. Goniometers are available in various sizes, for measuring joints of correspondingly varying size. Goniometers are available from: Carolina Biological Supply Co., 2700 York Road, Burlington, North Carolina 27215.

    b. Flexometer (*Fig. A. 6-6*). This is sort of a mechanical plumb line which is strapped to the body part being tested. Flexometers are available from Leighton Flexometer, E. 1321 55th Ave., Spokane, WA 99203.

    c. Digital flexibility tester (*Fig. A. 6-7*). This instrument automatically records the distance the fingers can be extended beyond the toes when bending forward at the waist with legs straight. Available from Country Technology, Inc., P.O. Box 87, Gays Mills, WI 54631.

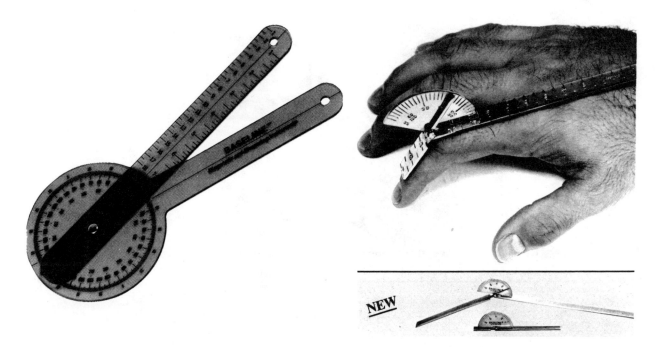

Fig. A. 6-5. **Goniometer**, courtesy, Lafayette Instrument Co.

Appendix A — Equipment

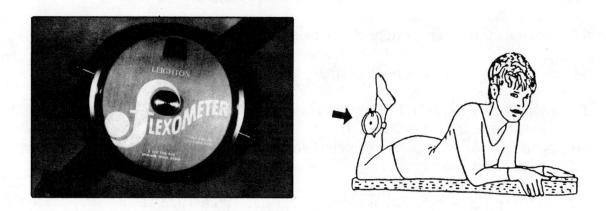

Fig. A. 6-6. **Leighton Flexometer**, courtesy Leighton Flexometer.

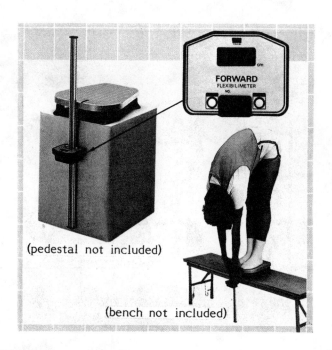

Fig. A. 6-7. **Digital Flexibility Tester**, courtesy Country Technology.

Equipment — Appendix A

6-9. Body weight scale.

6-10. Stopwatch.

OTHER SOURCES:

The above list of sources is not exhaustive. There are two directories containing comprehensive lists of manufacturers of medical devices. These directories are primarily designed for hospitals or large institutions. They are:

Medical Device Register, available from Medical Device Register, P.O. Box 50, Smithtown, NY 11787. $95.

ECRI Health Devices Sourcebook, available from ECRI, 5200 Butler Pike, Plymouth Meeting, PA 19462, $110.

Appendix B

BIOMARKER SUB-TESTS
with age-adjusted normal values

This Appendix includes age-adjusted normal values for all clinical laboratory tests used in the aging measurement systems described in this book. It is the most complete compilation of age-related physiological changes that has ever been compiled and published in a single volume. These biomarkers are presented in graphical form. The solid line indicates the mean value for the population studied in each case, and the shaded area indicates +/- 1 standard deviation.

Although the choice of the tests rests with the scientists who developed the test batteries, the choice of data showing the age-adjusted standard values associated with the tests is mine.

There were several somewhat arbitrary selection criteria for these data. Whenever possible, data from longitudinal studies were used, although most of the data have been derived from cross-sectional studies. In non-standard or infrequently performed tests, the only data available were often those of the test developer.

In other cases, in which there were conflicting data from many different studies—for example, systolic and diastolic blood pressure, and cholesterol levels; with no consensus on what should be the "norm"—an attempt was made to select representative American values.

If readers know of better data than are included in this Appendix, I would appreciate hearing from them.

An excellent discussion of the problems and methods of obtaining age-adjusted normal values is presented in the NIA's recent book—*Normal Human Aging—The Baltimore Longitudinal Study of Aging* (Shock, et al, 1985).

Appendix B — Sub-tests

1. CARDIOVASCULAR

1-1. Systolic blood pressure (SBP) (*Figs. B. 1-1 and 1-2*), recorded in mm Hg. The increase in SBP with age is a reflection of atherosclerosis-induced reduction in arterial elasticity (Shock, et al). SBP is usually considered "normal" if less than 140 mm Hg. However, longevity is shortened progressively in adults whose SBP exceeds 100 mm Hg (Engelman and Braunwald).

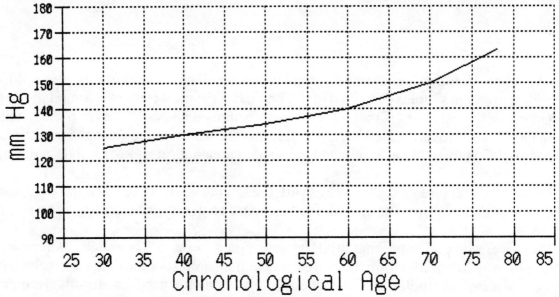

Fig. B. 1-1. **Systolic blood pressure — men** (Framingham).

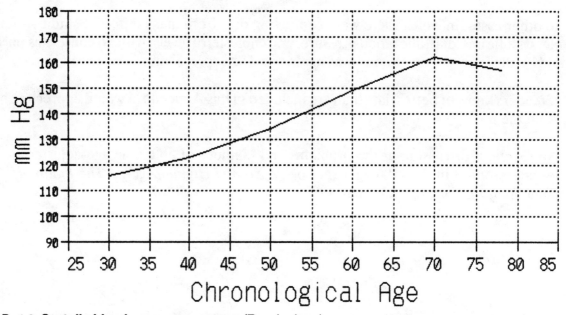

Fig. B. 1-2. **Systolic blood pressure — women** (Framingham).

1-2. Maximum systolic pressure (*Fig. B. 1-3*), the highest pressure attained during the last completed period of a progressive exercise test, as described in Appendix B. 1-5.

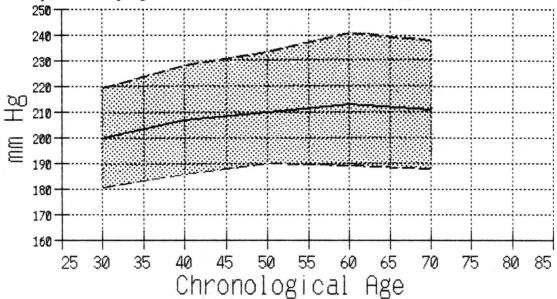

Fig. B. 1-3. **Maximum systolic pressure during the last completed minute of an exercise stress test** (Dirken).

1-3. Diastolic blood pressure (DBP) (*Figs. B. 1-4 and 1-5*). DBP is considered "normal" if less than 90 mm Hg. DBP consistent with longest life is about 60 mm Hg (Engelman and Araunwald).

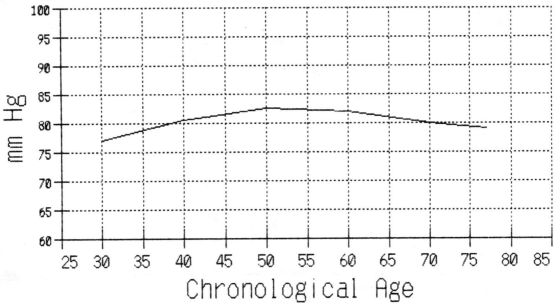

Fig. B. 1-4. **Diastolic blood pressure — men** (Framingham).

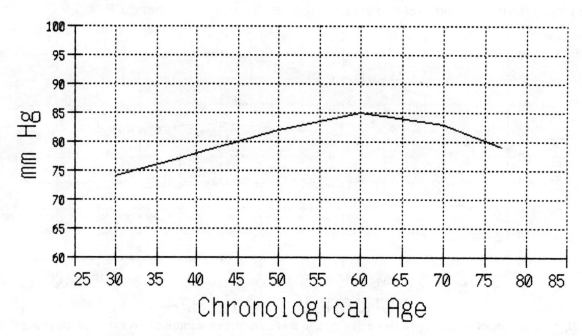

Fig. B. 1-5. **Diastolic blood pressure – women** (Framingham).

1-4. Pulse pressure (PP) (*Figs. B. 1-6 and 1-7*)--the difference between systolic and diastolic pressure.

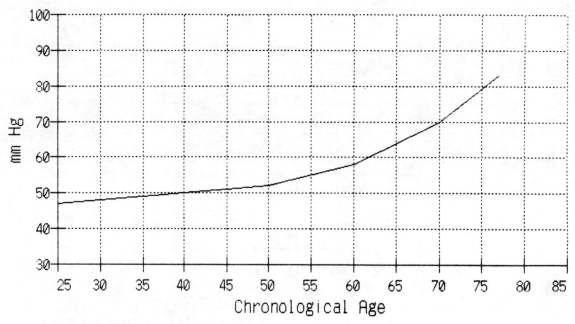

Fig. B. 1-6. **Pulse pressure – men** (Framingham).

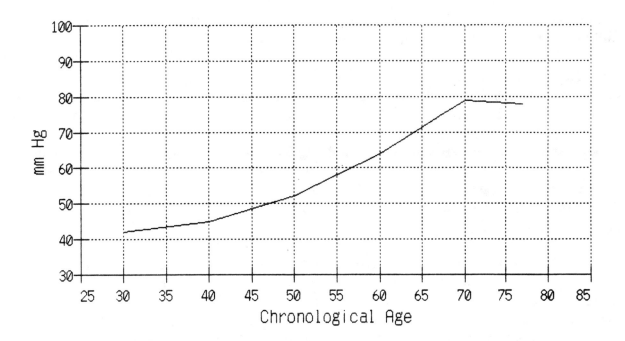

Fig. B. 1-7. **Pulse pressure — women** (Framingham)).

1-5. Maximal oxygen uptake (VO₂max) (*Figs. B. 1-8 to 1-10*). VO₂max measures the oxygen consumed during maximal prolonged exercise. It is an international reference standard for physical fitness (Shephard and Kavanaugh). There are two standard units of measurement (liters or ml per minute; and ml per kg per minute). There are also several methods for testing and numerous protocols for each particular method. The value in liters or ml per minute can be easily converted to ml/kg min by dividing by the subject's bodyweight in kg.

The most accurate values for VO₂max are obtained by direct measurement using a treadmill (Appendix A. 1-3) and physiological monitoring system (Appendix A. 1-4). VO₂max can also be estimated by several indirect methods using either the treadmill, a bicycle ergometer (Appendix A. 1-2), a two-step staircase (Appendix A 1-5), or a "field test" (Table B. 1-III). The other methods give values varying from 5-25% from those obtained directly on a treadmill. While such values are not exactly comparable, they do provide reproducible values which can be used for longitudinal comparisons.

a. Treadmill: There are a number of standard protocols. Nakamura's (Chapter 13) is satisfactory, and is conducted as follows: The subject warms up for several minutes by walking on the treadmill at 80 meters/minute with a slope of 0%. Thereafter, the slope is increased by 2.5% each minute until exhaustion. The VO₂max is calculated directly with a metabolic cart, or estimated using a nomogram (*Fig. B. 1-11*) based on the speed and the slope of the treadmill for the last completed minute of exercise.

b. Bicycle ergometer: The subject warms up for two minutes pedaling with no load at 60 cycles per minute. The starting load is 100 Watts for men and 50 Watts for women. Thereafter, the load is increased 10-20 watts every two minutes. The test continues until the subject is exhausted, or the physician considers further testing inadvisable. The heart rate is recorded every minute from a heart rate monitor (Appendix A. 1-6). The heart rate and maximum load in Watts during the last full minute completed before termination of the test are used to determine maximal oxygen uptake from the Astrand-Rhyming nomogram (*Fig. B. 1-12*). Some ergometers register resistance in kilopond meters/min (kpm) or kgm/min. Kpm and kgm/min are equivelant terms, and can be converted to Watts by dividing by 6.

c. Bench stepping: The Astrand-Rhyming nomogram can also be used to predict VO_2max from the postexercise heart rate and body weight during bench stepping, using the Master's staircase. The subject steps at a rate of 90 steps per minute, using a metronome to maintain the pace. At the count one-two-three, the participant steps up on the platform until completely erect with both feet on the platform. Counts four-five-six bring the participant back down to the starting position. To help avoid muscle fatigue, the lead leg can be changed at any time. The test is terminated at volitional fatigue or when the participant cannot keep up the proper rhythm. The post-exercise heart rate is obtained from the heart rate monitor between 15 and 30 sec immediately after exercise.

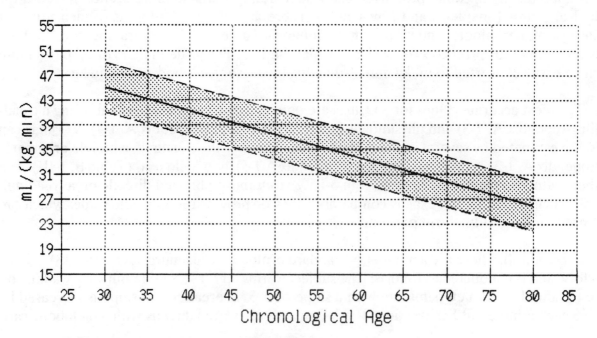

Fig. B. 1-8. **Maximal oxygen uptake — men, in ml/kg min** (Dehn and Bruce).

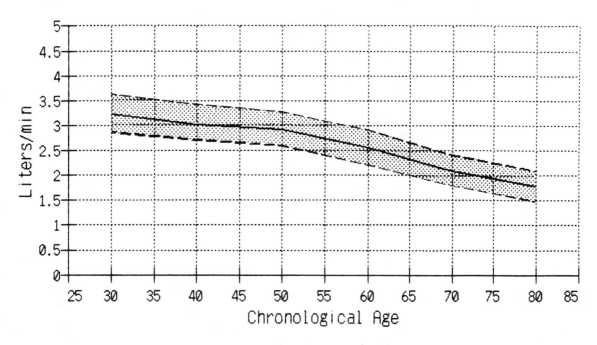

Fig. B. 1-9. **Maximal oxygen uptake – men, in liters/min** (Andersen, et al).

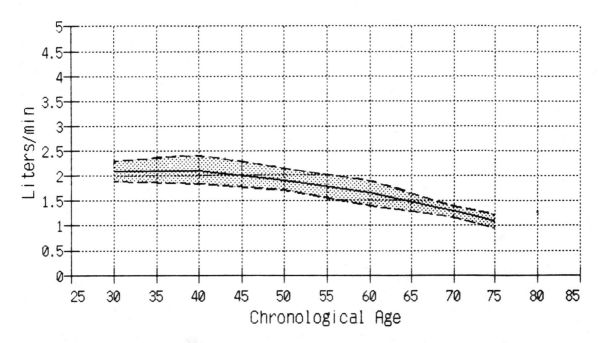

Fig. B. 1-10. **Maximal oxygen uptake – women, in liters/min** (Andersen, et al).

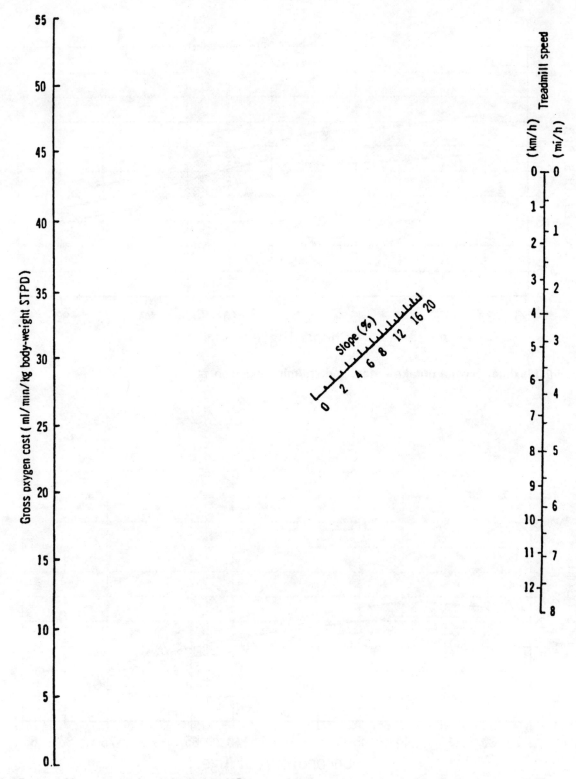

Fig. B. 1-11. **Nomogram for calculating VO₂max while running on a treadmill** (Andersen, et al).

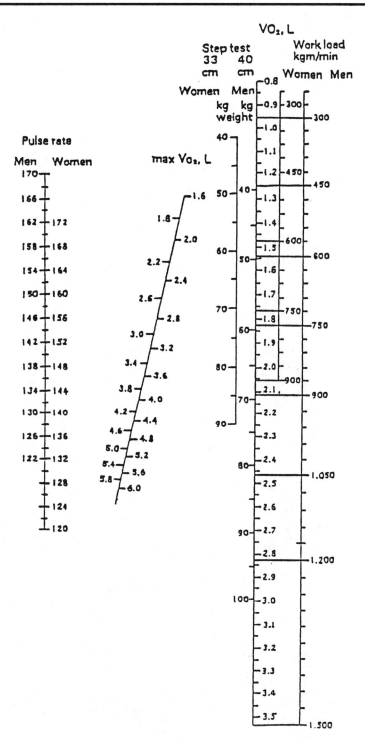

Fig. B. 1-12. **Modified Astrand-Rhyming nomogram.** The VO2max is determined by drawing a line with a ruler between the pulse rate and the work intensity--in kpm if using the bicycle ergometer, or the subject's body weight in kg if using the step test--and noting the point where the ruler and center scale intersect. The value from the nomogram is valid only for persons 20 to 25 years old. The scores of those over 25 should be multiplied by a correction factor, obtainable from *Fig. B. 1-13* (Astrand, 1960).

TABLE B. 1-I. Conversion from KPM to Watts.

WORK LOAD	
Watts	kpm
50	300
100	600
150	900
200	1200
250	1500
300	1800
350	2100
400	2400

TABLE B. 1-II. Field Test for Measurement of VO$_2$max

Maximum oxygen uptake ml/kg.min	Time to cover 1.5 miles (min:sec)
27.0	19:00
29.0	18:30
31.5	16:30
35.0	15:00
37.0	13:30
39.0	13:00
41.0	12:30
42.5	12:00
45.0	11:00
46.5	10.45
48.0	10:30
49.5	10:00
51.5	9:45
53.0	9:30
55.0	9:15
56.5	9:00
58.0	8:30
60.0	8:15
63.5	7:45
66.0	7:15
68.0	7:00
71.5	6:45
74.0	6:30
77.5	6:10

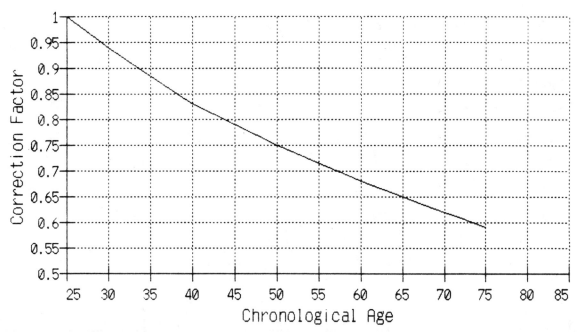

Fig. B. 1-13. **Astrand-Rhyming nomogram age correction factor**. The maximal oxygen uptake calculated from the Astrand nomogram (*Fig. B. 1-12*) should be be multiplied by the correction factor for the subject's chronological age, to obtain a more accurate value.

1-6. Maximum Heart rate (*Fig. B. 1-14*) during an exercise stress test. It is the highest stable heart rate measured during the last completed minute.

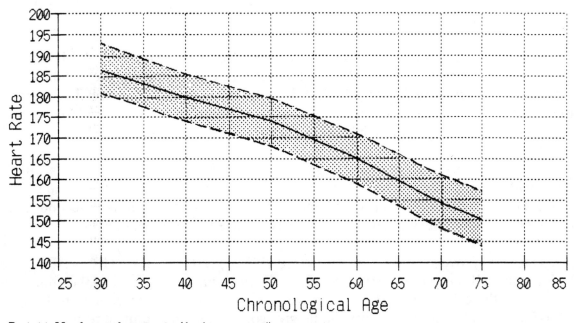

Fig. B. 1-14. **Maximum heart rate** (Anderson, et al).

1-7. Maximum load in Watts during a bicycle ergometer stress test (Appendix B. 1-5. b.) (*Fig. B. 1-15*). This is the maximum load sustained for the last completed minute. This value can also be extrapolated using data from other exercise tests and the Astrand-Rhyming nomogram (*Fig. B. 1-12*).

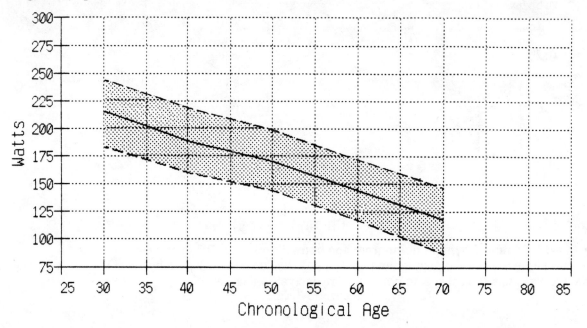

Fig. B. 1-15. **Maximum load in Watts during a bicycle ergometer stress test — men** (Dirken).

1-8. Other exercise tests:

a. Heart rate recovery after exercise — Furukawa (*Figs. B. 1-16 to 1-18*). A Master's two-step test is performed (Appendix B. 1-5. c). The heart rate is recorded while standing before exercise and at intervals of 30 seconds, 1, 2, 3, and 4 minutes after exercise. The maximum heart rate attainable with exercise decreases, with age, but the period required for the return of the resting heart rate to normal increases (*Figs. B. 1-16 to 1-18*).

b. Pulse-rate after exercise — Ries (*Figs. B. 1-19 and 1-20*). The subject stands with feet shoulder width apart, hands on hips. The resting pulse rate is recorded. At the signal to begin, the subject does 20 complete deep knee bends as fast as possible. The time in seconds to perform the exercises and the immediate post-exercise pulse rate are recorded.

c. Heart rate recovery ratio — Nakamura (*Fig. B. 1-21*) $(HR_e - HR_a)/(HR_e - HR_r)$, where HR_r, HR_e, and HR_a represent the heart rate at the beginning of exercise, at the end of exercise, and after three minutes of rest, respectively. Nakamura used the treadmill test (Appendix B. 1-5 a). Any of the exercise tests should give comparable longitudinal results.

d. Rate of oxygen removal, in ml/min – Nakamura (*Fig. B. 1-22*). This is another non-standard test to evaluate aerobic power and cardio-vascular efficiency. It is determined by dividing the maximal oxygen uptake in ml/min (Appendix B. 1-5) by the maximal voluntary ventilation (Appendix B. 2-4).

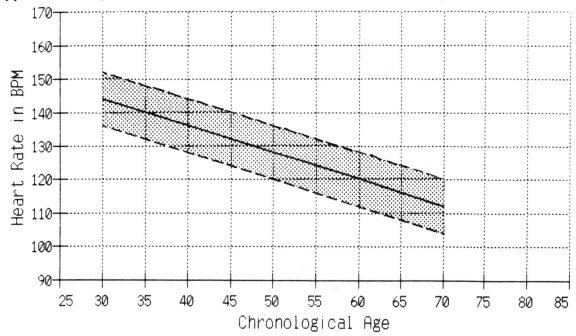

Fig. B. 1-16. **Heart rate 30 seconds after exercise – men** (Furukawa, 1975).

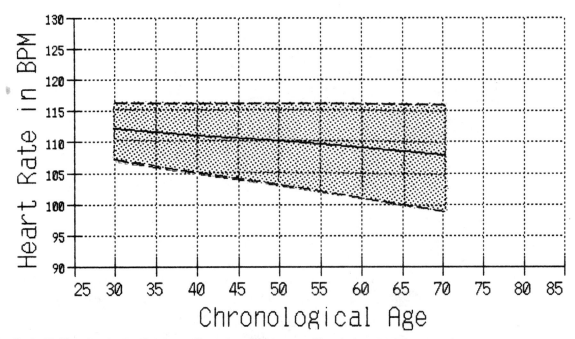

Fig. B. 1-17. **Heart rate 2 minutes after exercise – men** (Furukawa, 1975).

Appendix B   **Sub-tests**

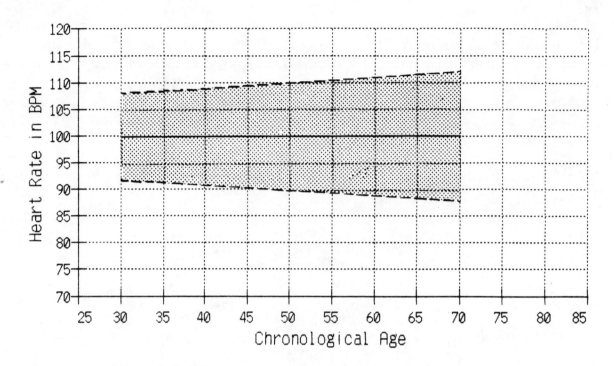

Fig. B. 1-18. **Heart rate 4 minutes after exercise — men** (Furukawa, 1975)

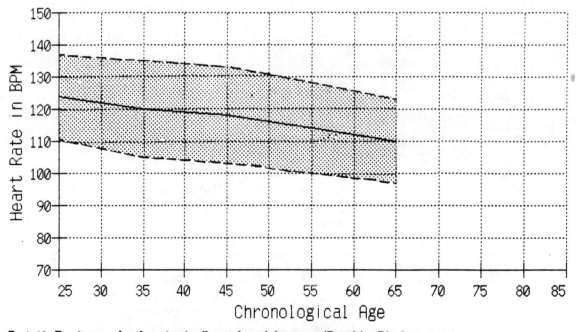

Fig. B. 1-19. **Post-exercise heart rate (knee-bends) — men** (Poethig; Ries).

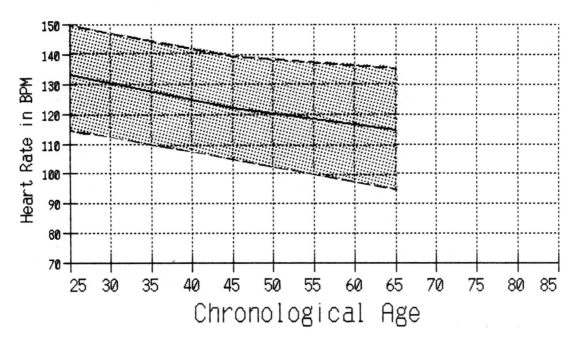

Fig. B. 1-20. **Post-exercise heart rate (knee-bends) – women** (Poethig; Ries).

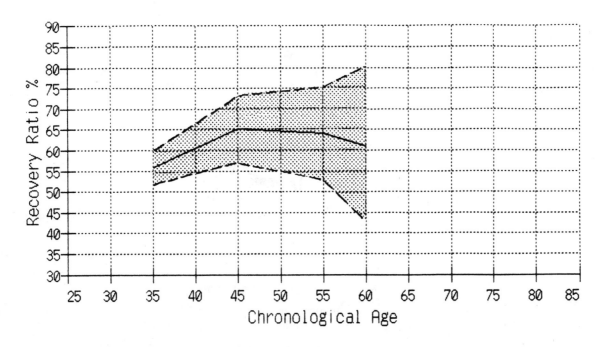

Fig. B. 1-21. **Heart rate recovery ratio – men** (Nakamura, Kyoiku Igaku).

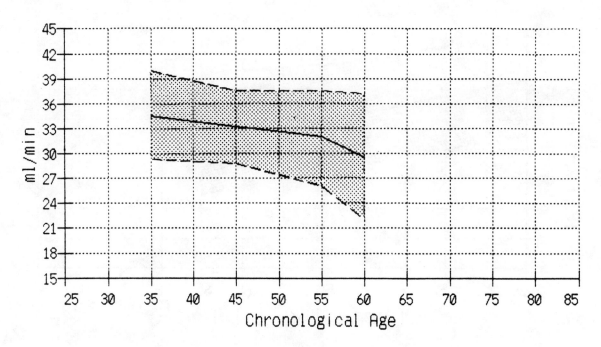

Fig. B. 1-22. **Rate of oxygen removal — men** (Nakamura, *Kyoiku Igaku*).

1-9. T-wave deflection in lead V5 of a 12 lead electrocardiogram (*Figs. B. 1-23 and 1-24*).

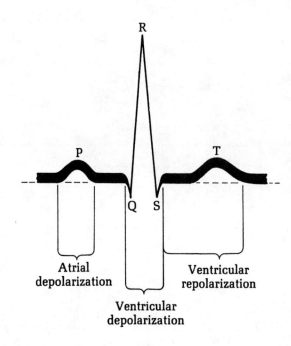

Fig. B. 1-23. **Normal QRS complex**. The T-wave represents ventricular repolarization.

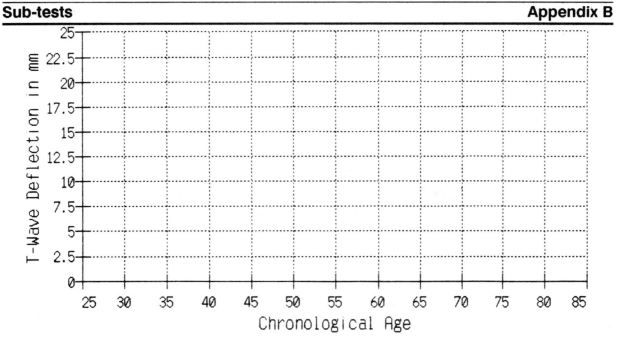

Fig. B. 1-24. **T-wave deflection in mm in lead V5 of a standard 12-lead electrocardiogram.** No data are available for this test used in Chapter 16.

1-10. Arterial pulse-wave velocity (APWV) in meters/second (*Figs. B. 1-25 and 1-26*). This time-honored test is used to quantitatively evaluate the aging-induced reduction in arterial elasticity (Hallock). It can be measured with equipment described in Appendix A. 1-8. The pulse wave is recorded at two different points in the peripheral arterial system. The APWV is obtained by dividing the distance between the two sites by the time difference in seconds between the pulse waves.

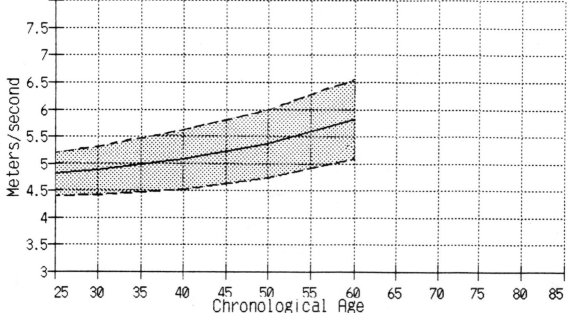

Fig. B. 1-25. **Arterial pulse-wave velocity from the femoral to posterior tibial arteries** (Wezler and Standl).

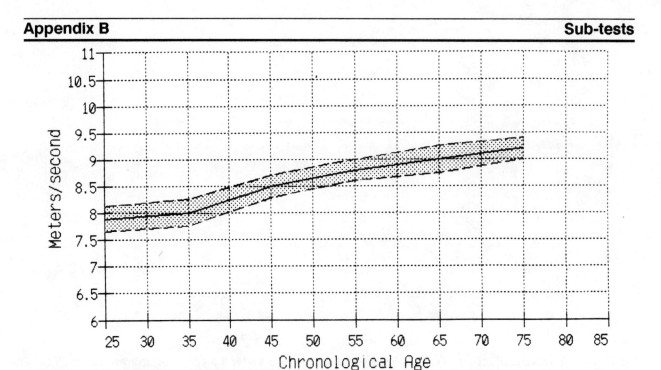

Fig. B. 1-26. **Arterial pulse-wave velocity from the axillary to radial arteries** (Mints, 1985).

1-11. Arterial oxygen tension (pO$_2$) (*Fig. B. 1-27*), in mm Hg. This measures the pressure exerted by O$_2$ dissolved in plasma. Usually an arterial puncture is required, which is painful and entails some risk. Fairly accurate values for pO$_2$ can be obtained noninvasively with an ear oximeter (Appendix A. 1-9). The ear oximeter painlessly measures tissue pO$_2$ with a sensitive electrode, giving a value nearly identical to arterial pO$_2$.

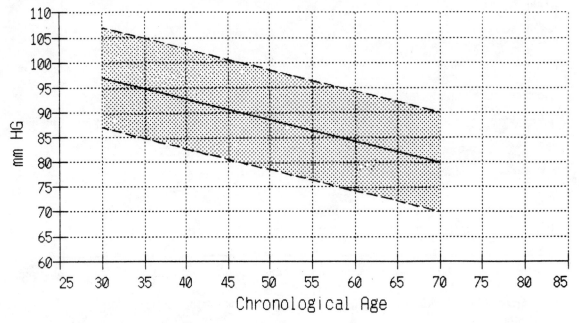

Fig. B. 1-27. **Arterial oxygen tension** (Muiesan, et al).

| Sub-tests | Appendix B |

2. PULMONARY

2-1. Forced expiratory volume in one second (FEV$_1$) (*Figs. B. 2-1 and 2-2*). This is the volume of air forcibly expelled from the lungs in one second, measured with a spirometer (Appendix A. 2-1) and recorded in ml or liters. These data are closely correlated with age and height.

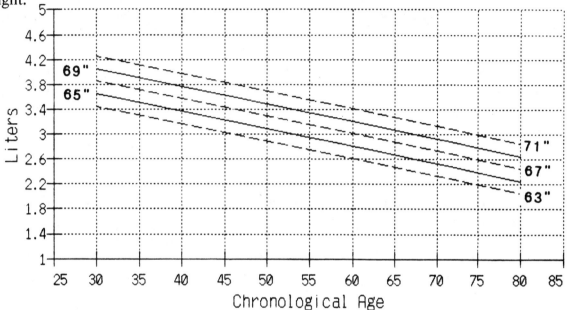

Fig. B. 2-1. **FEV$_1$ – men**. Mean values for height (Halsted). The normal range is from +/- 0.62 liters in young men, to +/- 0.36 liters in the elderly (Morris, et al).

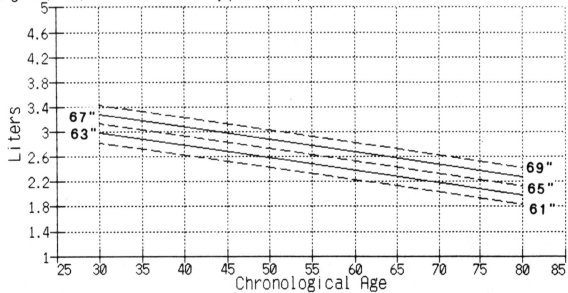

Fig. B. 2-2. **FEV$_1$ – women**. Mean values for height (Halsted). The normal range is from +/- 0.60 liters in young women, to +/- 0.32 liters in the elderly (Morris, et al).

2-2. Vital capacity (VC) (*Figs. B. 2-3 and 2-4*) and forced vital capacity (FVC). Vital capacity is the total volume of air expelled from the lungs by a maximal expiration after a maximal inspiration.

Forced vital capacity differs from "slow" vital capacity in that the subject exhales as hard and as fast as he can. In persons with small airway disease, the FVC will be somewhat less than the "slow" VC due to early airway closure. Both functions are measured with a spirometer (Appendix A. 2-1).

Based on data from the Framingham study, vital capacity has been found to be the *best predictor of subsequent longevity* (Kannel and Hubert). Nevertheless, vital capacity was not included as a recommended part of routine screening exams by *any* of the major orthodox medical groups that contributed to the studies summarized in Table 3-I. The importance of measurements of vital capacity has not gone unnoticed by those involved in aging measurement, however, as it is one of the most commonly used tests.

A problem with regard to the use of absolute values of pulmonary function tests in estimates of biological age is that none of the investigators (except Ries) have corrected for height. A tall person will tend to score younger due to a larger lung capacity, and a short person will score older. Although this may cause the absolute value of biological age to be less accurate, the rate of change should not be affected, due to the uniform linear decline with age.

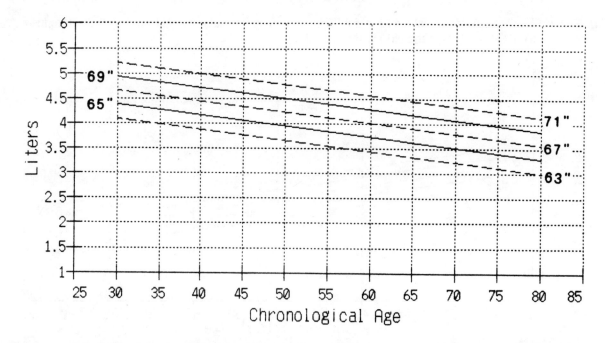

Fig. B. 2-3. **Vital capacity — men.** Mean values for height (Halsted). The normal range is from +/- 0.89 liters in young men to +/- 0.85 liters in the elderly (Morris, et al).

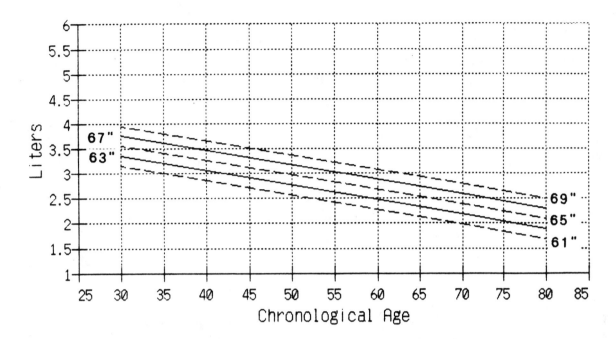

Fig. B. 2-4. **Vital capacity — women**. Mean values for height (Halsted). The normal range is from +/- 0.70 liters in young women to +/- 0.47 in the elderly (Morris, et al).

2-3. Maximum respiratory rate (*Fig. B. 2-5*). This is the maximum respiratory rate during the bicycle ergometer or other cardiovascular stress test.

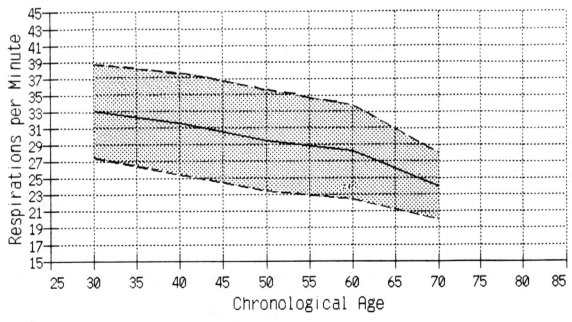

Fig. B. 2-5. **Maximum respiratory rate — men** (Dirken).

2-4. Maximum voluntary ventilation in one minute (MVV$_1$) (*Figs. B. 2-6 and 2-7*) is the maximum volume of air that can be breathed per minute, measured with a spirometer, and recorded in liters/minute. If this is used to calculate the rate of oxygen removal (Appendix B. 1-8. d), the test should be conducted immediately upon termination of the exercise stress test.

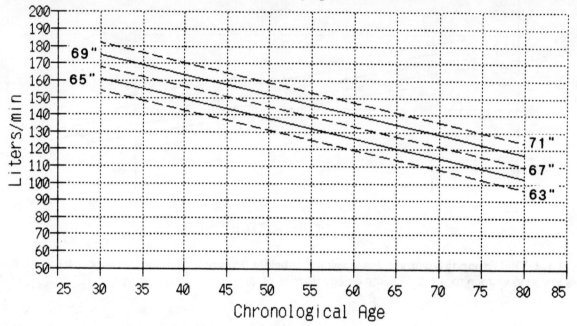

Fig. B. 2-6. **Maximum voluntary ventilation — men.** Mean values for height (Halsted).

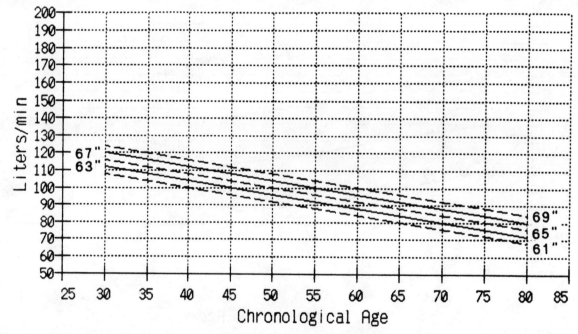

Fig. B. 2-7. **Maximum voluntary ventilation — women.** Mean values for height (Halsted).

3. AUDIOMETRIC

3-1. Audiometric exam (*Figs. B. 3-1 and 3-2*). Using an audiometer (Appendix A. 3-1), the decibel loss for each ear at 500, 1,000, 2,000, 4,000 and 6,000 Hz is assessed. Depending on the test used, the score is expressed either as the dB loss in the better ear, or as a percentage of hearing loss (Table B. 2-1). The "better ear" score is the lowest volume in dB heard in either ear.

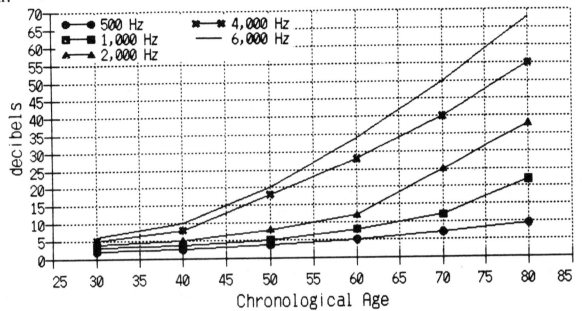

Fig. B. 3-1. **Auditory acuity at various frequencies — men** (Ordy, et al).

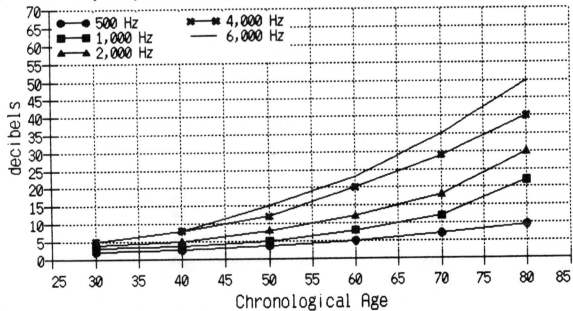

Fig. B. 3-2. **Auditory acuity at various frequencies — women** (Ordy, et al).

Appendix B — Sub-tests

TABLE B. 3-I. Hearing loss at various frequencies as a %*

loss in dB	% at 500 Hz	1,000 Hz	2,000 Hz	4,000 Hz
10	0.2	0.3	0.4	0.1
15	0.5	0.9	1.3	0.3
20	1.1	2.1	2.9	0.9
25	1.8	3.6	4.9	1.7
30	2.6	5.4	7.2	2.7
35	3.7	7.7	9.8	3.8
40	4.9	10.2	12.9	5.0
45	6.3	13.0	17.3	6.4
50	7.9	15.7	22.4	8.0
55	9.6	19.0	25.7	9.7
60	11.3	21.5	28.0	11.2
65	12.8	23.5	30.2	12.5
70	13.8	25.5	32.2	13.5
75	14.6	27.2	34.0	14.2
80	14.8	28.8	35.8	14.6
85	14.9	29.8	37.5	14.8
90	15.0	29.9	39.2	14.9
95	15.0	30.0	40.0	15.0

*Fowler and Sabine.

3-2. **High Frequency Audiometry** (*Fig. B. 3-3*) evaluates the ability to hear loud sounds at very high frequencies, using a special high frequency audiometer (Appendix A. 3-2). The test begins with a tone at 20 kHz and a constant volume of 80 decibels. The frequency is gradually decreased until the subject signals that he hears something.

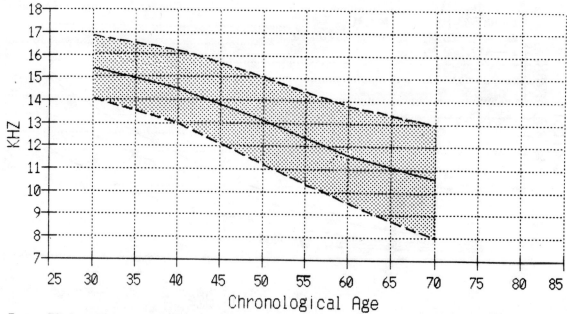

Fig. B. 3-3. **Pitch ceiling — men** (Dirken).

4. VISUAL

4-1. Near vision (*Figs. B. 4-1 and 4-2*). With age, the lens of the eye becomes progressively less elastic, resulting in *presbyopia*.

To measure near vision, use either a Krimsky-Prince rule (to age 44); Beren's rule (to age 50); or a yard stick and test card (Appendix A. 4-1). Position the base of the rule on the cheek bone directly below the eye being tested (inferior orbit) and slowly move the test card toward the subject from a distance at which the card can be easily read, until it blurs. Note the closest distance at which the test card can be clearly read. Glasses or contact lenses for nearsightedness *should* be worn, but reading glasses *should not* be used. There is a variation between various conversion scales, and there is no consensus as to which scale is the most accurate. Therefore, I recommend using a simple yard stick, and determining all parameters from Figs. B. 4-1 to 4-3. Longitudinal measurements should be made consistently with the same scale.

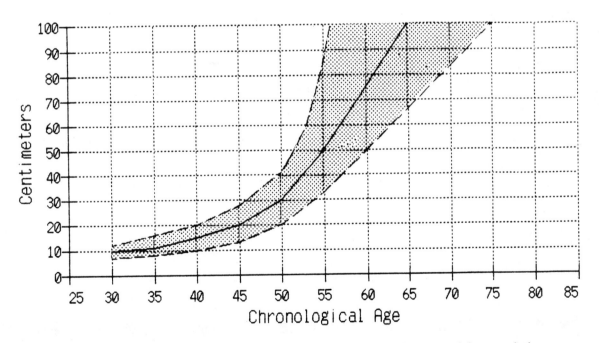

Fig. B. 4-1. **Near vision, in cm**. The area represents the distance at which 90% of the population can see near objects clearly (Combined data from: Morgan and Wilson; Duane; and Sekuler).

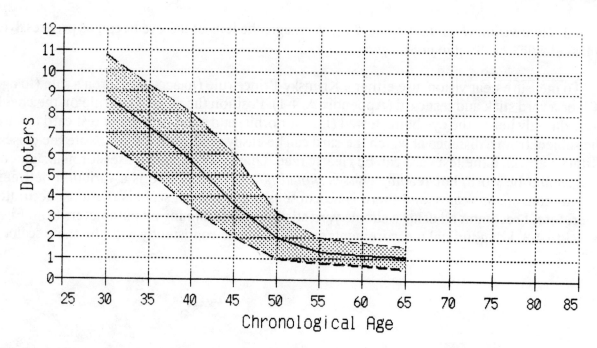

Fig. B. 4-2. **Near vision, in diopters** (Duane).

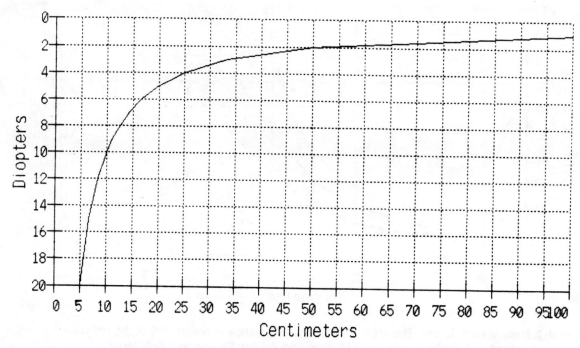

Fig. B. 4-3. **Conversion scale for converting near point of vision in centimeters to diopters** (Duane).

4-2. Distance visual acuity (*Fig. B. 4-4*), determined from the last row read correctly on a visual acuity chart. It is scored as a decimal, calculated by dividing the distance from the subject to the chart (d) by the distance from which the normal eye can distinguish the letters (D) (i.e., 20/20 = 1.0, 20/40 = 0.5, 20/200 = 0.1, etc). Glasses or contact lenses should be worn.

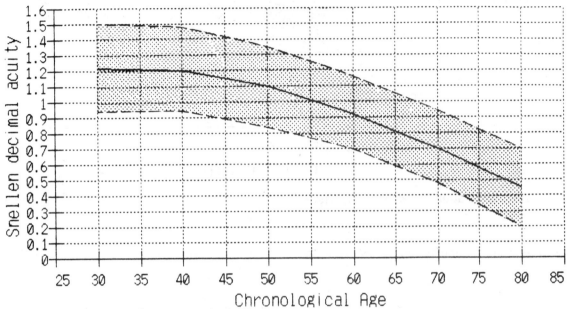

Fig. B. 4-4. **Visual acuity** (best correction) (Pitts).

4-3. Dark adaptation (*Fig. B. 4-5*). This test is made in a darkened room, using a Friedmann visual field analyzer (Appendix A, 4-3) with a 0.6 filter. Prior to the test, the eyes are exposed to a light of 1,000 lux for 2 minutes, with a wave length between 369-611 Nm. The test is scored in seconds.

Appendix B   Sub-tests

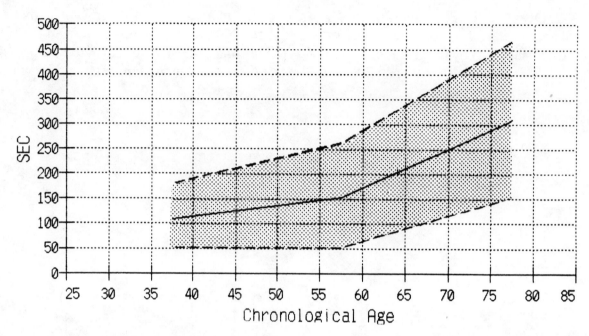

Fig. B. 4-5. **Dark adaptation** (Heikkinen, et al., 1984).

4-4. Near visual acuity (*Fig. B. 4-6*), as a decimal, obtained using an FAA Vision Tester (Appendix A. 4-4).

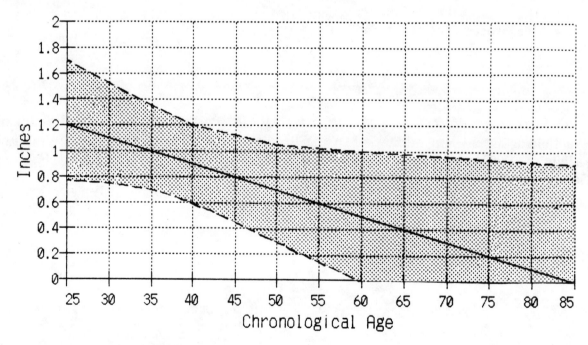

Fig. B. 4-6. **Near visual acuity** (Shimokata).

5. NEUROPSYCHOLOGICAL

5-1. Finger dexterity.

a. O'Connor pegboard test (*Fig. B. 5-1*). An O' Connor Pegboard (Appendix A. 5-1) is used. The object is to place three pins in each hole. The score is the total number of holes correctly filled in four minutes.

b. Purdue pegboard test (*Figs. B. 5-2 to 5-3*). A modified (all but the first 10 holes are covered with tape) Purdue pegboard (Appendix A. 5-2) is used. The subject fills the 10 holes with a pin, sleeve and washer. The score is the time required in seconds to fill the holes.

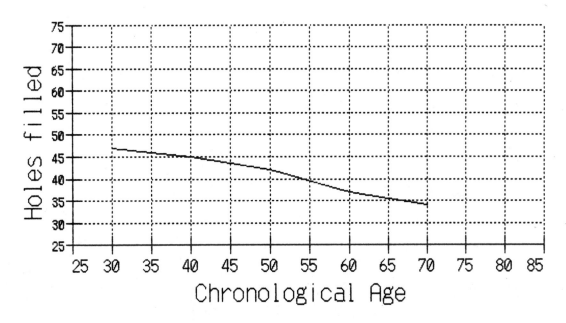

Fig. B. 5-1. **O'Connor pegboard test of finger dexterity – men and women** (Morgan and Wilson).

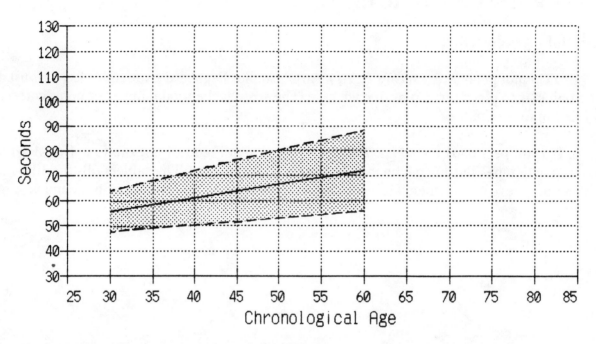

Fig. B. 5-2. **Modified Purdue pegboard test of Finger dexterity — men** (Suominen, 1 Apr 1986).

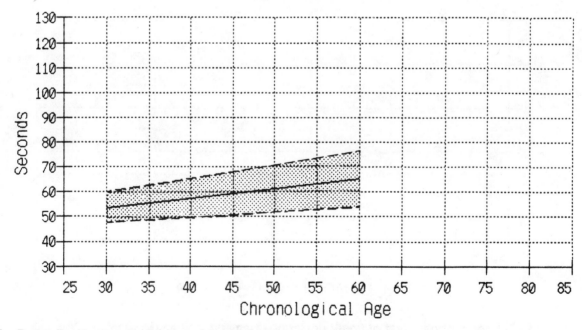

Fig. B. 5-3. **Purdue pegboard test of finger dexterity — women** (Suominen, 1 Apr 1986).

5-2. Hand steadiness (*Fig. B. 5-4*). Using the hand steadiness measuring device (Appendix A. 5-3), the subject stands with the arm unsupported, holding the brass pin like a pencil. Beginning at the largest hole, he inserts the pin into progressively smaller holes. Contact between the pin and brass plate causes a light to flash. The test continues until two consecutive holes are missed. The score is the number of the last correctly performed hole.

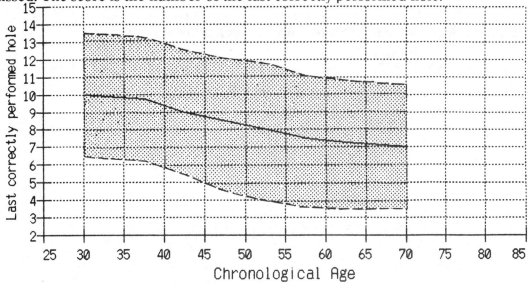

Fig. B. 5-4. **Hand steadiness — men** (Dirken).

5-3. Picture recognition (GIT pictures) (*Fig. B. 5-5*). This test uses 20 GIT test cards from the Dutch Intelligence Test (Appendix A. 5-4). The picture must be correctly identified within 30 seconds. The test is stopped after two consecutive pictures are missed. The score is the number of the last correctly identified picture.

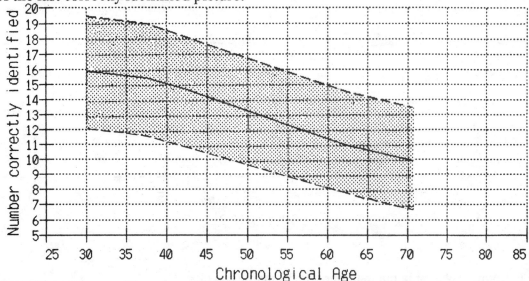

Fig. B. 5-5. **Picture recognition — men** (Dirken).

5-4. Concentration:

a. Bourdon-Wiersma test (*Fig. B. 5-6*). Using the Bourdon-Wiersma test sheets (Appendix A. 5-5), the subject strikes out the 4 and 5 dot groups, with horizontal lines for the 4-dot groups, and vertical lines for the 5-dot groups. A trial with a practice sheet is conducted, completing only two lines. The subject is then given a test sheet and works as fast as possible until told to stop. The score is the number of lines completed in 4 minutes.

b. Landolt "C" test (*Figs. B. 5-7 and 5-8*). Using the Landolt test sheet (Appendix A. 5-6), the subject marks all "Cs" with the opening at the top. The score is the time in seconds needed to complete the sheet, and number of errors.

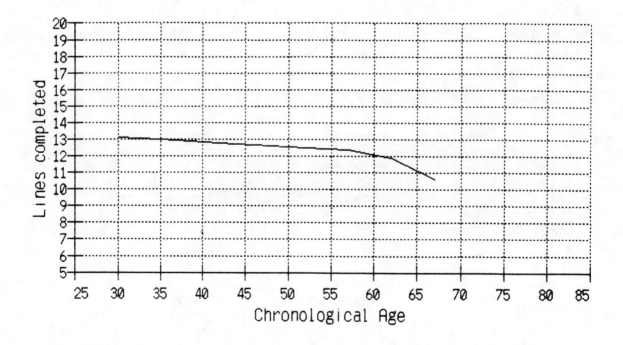

Fig. B. 5-6. **Bourdon-Wiersma concentration test — men** (Dirken).

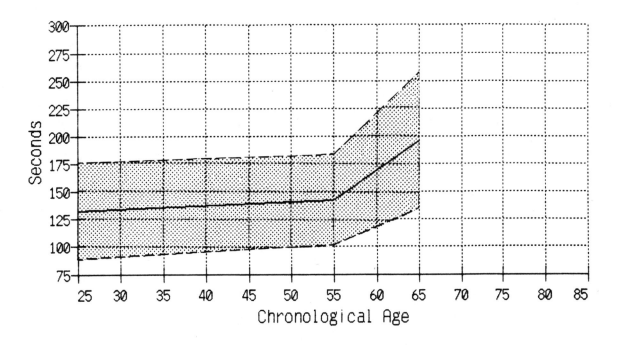

Fig. B. 5-7. **Landolt concentration test — men** (Ries; Poethig).

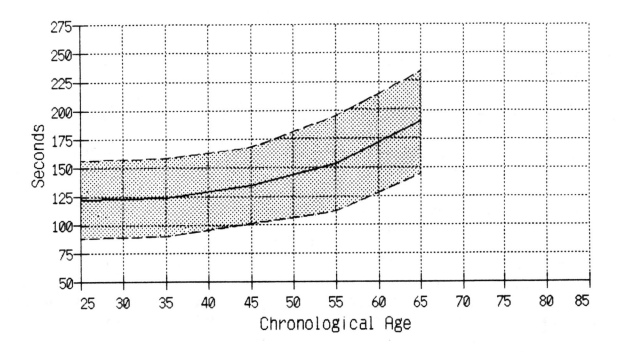

Fig. B. 5-8. **Landolt concentration test — women** (Ries; Poethig).

5-5. Categorization (*Fig. B. 5-9*). This test assesses ability to classify nouns according to subject (Table 7-1). Categories are: animals, objects, professions, and towns. The test device in Appendix A. 5-7, and a tape recorder are used. The words are played back at intervals varying from 4-8 seconds. The object is to categorize them by pressing one of the 4 buttons. An electronic timer starts as each word is spoken, and reaction times are recorded. Reactions taking longer than 2 seconds are counted as wrong. The score is the number of wrong answers.

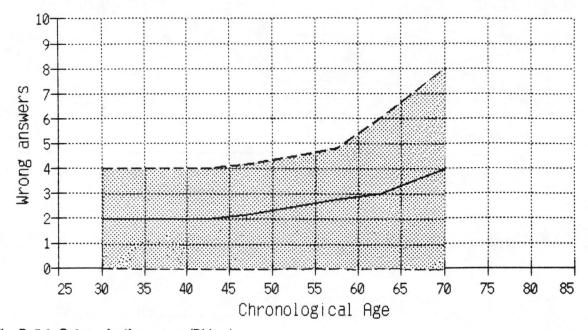

Fig. B. 5-9. **Categorization — men** (Dirken).

5-6. Vibratory sensitivity, measured using a vibrometer (Appendix A. 5-8) and recorded in volts or decibels (depending on the test) (*Figs. B. 5-10 to 5-13*). In addition to the aging-induced decrease in vibratory sensitivity, other causes of decreased sensation include diseases such as diabetes, and some occupational conditions from long-term use of vibrating machines like jack-hammers or motorcycles.

With the subject lying comfortably on an examining table, the vibrometer is turned to 20 volts. The tip is placed on the left great toe to demonstrate the vibratory sensation. The vibrometer tip is held lightly on the left medial or lateral malleolus (left inner or outer ankle), or index finger (depending on which test battery is being used). The amplitude of vibration is then slowly increased from zero to the point at which vibration is just perceptable. This point is recorded from the scale on the vibrometer in volts. The value in decibels or arbitrary unts can be obtained (if required) from the conversion chart in *Figs. B. 5-10 and 5-11*, respectively.

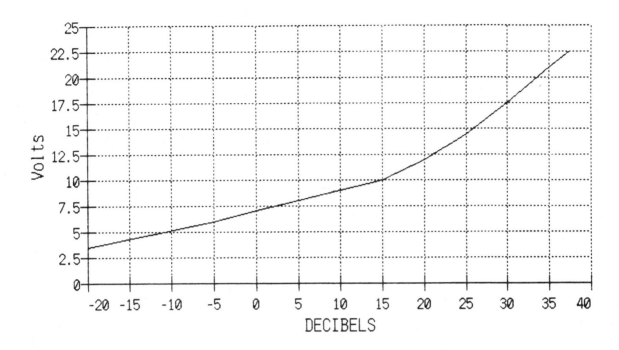

Fig. B. 5-10. **Conversion chart for transforming vibratory thresholds in volts to decibels**, based on comparitive data from Furukawa, et al, and Bloom, et al.

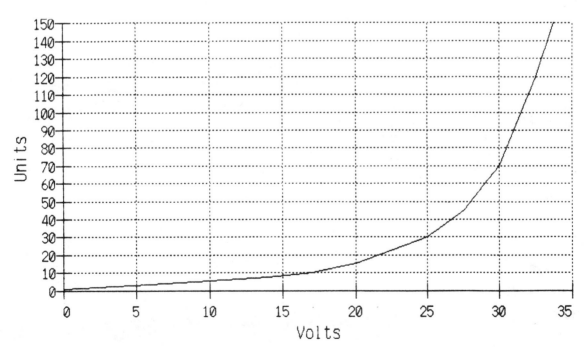

Fig. B. 5-11. **Conversion chart for transforming vibratory theresholds in volts to arbitrary units**, based on comparitive data from Heikkinen, et al, and Bloom, et al.

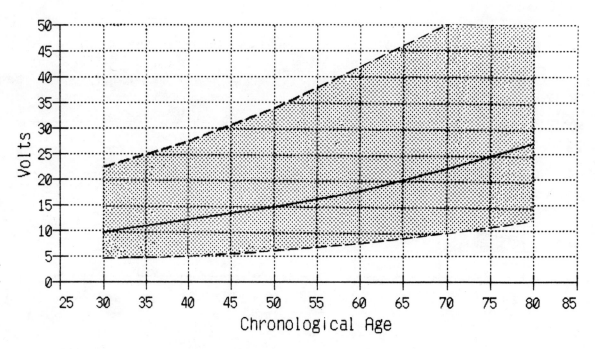

Fig. B. 5-12. **Vibratory sensitivity of the medial malleolus** (Bloom, et al).

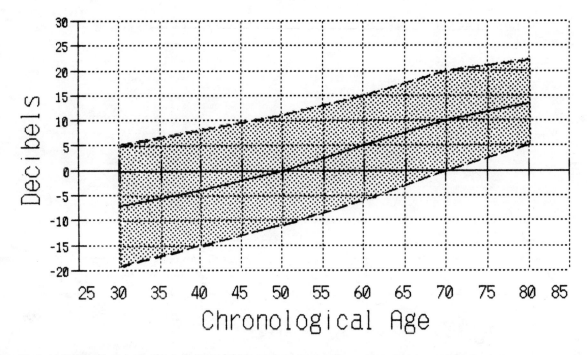

Fig. B. 5-13. **Vibratory sensitivity of the index fingers – men – in decibels** (Furukawa).

5-7. Tapping rate:

a. Hand tally counter (*Fig. B. 5-14*). This test measures nerve conduction velocity and neuro-muscular coordination using the hand tally counter (Appendix A. 5-9). The score is the maximum number of taps in 30 seconds, using the index finger of the dominant hand.

b. GRC tapping test (*Figs. B. 5-15 and 5-16*). A special tapping board (Appendix A. 5-11) is used in this test. At the signal to start, the subject taps with the metal stylus from one target to the other until a total of 50 taps are made on each target. The unit of measure is the time in minutes required to complete the 100 taps.

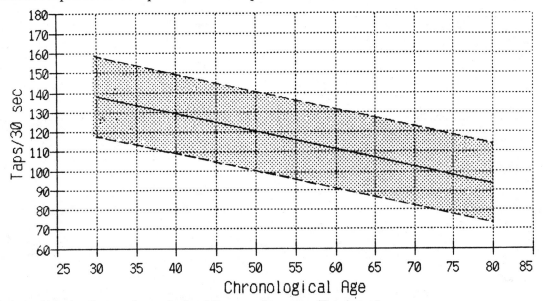

Fig. B. 5-14. **Hand tally tapping rate for 30 seconds—men** (Furukawa).

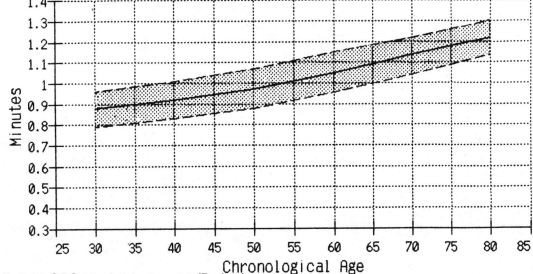

Fig. B. 5-15. **GRC tapping test—men** (Borkan).

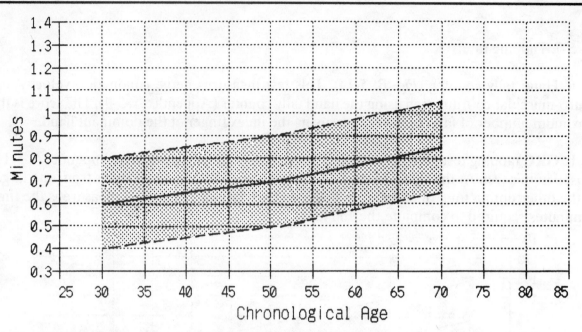

Fig. B. 5-16. **GRC tapping test — women** (Dean, unpublished data).

5-8. Digit Symbol test (*Fig. B. 5-17*), a subtest of the Wechsler Adult Intelligence Scale (Appendix A. 5-11). It consists of a set of symbols (such as: -, o, _, u, o, x, =), each of which represents a number. The score sheet displays the numbers and their symbols, and a series of numbers in random order. The subject writes the symbols adjacent to the numbers they represent during 90 seconds. The score is the number of correct responses.

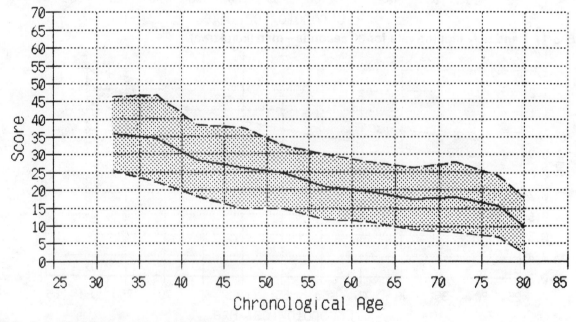

Fig. B. 5-17. **Digit Symbol test** (Berkowitz).

5-9. Short term memory (*Fig. B. 5-18*). This is a nonstandard memory test similar to the Rey Auditory Verbal Learning Test (Taylor). The examiner reads a series of ten words (selected from Table 14-I) to the subject. This is repeated ten times. Immediately after each repetition, the subject writes down as many words as he can recall (each repetition on a separate sheet of paper). The score is the total number of words recalled.

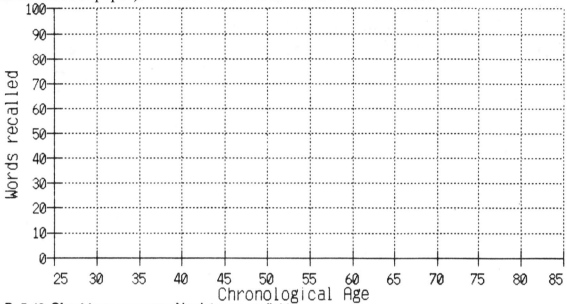

Fig. B. 5-18. **Short term memory.** No data are available.

5-10. Block design (*Fig. B. 5-19*). This is a subtest of the Wechsler Adult Intelligence Scale (WAIS). Colored blocks (Appendix A. 5-15) are arranged to form designated designs.

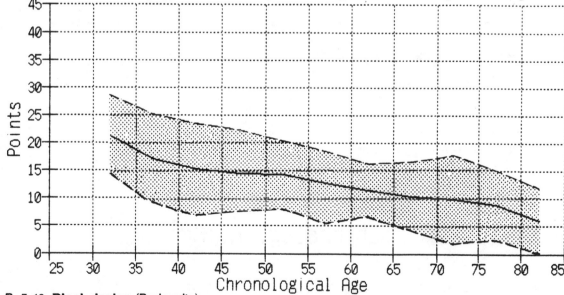

Fig. B. 5-19. **Block design** (Berkowitz).

5-11. Static Balance Test:

a. Standing unsupported on the left leg (Fig. B. 5-20). The subject stands on his left leg, hands on hips, with eyes closed. The test is repeated three times at 5 minute intervals. The score is the longest duration in seconds that he can stand without losing his balance.

b. Biomechanical force platform (Appendix A. 5-14) (*Fig. B. 5-21*). The subject stands on the platform in bare feet, feet slightly apart, hands extended to the front, eyes closed, standing as steady as he can. The force platform senses forward and sideward sway. The value in the equation is: total extent of sway in mm for 8 seconds, multiplied by 175 cm, divided by the subject's height in cm.

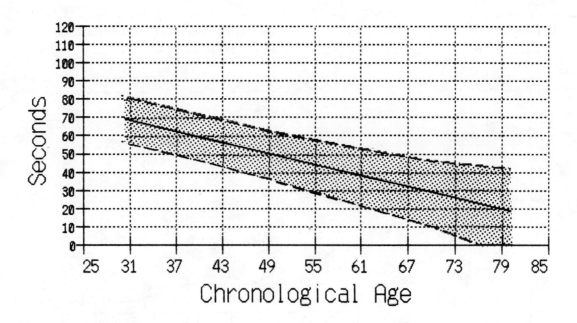

Fig. B. 5-20. **Static Balance test on one leg** (Shimokata).

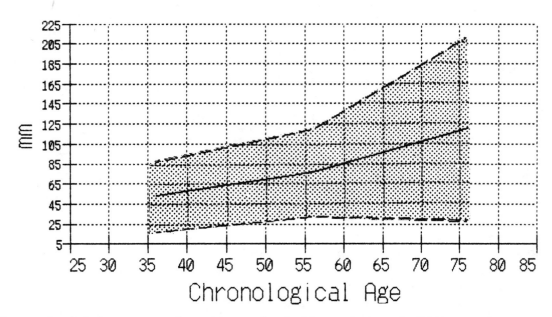

Fig. B. 5-21. **Static balance test using a bio-mechanical force platform** (Heikkinen, et al).

5-12. Stroop color-word test (*Figs. B. 5-22 and 5-23*). This is a test of mental flexibility involving "color-word" reading and color-naming, using a color-word test set (Appendix A. 5-16). The task is to name the color of the ink of each word as quickly as possible. The three cards comprising the test are administered in order--card A, card B, and card C. The score is the total time in seconds for responding to the 30 items on each card (Comalli, et al).

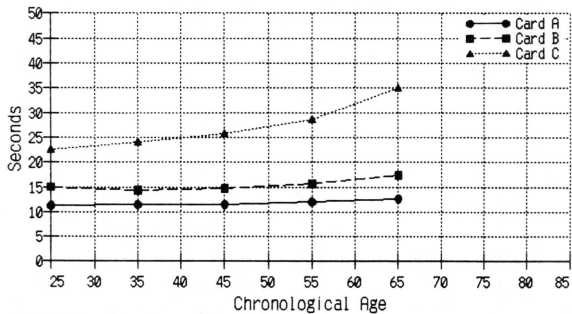

Fig. B. 5-22. **Color-word test — men** (Ries; Poethig).

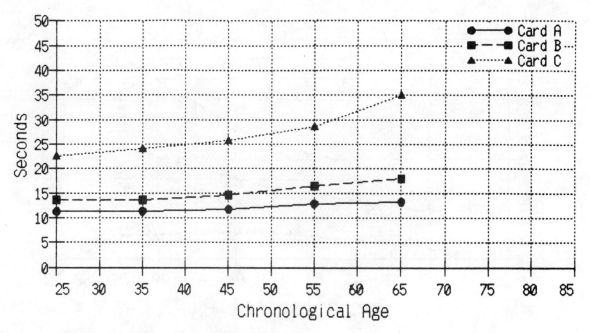

Fig. B. 5-23. **Color-word test — women** (Ries; Poethig).

5-13. Reaction time:

a. 3 and 4-choice reaction time (*Figs. B. 5-24 to 5-26*). Using the choice reaction test device (Appendix A. 5-12), lights are automatically turned on randomly, one at a time. An electronic timer starts when each light is turned on, and stops when the corresponding button is pressed, turning the light off. The test is repeated 5 times, and the score is the average of the reaction times in each trial.

b. "Bogitch" light extinction time (*Figs. B. 5-27 and 5-28*). The Bogitch light extinction device is used (Appendix A. 5-13). The test begins with one light already turned on. When the subject presses the switch beneath the light, turning it off, the timer begins and another light turns on. The sequence is repeated ten times, and the total time necessary to extinguish all the lights is measured, in seconds.

Sub-tests Appendix B

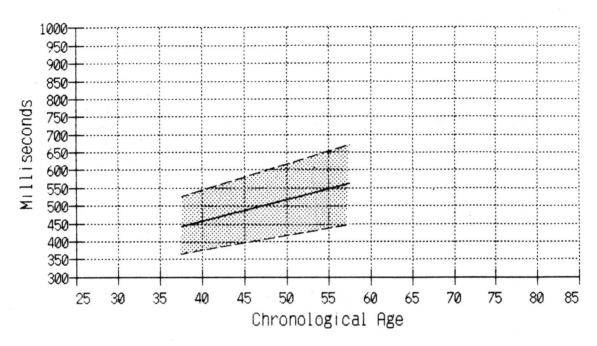

Fig. B. 5-24. **3-choice reaction time – men** (Heikkinen, 26 June 1985).

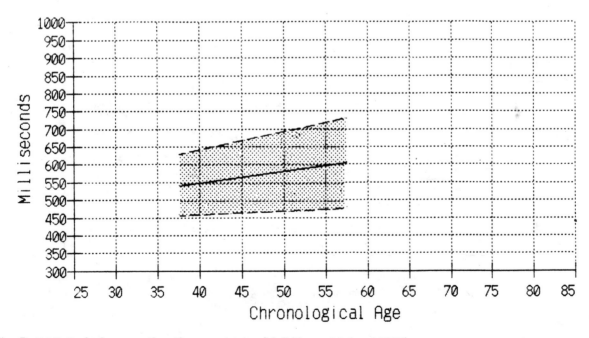

Fig. B. 5-25. **3-choice reaction time – women** (Heikkinen, 26 June 1985).

Appendix B   **Sub-tests**

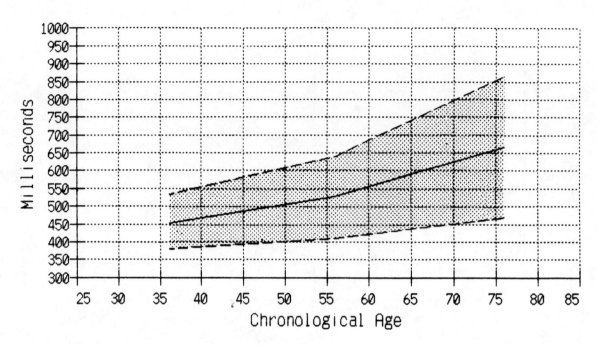

Fig. B. 5-26. **4-choice reaction time — men** (Dirken).

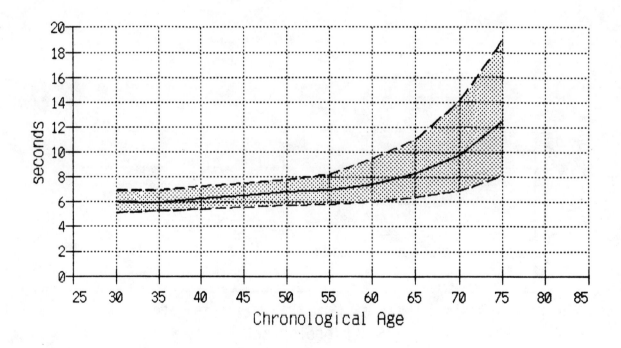

Fig. B. 5-27. **Light extinction time — men** (Hollingsworth).

340

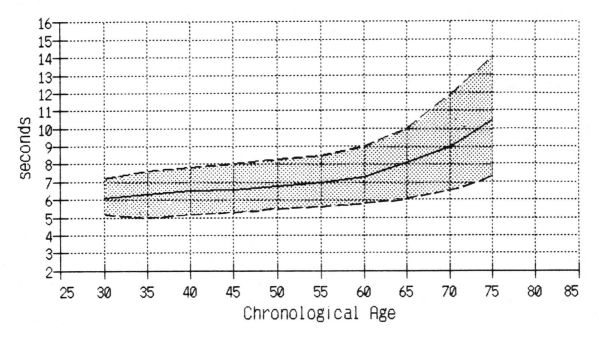

Fig. B. 5-28. **Light extinction time – women** (Hollingsworth).

5-14. Geromat™ tests: The following tests are conducted with a Geromat™, described in detail in Chapter 17.

a. Light reaction time (RTL). The subject extinguishes a light by pressing a button as soon as the light is turned on. The score is the mean value in msec of ten trials.

b. Clock reaction time (RTC). A clock second hand is set in motion. The subject stops the hand at zero by pressing a button. The score is the deviation from zero (left or right) in msec.

c. Auditory reaction time (RTA). The subject switches off a sound as quickly as possible by pressing a button. The score is the mean value in msec of ten trials.

d. Hand-eye coordination. Using a writing table with a meandering engraved guide line, the subject follows the line with an electronic pen. The values scored are the time in seconds (Vt) and number of errors (Ve).

e. Stepping-stone maze. This test uses a special keyboard with an array of 10 rows of 10 buttons. The object of the test is to travel from the start button to a fixed final button, over an irregular path. Three different "trails" are used. The Geromat™ records the total time required (Maz_{t1}) in seconds, the total number of buttons required to complete the three pathways (without repeating wrong buttons) (Maz_A), sum of repeated errors (Maz_B), and the mean time needed for one step (Maz_{t2}) in seconds. $Maz_{t2} = Maz_{t1}/Maz_A + Maz_B$.

f. Tapping rate. Using a Geromat™, the subject taps continuously with a "telegraph key" type counter for two minutes. The tapping rate is determined over a series of 10-second intervals, with 8.33-second pauses interspersed between the test periods. The mean tapping rate in taps per second is recorded for the first (TR_1), second (TR_2), sixth (TR_6) and seventh (TR_7) periods.

6. ANTHROPOMETRIC

6-1. Grayness of hair (*Figs. B. 6-1 and 6-2*). For the population as a whole grayness is the anthropometric parameter having the best correlation with chronological age. Unfortunately, it is also one of the most difficult to quantify precisely. There is no standard measurement scale.

For Damon's test battery (Chapter 6), grayness is rated on an arbitrary scale from 0 to 5. No gray hair whatsoever is "0", slight presence of gray is "1", and grayness in the amounts of 1/4, 1/2, 3/4, and complete, are "2" through "5", respectively.

For Shimokata's test battery (Chapter 18), grayness is rated "1" (less than 10%, "2" (10-50%), or "3" (more than 50%).

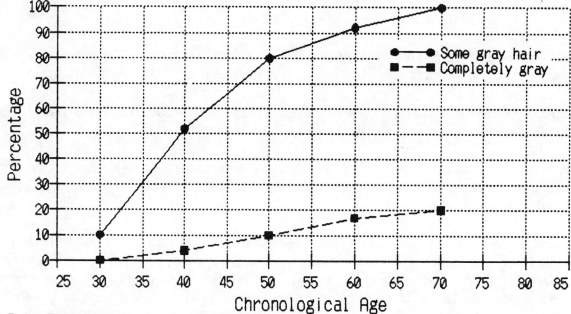

Fig. B. 6-1. **Rate of hair graying for 3872 Australian men and women** (Keogh and Walsh).

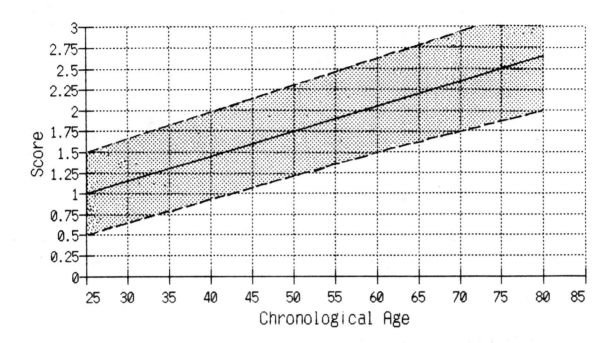

Fig. B. 6-2. **Rate of hair graying** (Shimokata).

6-2. Handgrip strength (*Figs. B. 6-3 to 6-5*), measured with a dynamometer (Appendix A. 6-1), and recorded in kg. It reflects overall muscle mass and strength.

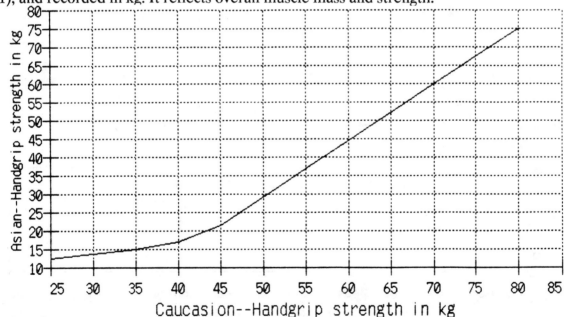

Fig. B. 6-3. **Handgrip strength conversion scale**, based on comparative age-adjusted data from Furukawa, et al, and Borkan and Norris.

Appendix B — Sub-tests

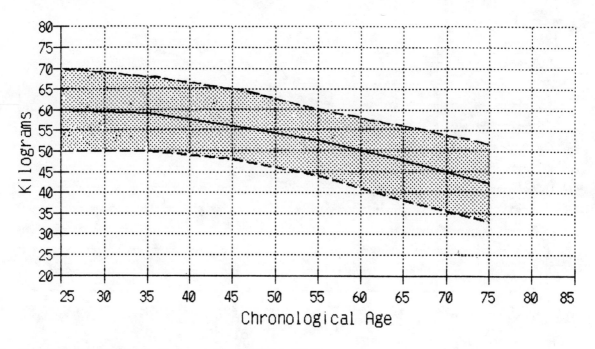

Fig. B. 6-4. **Handgrip strength — men** (Damon et al, 1972).

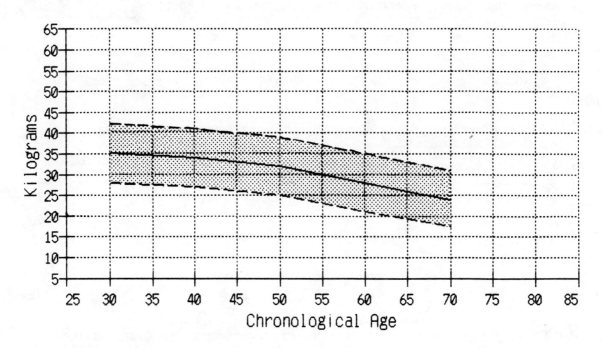

Fig. B. 6-5. **Handgrip strength — women** (Dean, unpublished data).

6-3. Ear breadth (*Figs. B. 6-6 and 6-7*) measures cartilage growth, which continues throughout life. With the subject sitting, the fixed arm of a sliding caliper (Appendix A. 6-2) is placed parallel to the long axis of the ear, and the maximum breadth of the ear is measured, in mm.

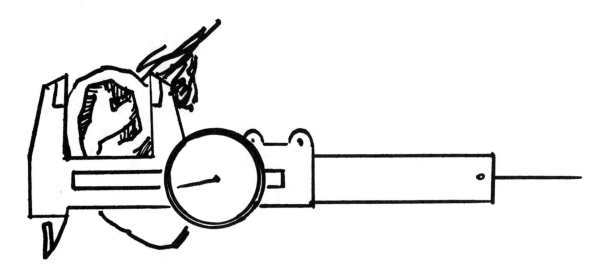

Fig. B. 6-6. **Technique for measuring ear breadth** (Redrawn from Herzberg).

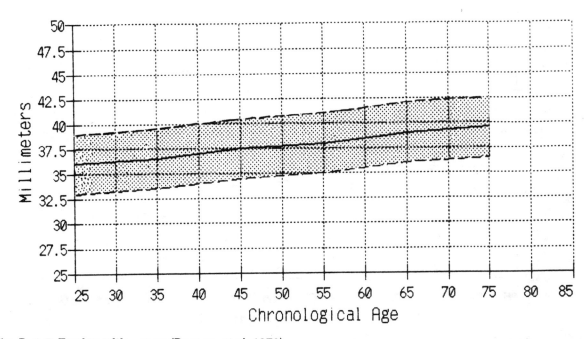

Fig. B. 6-7. **Ear breadth—men** (Damon, et al, 1972).

6-4. Sitting height (*Figs. B. 6-8 and 6-9*) decreases with age as the intervertebral disks lose water and shrink. The subject sits erect on a wooden bench, with buttocks, shoulders and back of the head against the wall. Use a tape measure and draftsman's triangle to measure the vertical distance from the sitting surface to the top of the head, in mm.

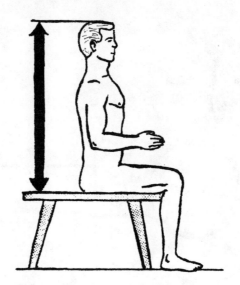

Fig. B. 6-8. **Technique for measuring sitting height** (Redrawn from Herzberg).

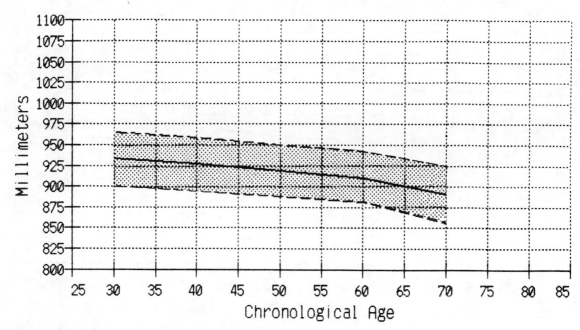

Fig. B. 6-9. **Sitting height — men** (Friedlander, et al).

6-5. Ear length (*Figs. B. 6-10 and 6-11*). This is another measurement of the growth of cartilage. Use the sliding caliper to measure the maximum length of the subject's right ear along its long axis, in mm.

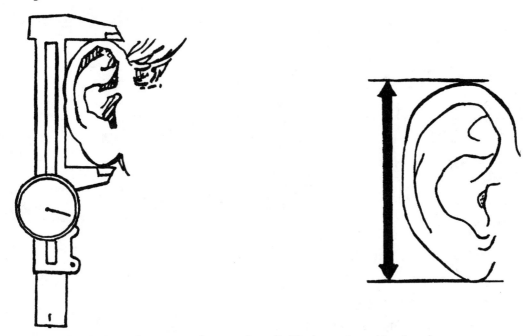

Fig. B. 6-10. **Technique for measuring ear length** (Redrawn from Herzberg).

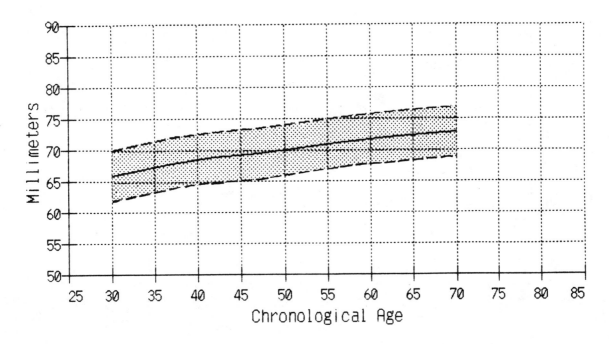

Fig. B. 6-11. **Ear length — men** (Friedlander, et al).

6-6. Nose breadth (*Figs. B. 6-12 and 6-13*) is another measurement of cartilage growth. Use the sliding caliper to measure the maximum horizontal breadth of the nose, in mm.

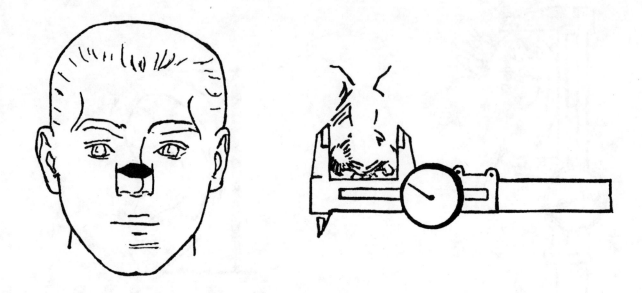

Fig. B. 6-12. **Technique for measuring nose breadth** (Redrawn from Herzberg).

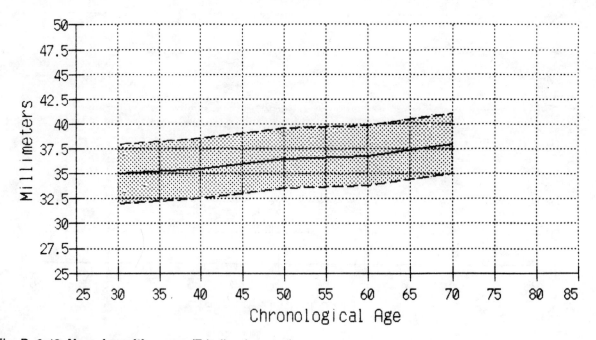

Fig. B. 6-13. **Nose breadth — men** (Friedlander, et al).

6-7. **Bideltoid breadth (shoulder breadth)** (*Figs. B. 6-14 and 6-15*) decreases with age, reflecting a loss of fat and muscle mass. The subject sits erect with his upper arms hanging at his sides and his lower arms extended forward horizontally, hands resting on the thighs. Measure the horizontal distance across the maximum lateral protrusions of the right and left deltoid muscles with the anthropometric caliper (Appendix A. 6-2), in mm.

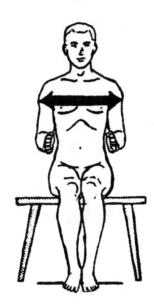

Fig. B. 6-14. **Technique for measuring bideltoid breadth** (Redrawn from Herzberg).

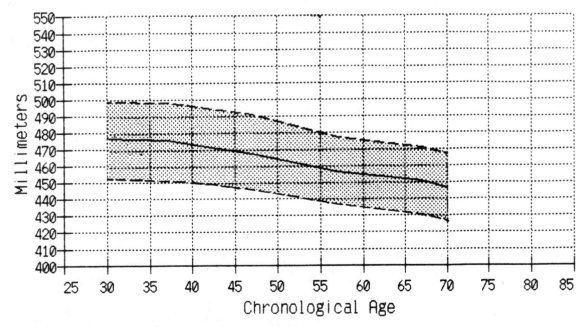

Fig. B. 6-15. **Bideltoid breadth — men** (Friedlander, et al).

6-8. Abdominal depth (*Figs. B. 6-16 and 6-17*) increases with age, due to the internal deposition of fat and loss of muscle tone of the abdominal musculature. The subject stands, with his abdomen relaxed, right hand on his left shoulder. Hold the anthropometer on the subject's right side, and measure the horizontal body depth at the level of the center of the umbilicus, in mm.

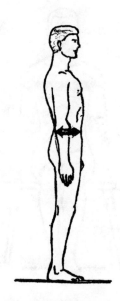

Fig. B. 6-16. **Technique for measuring abdominal depth** (Redrawn from Herzberg).

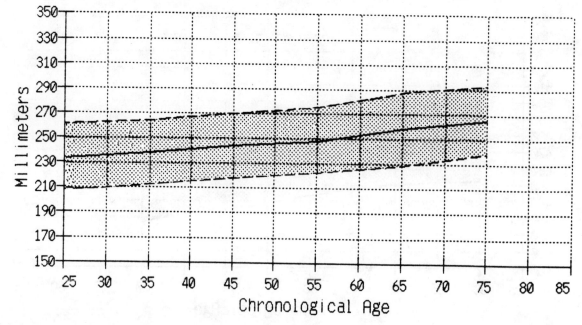

Fig. B. 6-17. **Abdominal depth — men** (Damon, et al, 1972).

6-9. Triceps skinfold thickness (*Figs. B. 6-18 and 6-19*) decreases with age, reflecting a loss of fat late in life. Use a standard skinfold caliper (Appendix A. 6-4), to measure a vertical skinfold of the right triceps, in mm.

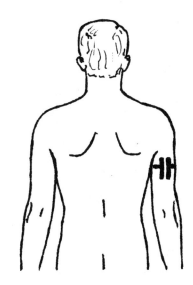

Fig. B. 6-18. **Technique for measuring triceps skinfold thickness** (Redrawn from Herzberg).

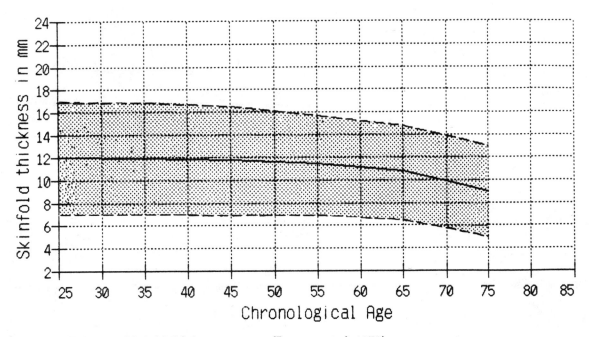

Fig. B. 6-19. **Triceps skinfold thickness — men** (Damon, et al, 1972).

Appendix B — Sub-tests

6-10. Baldness (*Figs. B. 6-20 and 6-21*). Like grayness, there is no universal standard of measurement. For Damon's test battery (Chapter 6), baldness is rated on an arbitrary scale from 0 to 5. No hair loss at all is "0", slight thinning is "1", and baldness in the amounts of 1/4, 1/2, 3/4, and complete, are "2" through "5", respectively. For Shimokata's test battery (Chapter 18), baldness is rated "1" (less than 10%), "2" (10-50%), or "3" (more than 50%).

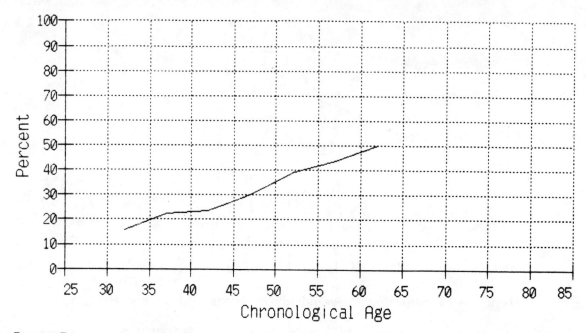

Fig. B. 6-20. **Percent of men showing some degree of baldness** (Hamilton).

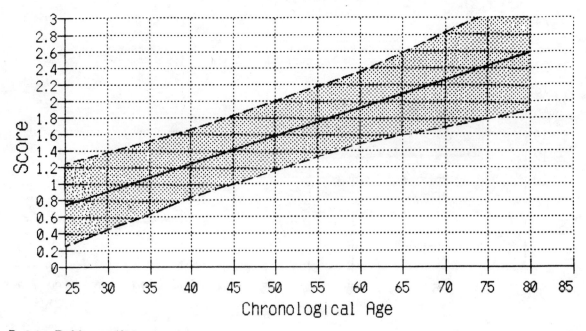

Fig. B. 6-21. **Baldness** (Shimokata).

6-11. Body flexibility, in degrees (*Figs. B. 6-22 to 6-25*), is determined for Furukawa's test batteries (Chapter 9) by measuring the angles of bending the trunk in the anterior (anteflexion), posterior (retroflexion), and lateral (sideflexion) directions, with a goniometer (Appendix A. 6-8).

Shimokata (Chapter 18) uses a different scale for anteflexion. The subject bends forward at the waist, and attempts to touch his toes. The score is the distance in cm the subject can extend his fingertips beyond his toes. A Digital Flexibility Tester (Appendix A. 6-7) can be used for this test. Inability to touch the toes is scored by a minus number.

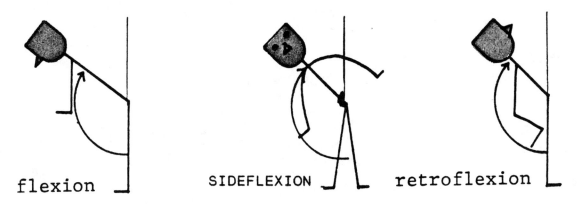

Fig. B. 6-22. **Body flexibility — angles to be measured**. (Furukawa, 1985).

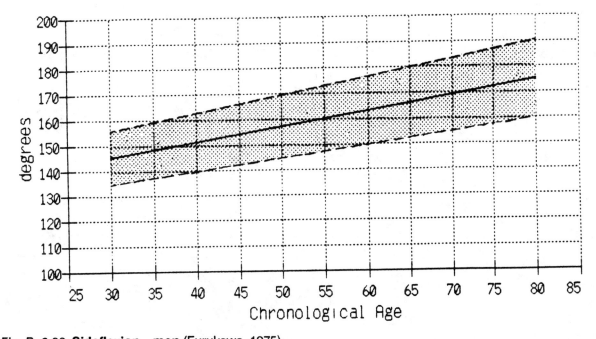

Fig. B. 6-23. **Sideflexion — men** (Furukawa, 1975).

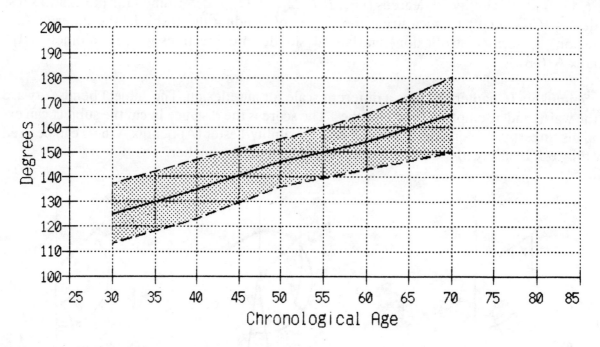

Fig. B. 6-24. **Retroflexion — men** (Furukawa, 1975).

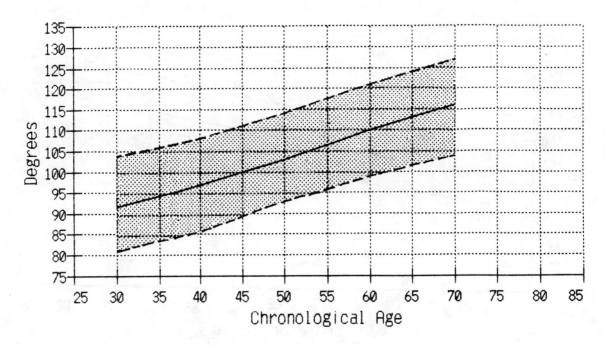

Fig. B. 6-25. **Anteflexion — men** (Furukawa, 1975).

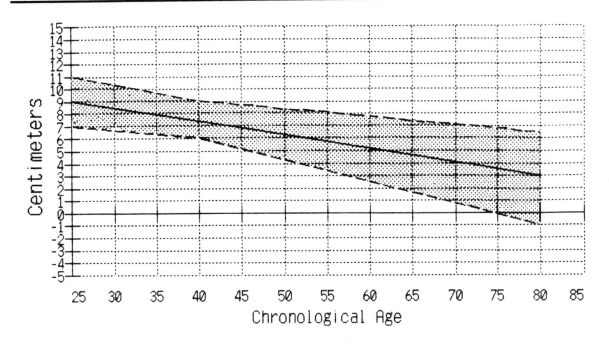

Fig. B. 6-26. **Anteflexion — men** (Shimokata).

6-12. Skin elasticity (*Figs. B. 6-27 and 6-28*). Pinch the skin on the back of the hand with a skinfold caliper (Appendix A. 6-4) for one minute, and measure the time for the skinfold to retract to the surrounding skin surface. The exact endpoint is sometimes difficult to measure in older people. If the fold does not retract completely in 90 seconds, this maximum time measurement is used.

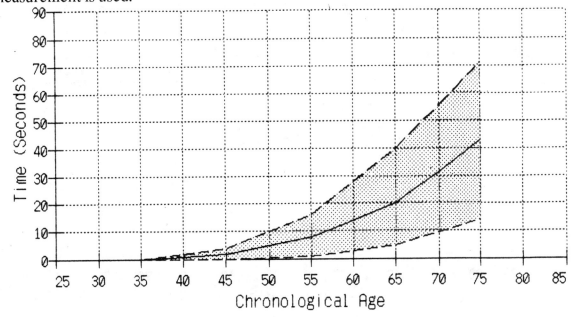

Fig. B. 6-27. **Skin elasticity — men** (Hollingsworth).

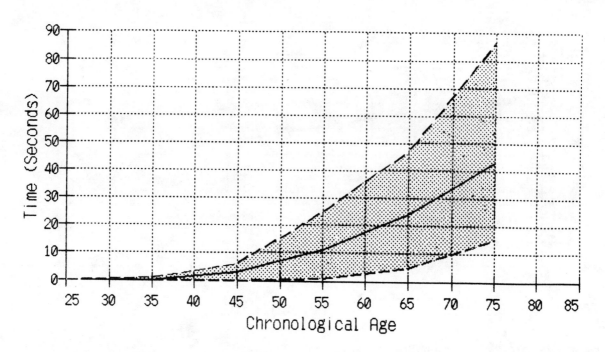

Fig. B. 6-28. **Skin elasticity — women** (Hollingsworth).

6-13. Height, in cm (*Fig. B. 6-29*).

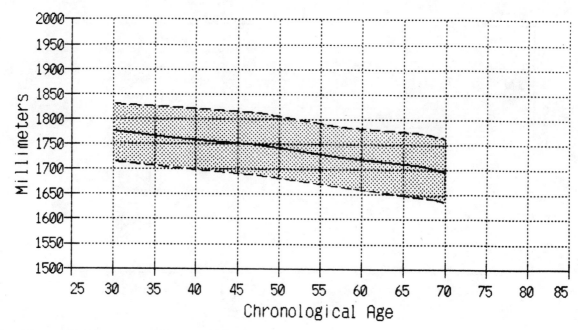

Fig. B. 6-29. **Height — men** (Friedlander, et al).

6-14. Weight, in kg (*Fig. B. 6-30*).

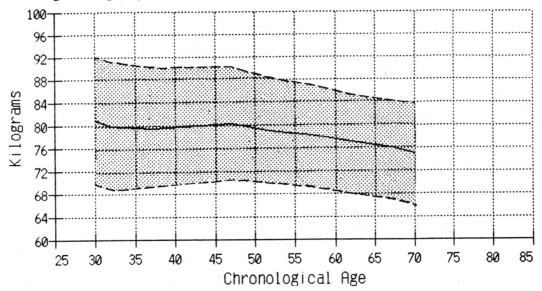

Fig. B. 6-30. **Weight — men** (Friedlander, et al).

6-15. Tendon extensibility (*Figs. B. 6-31 and 6-32*). The subject's forearm and hand (palm down) are placed on a table. A small-joint goniometer (Appendix A. 6-8) is held against the back of the hand, with the middle of the goniometer against the fifth metacarpo-phalangeal joint. The fifth finger is hyper-extended as far as possible, without causing pain. The angle between the extended finger and the table is determined. The test is repeated with both hands. The score is the sum of the values determined for both hands.

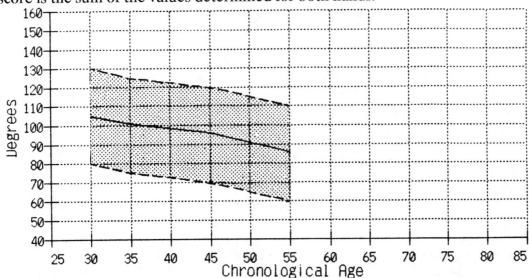

Fig. B. 6-31. **Sum of the tendon extensibility of the fifth fingers of both hands — men** (Emmrich and Schwarz).

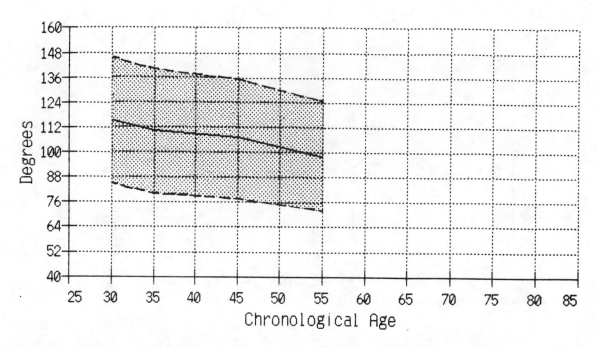

Fig. B. 6-32. **Sum of the tendon extensibility of the fifth fingers of both hands — women** (Emmrich and Schwarz).

7. DENTAL

7-1. Periodontal index (*Figs. B. 7-1 and 7-2*). This is a dental score, determined by a dentist. For this test, each tooth is scored on a scale according to the presence or absence of manifest signs of periodontal disease. When a portion of the free gingiva is overtly inflamed, a score of "1" is assigned. When completely circumscribed by inflammation, a tooth is scored "2". Teeth with frank periodontal pockets are scored "6" when their masticatory function is unimpaired, and "8" when it is impaired. In the absence of obvious signs of inflammation, pocket formation, and loss of function, teeth are given a score of "0". Each tooth in the mouth is scored, and the arithmetic average of all scores is the individual's Periodontal Index (Russel).

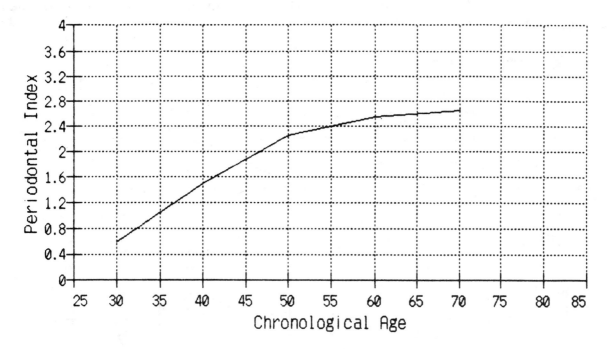

Fig. B. 7-1. **Periodontal Index – men** (Morgan and Wilson).

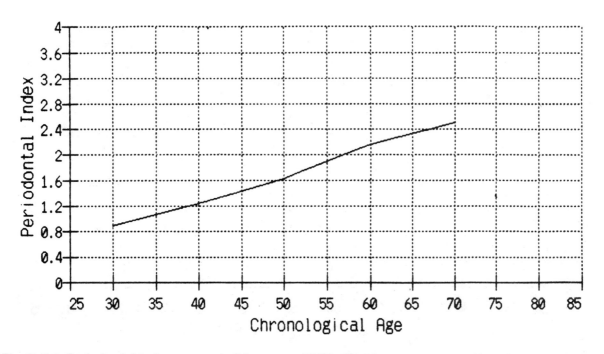

Fig. B. 7-2. **Periodontal Index – women** (Morgan and Wilson).

7-2. Caries index (*Figs. B. 7-3 and 7-4*). This is the total number of decayed, missing or filled teeth (DMF) (Morgan and Wilson).

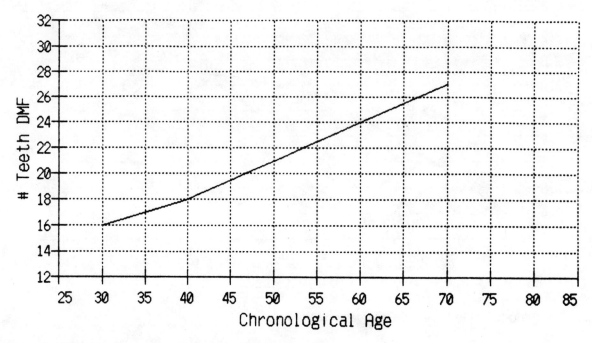

Fig. B. 7-3. **Caries Index — men** (Morgan and Wilson).

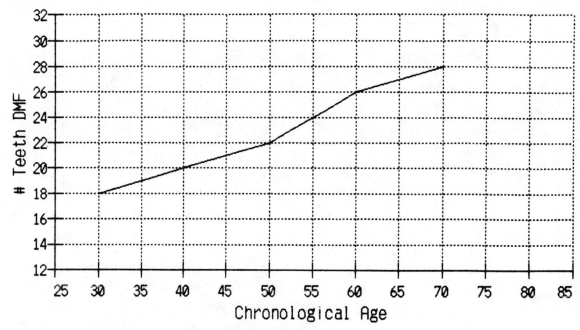

Fig. B. 7-4. **Caries Index — women** (Morgan and Wilson).

8. HEMATOLOGIC

8-1. Erythrocyte sedimentation rate (ESR) (*Figs. B. 8-1 and 8-2*), measured in mm per hour, using the Westergren technique. The ESR measures the rate at which red blood cells settle out of suspension in plasma during the first hour. It is a nonspecific reaction like fever or leukocytosis, and is a general manifestation of disease or tissue destruction. It can often supply objective evidence of disease at a time when other signs are lacking. It also measures the intensity of tissue destruction or repair. The cause of the sedimentation increase is not clear.

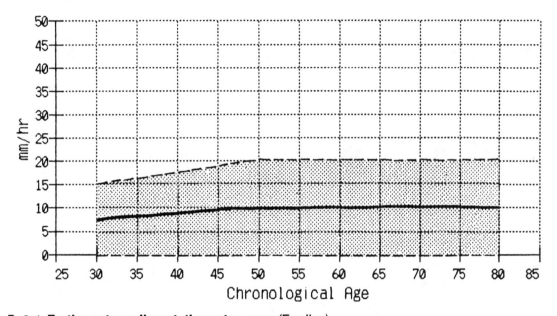

Fig. B. 8-1. **Erythrocyte sedimentation rate — men** (Fordice).

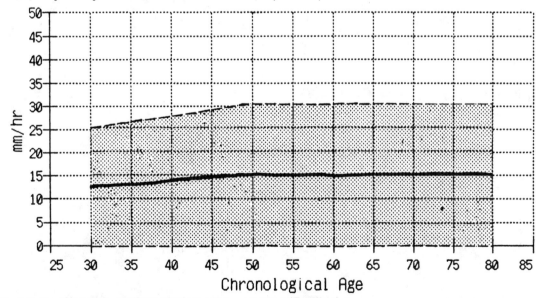

Fig. B. 8-2. **Erythrocyte sedimentation rate — women** (Fordice).

8-2. Hemoglobin (Hb) (*Figs. B. 8-3 and 8-4*).

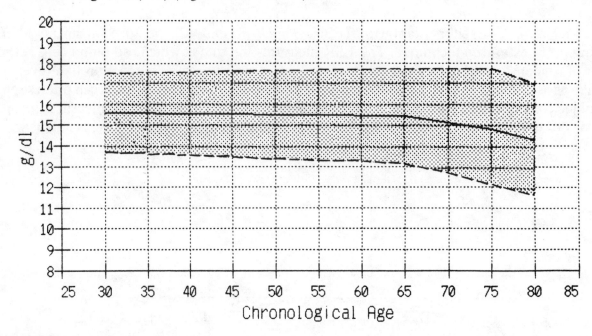

Fig. B. 8-3. **Hemoglobin — men** (Fordice).

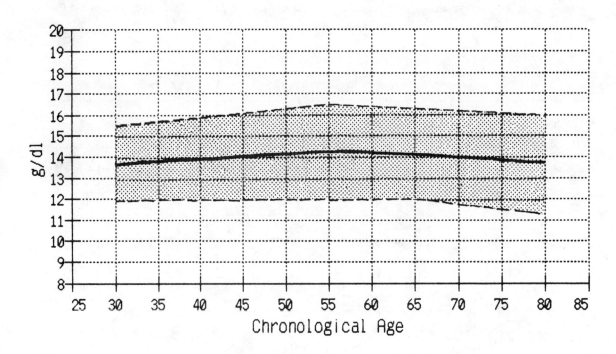

Fig. B. 8-4. **Hemoglobin — women** (Fordice).

8-3. Red blood cell count (RBC) (*Figs. B. 8-5 and 8-6*).

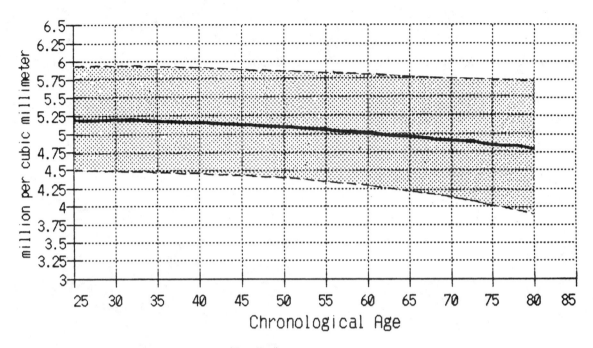

Fig. B. 8-5. **Red blood cell count — men** (Fordice).

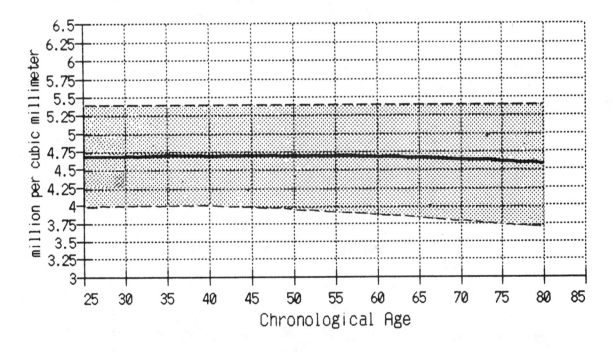

Fig. B. 8-6. **Red blood cell count — women** (Fordice).

Appendix B **Sub-tests**

9. BLOOD CHEMISTRY

9-1. Cholesterol (fasting) (*Figs. B. 9-1 and 9-2*). Cholesterol is manufactured by the liver, and is also supplied by the diet. Abnormally high levels have been implicated in heart disease, and abnormally low levels have been related to increases in mortality from other causes (Peterson, et al). Cholesterol is measured in mg per 100 ml (mg%). The optimum level appears to be about 160-180 mg% (Arends).

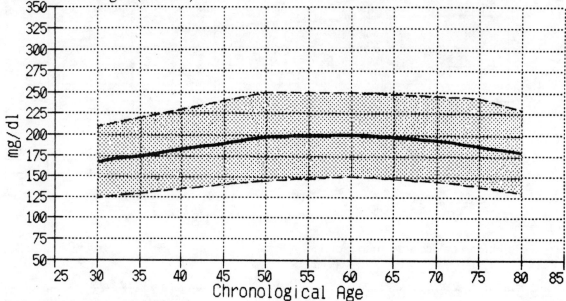

Fig. B. 9-1. **Cholesterol — men** (Fordice).

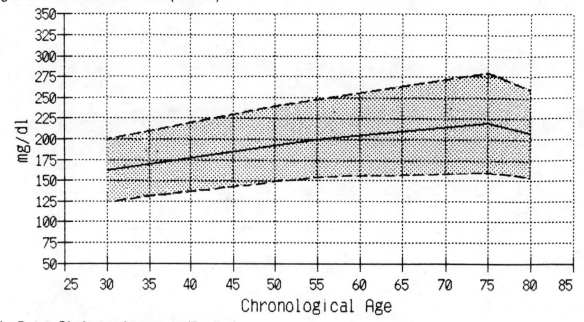

Fig. B. 9-2. **Cholesterol — women** (Fordice).

9-2. HDL cholesterol (*Figs. B. 9-3 and 9-4*). High Density Lipoprotein (HDL) cholesterol is a "good" type of cholesterol. Elevated HDL levels are protective against coronary artery disease. Normal levels for men are 30-65 mg/dl, and for women are 35-85 mg/dl.

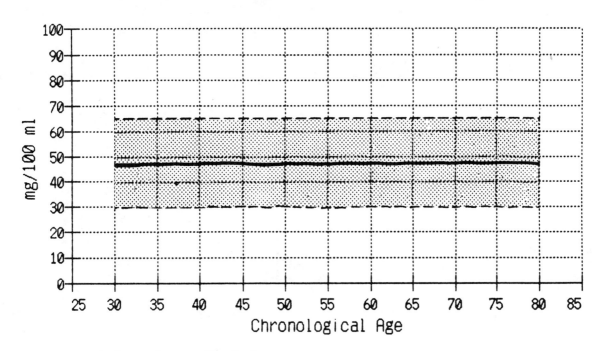

Fig. B. 9-3. **HDL cholesterol — men** (Fordice).

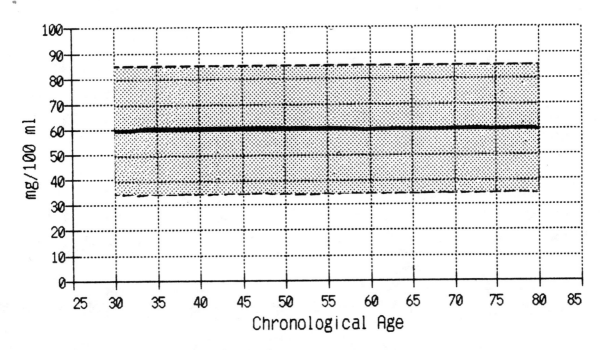

Fig. B. 9-4. **HDL cholesterol — women** (Fordice).

9-3. Triglycerides (*Figs. B. 9-5 and 9-6*). Triglycerides are a type of fat in the blood. Elevated levels are associated with an increased incidence of premature coronary artery disease and peripheral arterial disease. Normal levels should be less than 100 mg/100 ml, although some authors recommend less than 75 mg/100 ml as an optimum level (Arends).

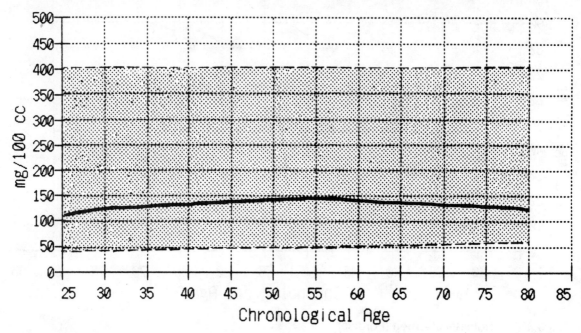

Fig. B. 9-5. **Triglycerides — men** (Fordice).

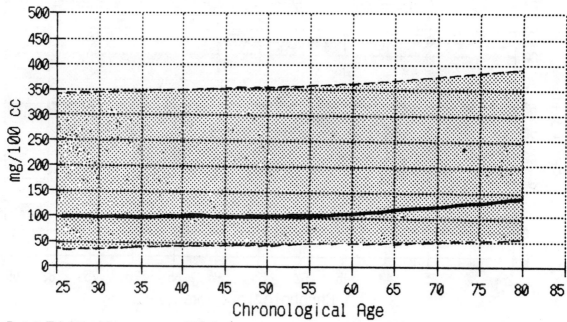

Fig. B. 9-6. **Triglycerides — women** (Fordice).

9-4. Glucose (*Figs. B. 9-7 and 9-8*). This should be conducted in the fasting state. Fasting glucose is an indicator of the body's ability to handle carbohydrates.

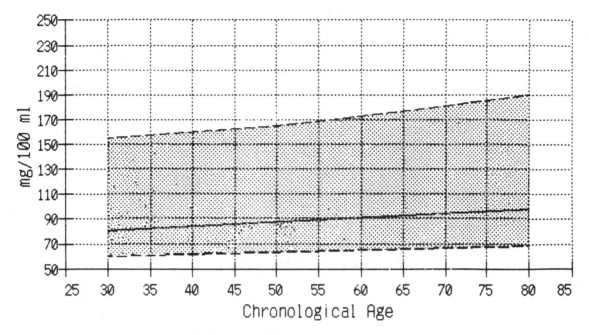

Fig. B. 9-7. **Glucose—men** (Gillibrand, et al).

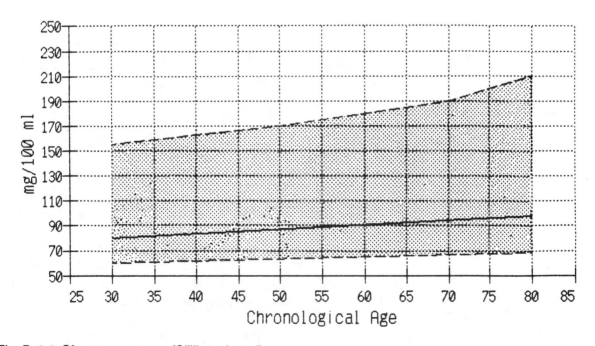

Fig. B. 9-8. **Glucose—women** (Gillibrand, et al).

9-5. Urea nitrogen (BUN) (*Figs. B. 9-9 and 9-10*). Urea is formed by the liver as a nitrogen excretion product. It is released into the blood and cleared by the kidneys. The concentration of urea nitrogen in the blood is thus a test of both liver and kidney function.

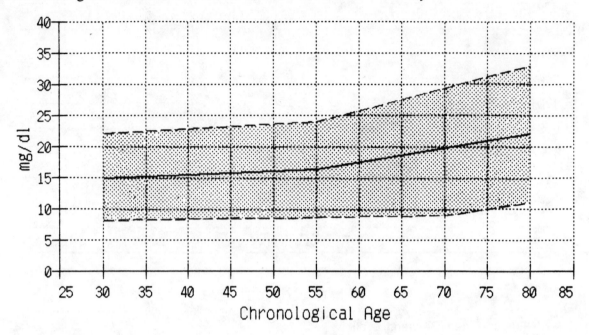

Fig. B. 9-9. **BUN — men** (Fordice).

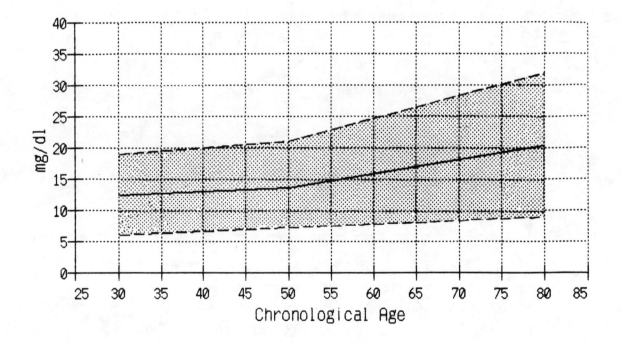

Fig. B. 9-10. **BUN — women** (Fordice).

9-6. Alkaline phosphatase (*Figs. B. 9-11 to 9-13*). This enzyme is normally measured in I.U. per liter, although Shimokata (Chapter 18) uses King-Armstrong units. Use the conversion scale in *Fig. B. 9-13* to convert from one system to the other. Alkaline phosphatase is made in the liver, bones, intestine and placenta, and may be increased or decreased in concentration in the blood as a result of bone or liver diseases.

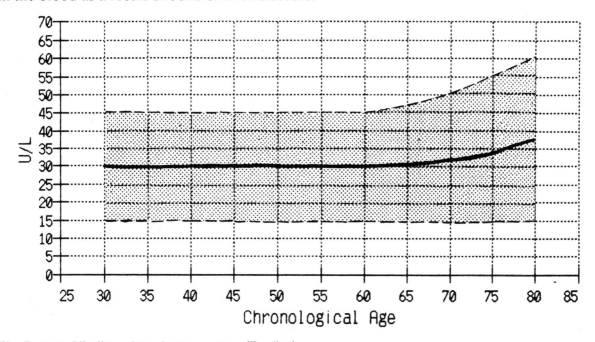

Fig. B. 9-11. **Alkaline phosphatase — men** (Fordice).

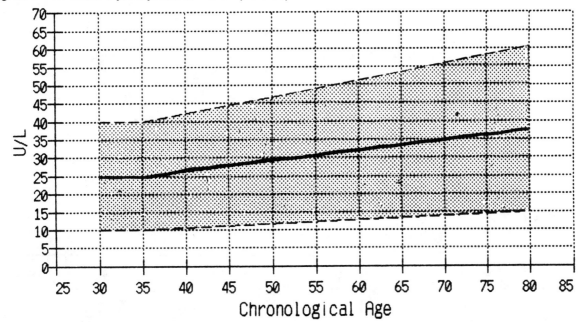

Fig. B. 9-12. **Alkaline phosphatase — women** (Fordice).

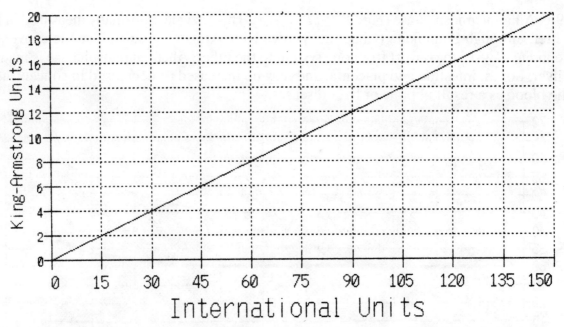

Fig. B. 9-13. **Conversion scale for converting King-Armstrong units** (for alkaline phosphatase) to International units.

9-7. Albumin (*Figs. B. 9-14 and 9-15*). Albumin is made in the liver, and is the most abundant of the plasma proteins. The plasma proteins comprise the major part of the solids of the blood plasma. An abnormally low albumin level generally indicates a reduction in the ability of the liver to synthesize plasma proteins.

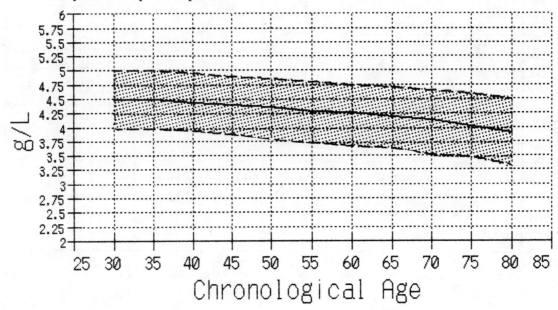

Fig. B. 9-14. **Albumin — men** (Fordice).

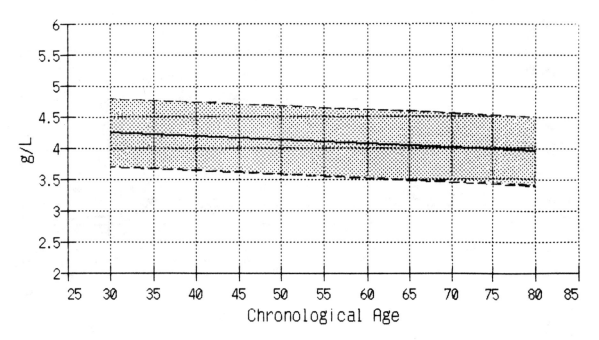

Fig. B. 9-15. **Albumin — women** (Fordice).

9-8. Glutamic Pyruvic Transaminase (SGPT) (*Figs. B. 9-16 and 9-17*), is an enzyme whose activity is elevated by liver diseases or myocardial infarction.

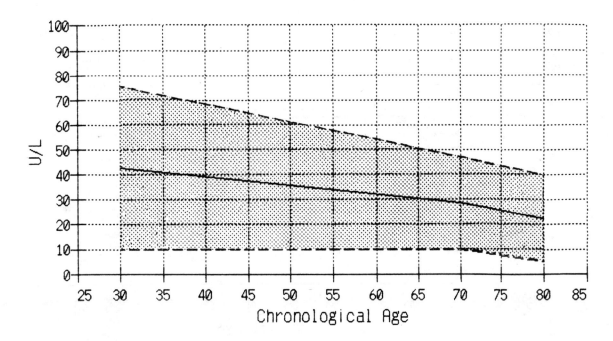

Fig. B. 9-16. **Glutamic pyruvic transaminase — men** (Fordice).

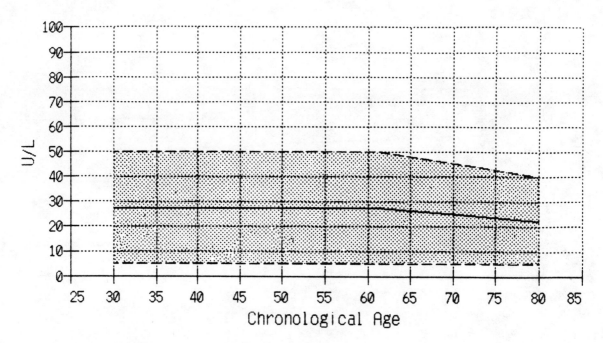

Fig. B. 9-17. **Glutamic pyruvic transaminase — women** (Fordice).

9-9. Calcium (*Fig. B. 9-18*).

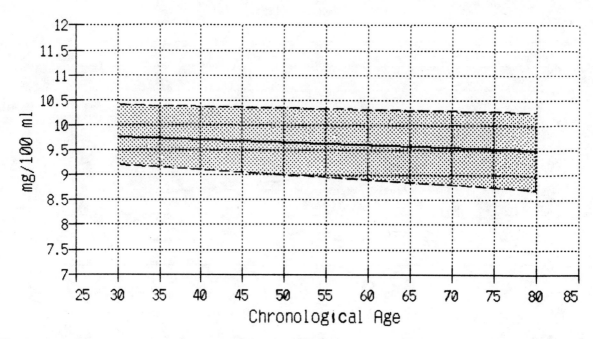

Fig. B. 9-18. **Calcium — men and women** (Gillibrand, et al).

9-10. Lecithin/cholesterol ratio (*Figs. B. 9-19 and 9-20*). The presence of polyunsaturated fatty-acid rich phospholipids (of which lecithin is the most abundant) assists in the mobilization of cholesterol, preventing it from being deposited in the arterial wall (Hall, pp 181-188). The relative concentration of phospholipids normally increases only slightly with age, compared with the greater increase in cholesterol. The ratio therefore decreases with age, becoming more atherogenic.

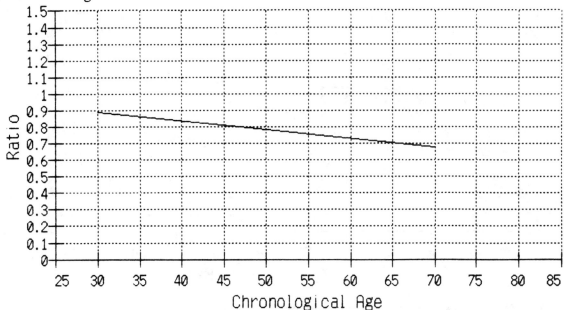

Fig. B. 9-19. **Lecithin/cholesterol ratio — men**, extrapolated from comparative data by Svanborg, et al, and Fordice.

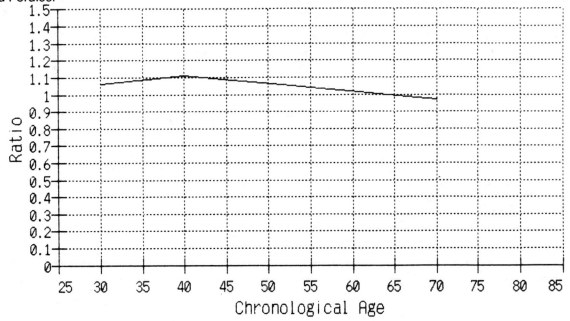

Fig. B. 9-20. **Lecithin/cholesterol ratio — women** (Svanborg, et al).

9-11. Glutamic oxaloacetic transaminase (SGOT) (*Figs. B. 9-21 and 9-22*). SGOT is an enzyme present in tissues of high metabolic activity such as the heart, liver, skeletal muscle, kidney, brain, pancreas, spleen, and lungs. The enzyme is released following injury or death of cells. Any disease that causes change in these highly metabolic tissues results in a rise in SGOT.

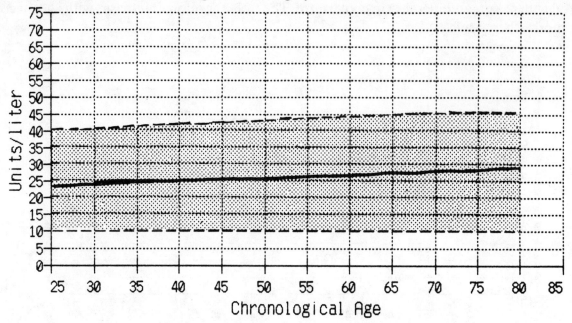

Fig. B. 9-21. **Glutamic oxaloacetic transaminase (SGOT) — men** (Fordice).

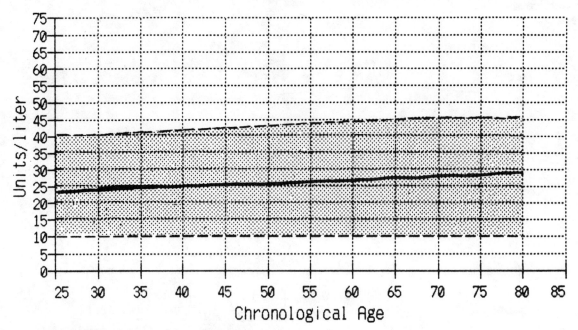

Fig. B. 9-22. **Glutamic oxaloacetic transaminase (SGOT) — women** (Fordice).

9-12. Albumin/globulin (A/G) ratio (*Fig. B. 9-23*). The serum globulins act mainly as immunologic agents. They also contribute to the osmotic pressure of the blood. Their osmotic effect is less than albumin, however, because the globulin molecule is much larger than the albumin molecule. Therefore, the osmotic pressure may be below normal even though the total protein level (albumin + globulin) is normal. Thus, the ratio of albumin to globulin becomes an important indicator of certain disease states.

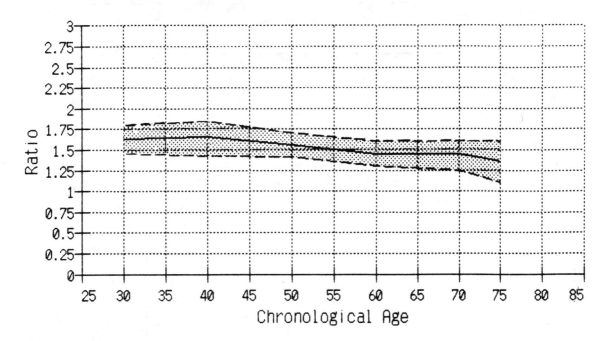

Fig. B. 9-23. **Albumin/globulin ratio — men** (Nakamura).

9-13. Total Protein (*Figs. B. 9-24 and 9-25*). Amino acids are the building blocks of protein. Plasma proteins serve as a source of nutrition for the body tissues and function in body buffering ability by combining with hemoglobin to exert an effect comparable to that of bicarbonate and other inorganic blood buffer systems.

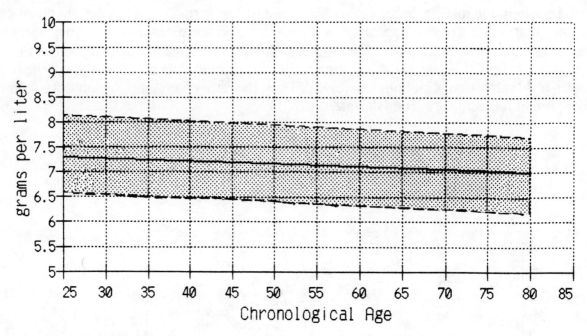

Fig. B. 9-24. **Total protein — men** (Fordice).

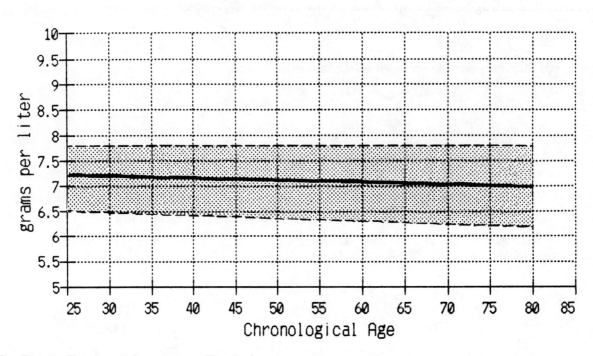

Fig. B. 9-25. **Total protein — women** (Fordice).

9-14. Fibrinogen (*Fig. B. 9-26*). Fibrinogen is a high-molecular weight plasma protein which is converted to fibrin through the action of thrombin. Fibrinogen increases slightly with age, possibly contributing to the increased risk of thromboembolic disease in the elderly.

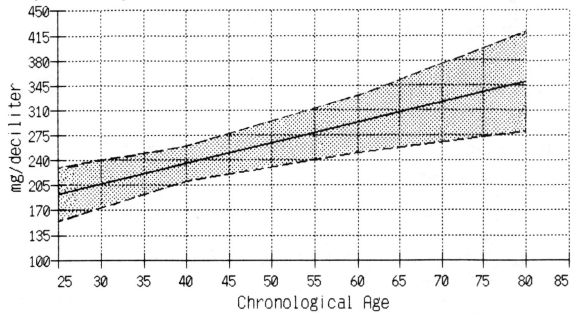

Fig. B. 9-26. **Fibrinogen — men** (Shimokata).

9-15. Total phospholipids (*Fig. B. 9-27*). Phospholipids, on hydrolysis, yield fatty acids, glycerin, and nitrogenous compounds. Lecithin is the major fraction, comprising nearly 70% of the total. Other phospholipids include cephalins and sphingomyelins.

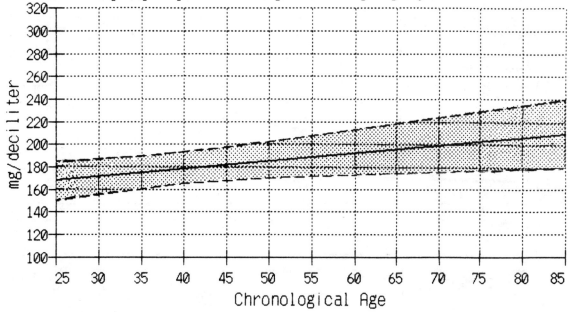

Fig. B. 9-27. **Total phospholipids — men** (Shimokata).

9-16. Uric acid (UA) (*Figs. B. 9-28 and 29*). Uric acid forms from the breakdown of nucleonic acids. It is an end product of purine metabolism. Two-thirds of the uric acid is excreted by the kidneys and the remaining one-third is excreted in the stool. An overproduction occurs in conditions characterized by excessive cell breakdown and catabolism of nucleonic acids (gout), excessive production and destruction of cells (leukemia), or an inability to excrete the substance (renal failure).

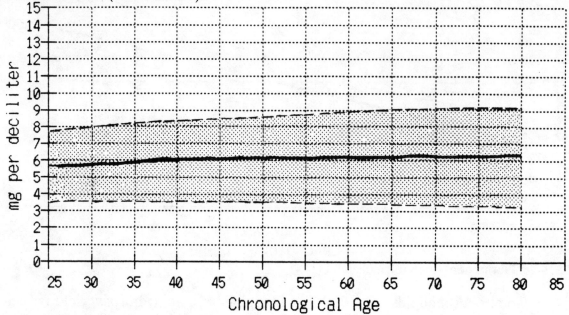

Fig. B. 9-28. **Uric acid — men** (Fordice).

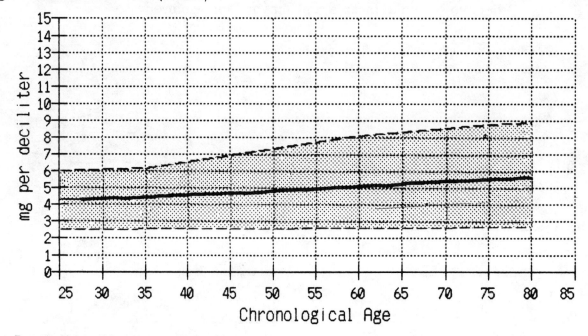

Fig. B. 9-29. **Uric acid — women** (Fordice).

10. RENAL

10-1. Phenolsulfonphthalein test (PSP) (*Fig. B. 10-1*). This test evaluates renal blood flow, and is conducted as follows: The subject drinks 400 ml of water. Twenty minutes later, 6 mg of phenolsulfonphthalein (a dye excreted unchanged by the kidneys) is given intravenously. Exactly 15 minutes later, the subject empties his bladder completely. Results are reported in the percentage of dye recovered, as determined by colorimetry. Less than 25% excretion of the dye at the 15 minute interval constitutes definite evidence of renal functional impairment.

The PSP test is now practically obsolete, and has largely been replaced by measurement of 24-hour creatinine clearance (Appendix B. 10-2). PSP clearance values can be determined from creatinine clearance, using the conversion table in *Fig. B. 10-2*.

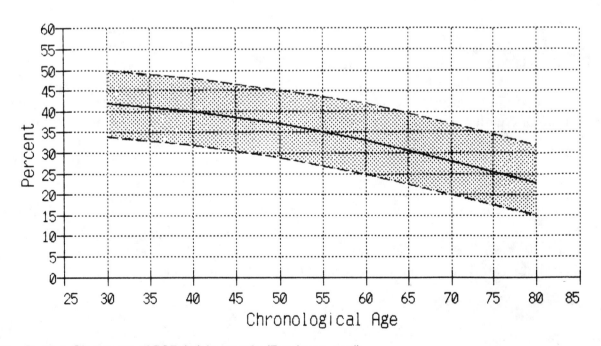

Fig. B. 10-1. **Clearance of PSP (%) in 15 min** (Furukawa, et al).

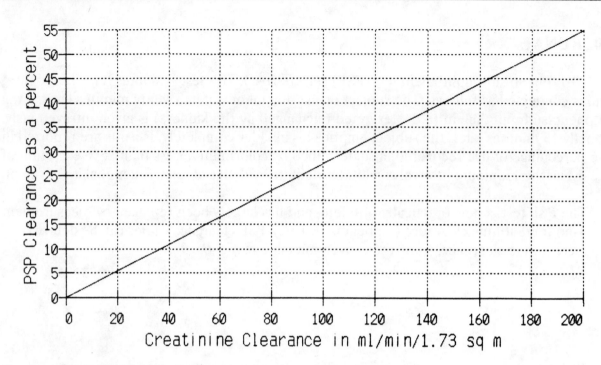

Fig. B. 10-2. **PSP Clearance / Creatinine Clearance conversion chart** (based on comparative data from Furukawa, et al; and Andres and Tobin).

10-2. Creatinine clearance (Creat Cl) (*Fig. B. 10-3*), measured in ml per minute. Creatinine is derived from protein metabolism. The rate of creatinine cleared by the kidneys and excreted in the urine is an indicator of kidney function.

The creatinine clearance is computed by the formula UV/P, where U is the average concentration of creatinine in the urine during a 24 hour collection period, and V is the volume of urine collected during this period. The product UV is the total amount of creatinine excreted in 24 hours. P is the average concentration of creatinine in the plasma during the same period. The quotient UV/P is the clearance, or the average amount of blood cleared of creatinine during a certain time period, in this case expressed in ml per minute.

An obvious inconvenient aspect of this measurement is the necessity to collect a 24-hour urine sample. A means of estimating creatinine clearance based on serum creatinine (*Fig. B. 10-4*) has been calculated by a group of Danish scientists (Siersbaek, et al).

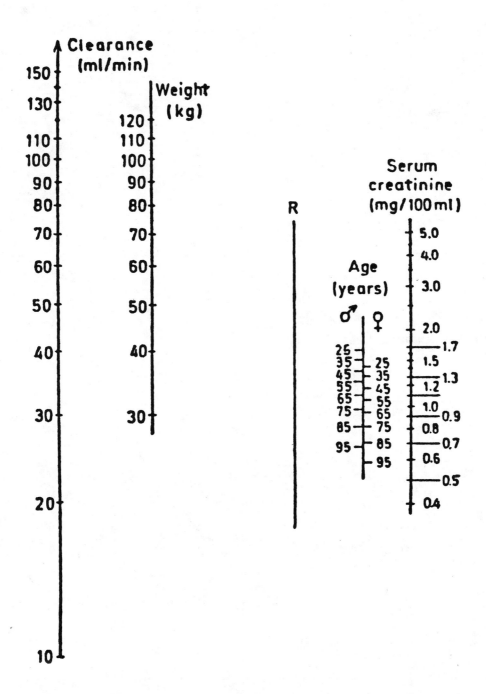

Fig. B. 10-3. **Nomogram for rapid evaluation of creatinine clearance**, based on serum creatinine (Siersbaek, et al). Draw a line with a ruler between weight and age in years. Then align the point at which the line crosses "R" with the serum creatinine, and read the subject's estimated creatinine clearance from the left side of the nomogram.

Appendix B — Sub-tests

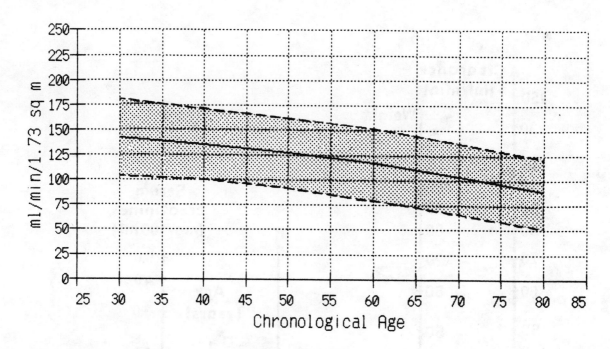

Fig. B. 10-4. **Creatine clearance** (Anres and Tobin).

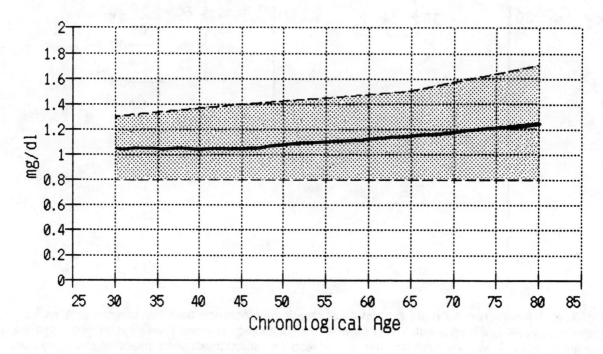

Fig. B. 10-5. **Serum creatinine — men** (Fordice).

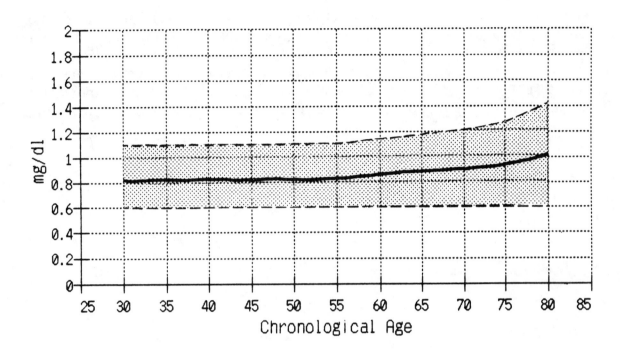

Fig. B. 10-6. **Serum creatinine — women** (Fordice).

11. ENDOCRINE/METABOLIC

11-1. Oral glucose tolerance test (OGTT) (*Figs. B. 11-1 to 11-3*). This tests the body's response to an oral carbohydrate challenge. It is used to diagnose diabetes, and is measured in mg per 100 ml. The test should be preceded by 3 days of adequate diet (150 gm of carbohydrate daily), and performed in the morning after an overnight fast. A fasting glucose level is drawn, 50 gm of glucose is given orally, and glucose levels are drawn at 30 minute intervals for two hours. If reactive hypoglycemia is suspected, the test can be continued for 5 hours.

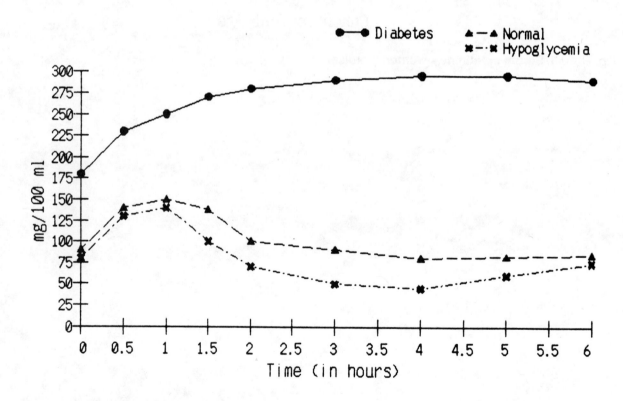

Fig. 11-1. **Glucose tolerance test**. Typical patterns in normal and various pathological states (Pinckney and Pinckney).

Sub-tests Appendix B

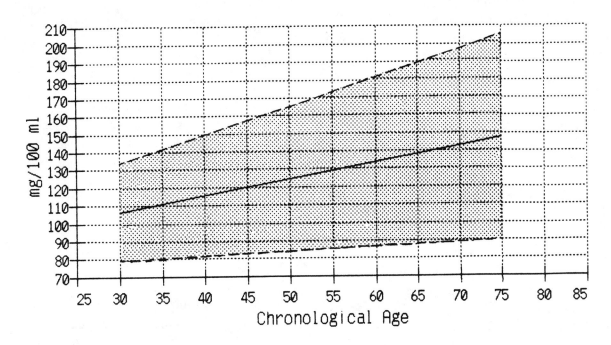

Fig. B. 11-2. **Glucose tolerance test at one hour — men** (Nakamura).

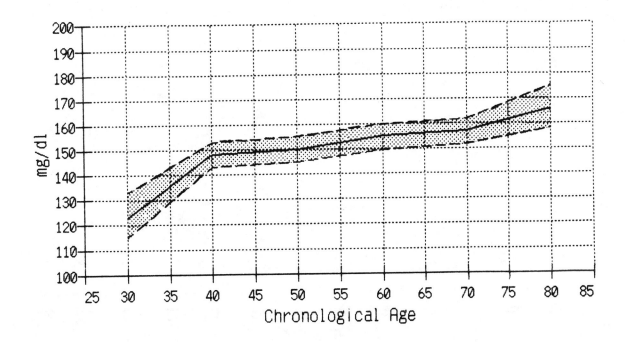

Fig. B. 11-3. **Glucose tolerance test at two hours — men** (Nakamura).

11-2. Basal metabolic rate (BMR) (*Fig. B. 11-4*). This is the sum of all the heat produced by chemical reactions within the body, measured under standardized conditions. BMR appears to decrease progressively with age after maturity (see Chapter 19 for a more complete discussion of BMR).

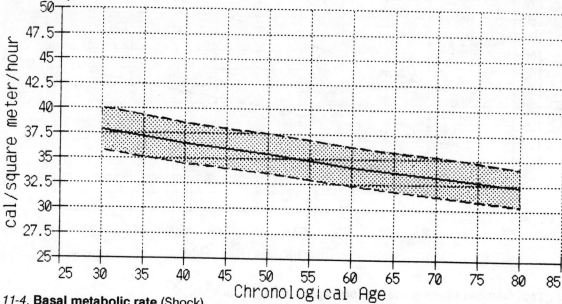

Fig. 11-4. **Basal metabolic rate** (Shock).

11-3. Luteinizing hormone (LH) (*Figs. B. 11-5 and 11-6*). This hormone regulates ovulation and helps maintain the corpus luteum in the female, and stimulates Leydig cells in the male.

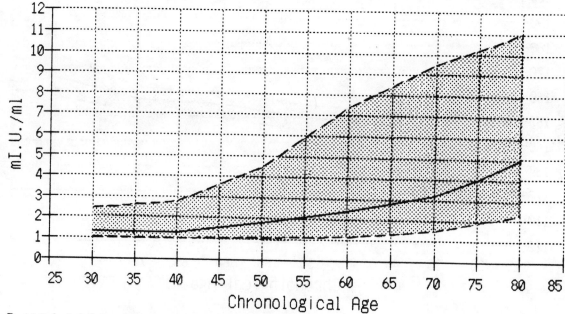

Fig. B. 11-5. **Luteinizing hormone (LH) — men** (Baker, et al).

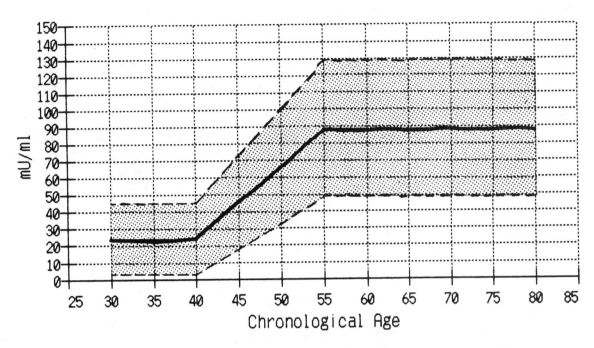

Fig. B. 11-6. **Luteinizing hormone (LH) – women** (Wills and Havard).

11-4. Follicle stimulating hormone (FSH) (*Figs. B. 11-7 and 11-8*). FSH stimulates the ovarian follicle in the female, and the formation of sperm in the male.

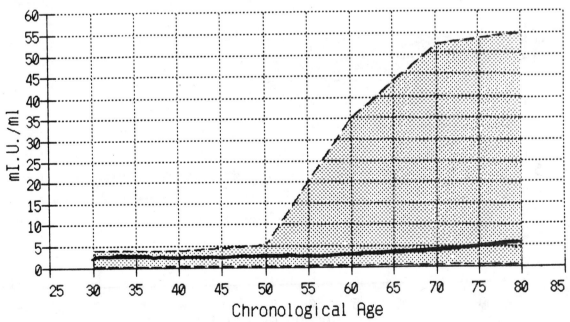

Fig. B. 11-7. **Follicle stimulating hormone (FSH) – men** (Baker, et al).

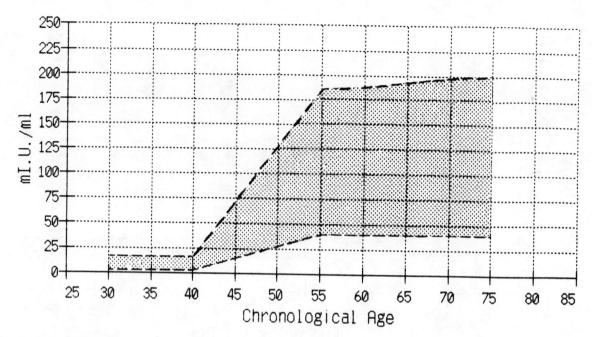

Fig. B. 11-8. **Follicle stimulating hormone – women** (Combined reference values from: Wills and Havard; and Kenny and Fotherby).

11-5. Testosterone (*Fig. B. 11-9*). Testosterone decreases markedly in men after age 50, although many men in their 60's and 70's are capable of maintaining levels in the high normal range of young men.

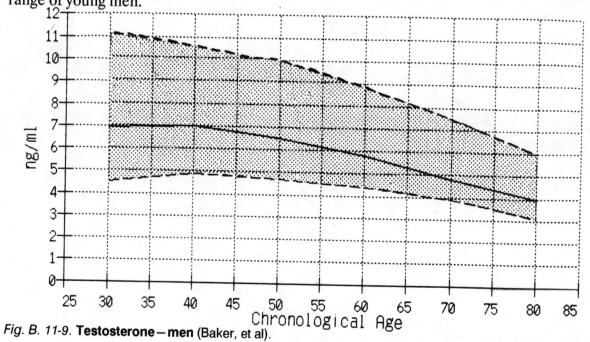

Fig. B. 11-9. **Testosterone – men** (Baker, et al).

11-6. Estradiol (*Figs B. 11-10 and 11-11*). Estradiol is produced by the ovaries and the placenta in females of reproductive age; a small amount of estrone is produced by the adrenal cortex and converted into estradiol. As nearly all of the estrogen produced in females of reproductive age is estradiol, measurement of its plasma concentration gives a valuable index of ovarian function (Wills and Havard). In the post-menopausal state, estradiol decreases by

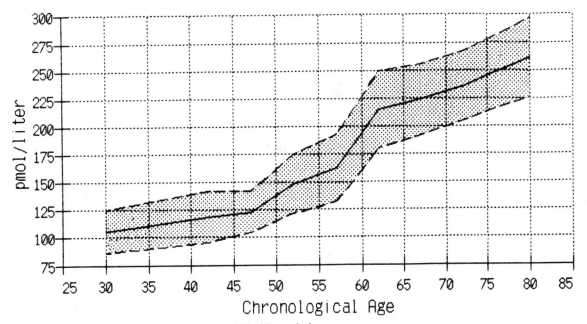

Fig. B. 11-10. **Estradiol — men** (Moroz and Verkhratsky).

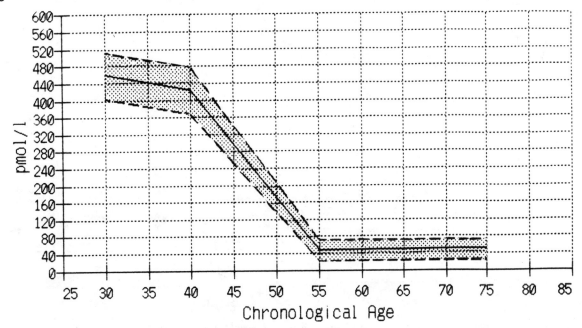

Fig. B. 11-11. **Estradiol — women** (Judd and Korenman).

as much as 95%. This results in an estrogen-androgen balance similar to a more male-oriented metabolism, accounting for the increasing masculinization of elderly females, characterized by the onset of male secondary sex characteristics (Hall).

LH, FSH, estradiol and testosterone levels fluctuate greatly during various times. Therefore, single determinations should not be relied upon to give average values (Baker).

11-7. Urinary excretion of total gonadotropins (LH and FSH) and total phenolsteroids (the sum of "classic" and "non-classic" phenolsteroids) (*Figs. B. 11-12 and 11-13*). The classic phenolsteroids are estradiol, estrone, and estriol. Non-classic phenolsteroids include 2-methoxy- estrone, 2-methoxyestradiol, 16-epiestriol, 17-epiestrone, 16, 17-epiestriol, 18-hydrosyestrone, and 16-hydroxyestrone. Nonclassic phenolsteroids are calculated by subtracting the classic phenolsteroids from the total phenolsteroids. The excretion of gonadotropins and phenolsteroids in the urine increases progressively with age. This is due to changes in the hypothalamic regulation of the reproductive system (Dilman).

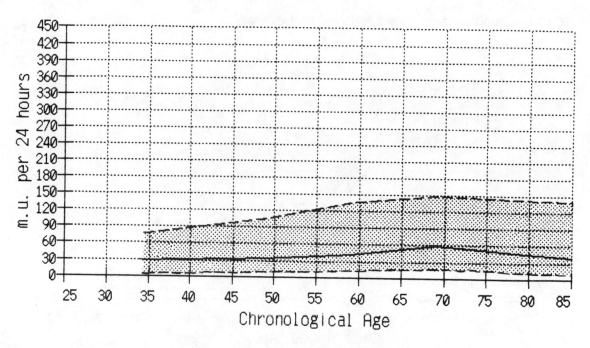

Fig. B. 11-12. **Urinary excretion of total gonadotropins—men** (Johnsen).

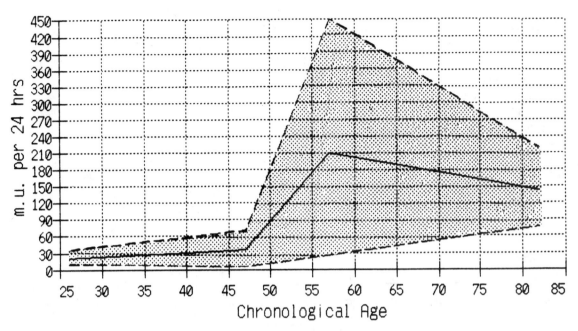

Fig. B. 11-13. **Urinary excretion of total gonadotropins— women** (Johnsen).

11-8. T3, T4, and Thyroid Stimulating Hormone (TSH) (*Figs. B. 11-14 to 11-16*). These are standard blood tests which evaluate thyroid gland function.

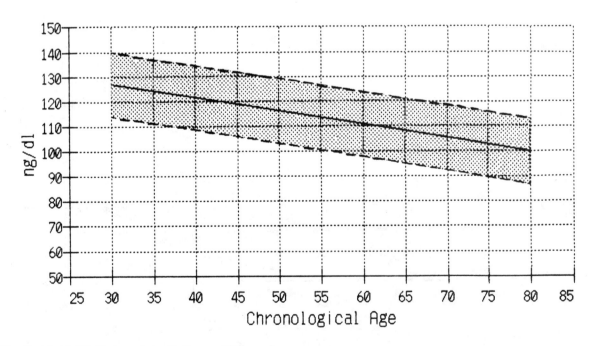

Fig. B. 11-14. **T3** (Rubenstein, Butler and Werner).

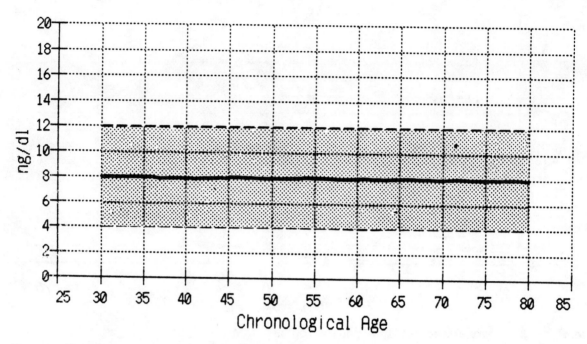

Fig. B. 11-15. **T4** (Wills and Havard).

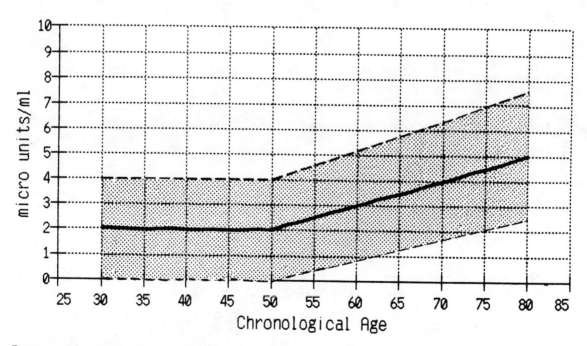

Fig. B. 11-16. **TSH** (Melmed and Hershman).

11-9. Prolactin (*Fig. B. 11-17*). The only known function of prolactin is to stimulate lactation in women. It has no known role in men. Its secretion is regulated by hypothalamic prolactin inhibiting factors like dopamine (primary) and throtropin releasing hormone (TRH). Surgery and physical stress cause rises in prolactin of unknown significance.

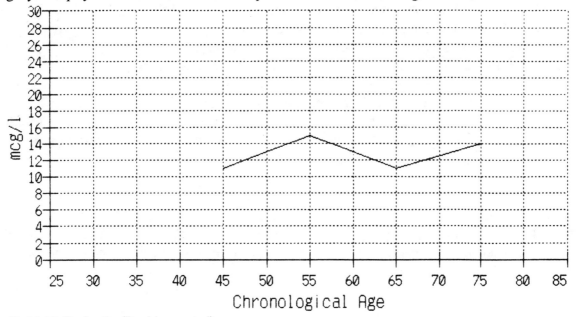

Fig. B. 11-17. **Prolactin** (Davidson, et al).

11-10. Melanocyte stimulating hormone (MSH) (*Fig. B. 11-18*). MSH exerts an effect on pigment metabolism. Normal values are 45-111 pg/ml.

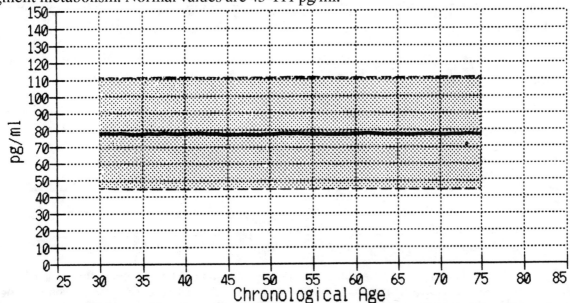

Fig. B. 11-18. **Melanocyte stimulating hormone (MSH)** (No age-adjusted data are available).

Appendix B — Sub-tests

11-10. Dexamethasone suppression test (DST) (*Fig. B. 11-19*). Dexamethasone is a potent synthetic glucocorticoid, which suppresses endogenous ACTH and cortisol production for up to 24 hours in normal subjects. The DST evaluates hypothalamic-pituitary-adrenal axis activity. It is used primarily to diagnose endogenous depression, but it is also abnormal in disorders such as Cushing's syndrome, alcoholism (during and after withdrawal), anorexia nervosa, prolonged hemodialysis, malignancies with ectopic ACTH secretion (mostly small cell bronchogenic carcinoma, obesity, protein-calorie malnutrition, renovascular hypertension, and uncontrolled diabetes mellitus) (Jenike, M. A.). It is also affected by age.

Dilman (1981) found that the hypothalamic threshold of sensitivity to inhibition by glucocorticoids is elevated with advancing age, resulting in failure of dexamethasone to inhibit endogenous cortisol production. This age-related change can be demonstrated by the "long DST." The "short DST" will not elicit this change.

The long dexamethasone test is conducted as follows: Blood for baseline cortisol determination is drawn in the morning. Dexamethasone 0.125 mg is then taken orally 4 times per day for two days. Blood is drawn again on the morning of the third day. Dilman also measures urine 17-ketosteroids on the day preceding dexamethasone adminstration and on the day three of the test.

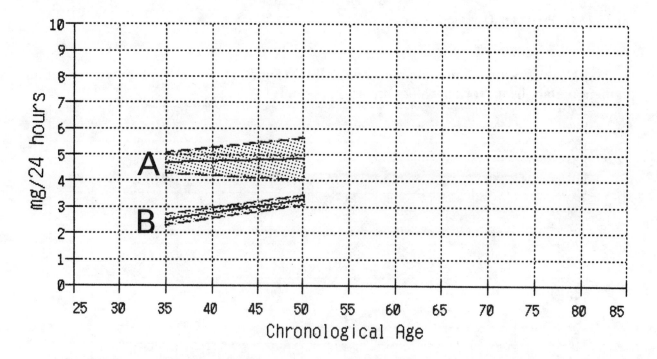

Fig. B. 11-19. **Dexamethasone suppression test.** This illustrates there is little change with age in urine 17-ketosteroid levels (**A**). However, there is a significant age-dependent difference in the efficiency of the suppression of 17-ketosteroid excretion by dexamethasone (**B**) (Dilman, 1981, pp. 36-37).

11-11. Diurnal blood cortisol levels (*Fig. B. 11-20*). Cortisol is the most important steroid secreted by the adrenal cortex, and estimation of its plasma concentration is the basis for most tests of adrenocortical function. Serum for this test is drawn at 9 AM and midnight. Normal values are between 5 and 25 µg/100 ml for the morning sample, and below 10 µg/100 ml for the evening sample. There is remarkably little change with age in cortisol concentrations.

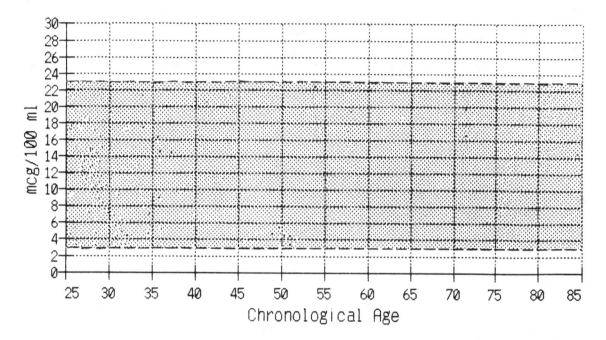

Fig. B. 11-20. **Cortisol**. The dashed lines are the upper and lower normal ranges of the morning (high) and evening (low) values.

11-12. 17-ketosteroid/17-hydroxycorticosteroid excretion ratio (*Fig. B. 11-21*). This test requires a 24-hour urine collection, and measures the breakdown products of adrenal hormones. It is a standard evaluation of adrenal gland function. There usually is no change in the output of 17-hydroxy-corticosteroids with age. However, there is a decrease of 17-ketosteroids. This consequently results in a decrease in the ratio of 17-ketosteroids to 17-hydroxycorticosteroids leading to the development of relative hypercorticism.

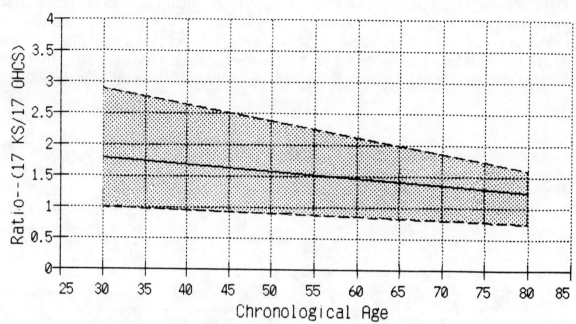

Fig. B. 11-21. **17-KS/17-OHCS ratio — men** (Abbo).

12. IMMUNOLOGICAL

12-1. Assay of T and B lymphocytes in peripheral blood. The major classifications of circulating lymphocytes are T-cells and B-cells. Normal immune function depends on the proper interactions of these lymphocyte subpopulations with all other components of the immune system.

To determine the T and B cell count, erythrocytes are lysed, leukocytes are suspended in saline and labeled with either polyclonal or monoclonal antibodies tagged with fluorescent molecules. Samples are analyzed by flow cytometry. Roche Biomedical Laboratories, Inc. can conduct this assay (P.O. Box 2230, Burlington, NC 27215 (919) 584-5171). They require 7 ml EDTA whole blood (lavendar top tube) and 7 ml heparinized whole blood (green top tube). The specimens should be maintained at room temperature, without refrigeration. They should be shipped to arrive in the laboratory within 48 hours of venipuncture on Monday through Thursday.

a. T lymphocytes (*Fig. B. 12-1*) (Jondal, et al).

b. B lymphocytes (*Fig. B. 12-2*) (Bianco, et al).

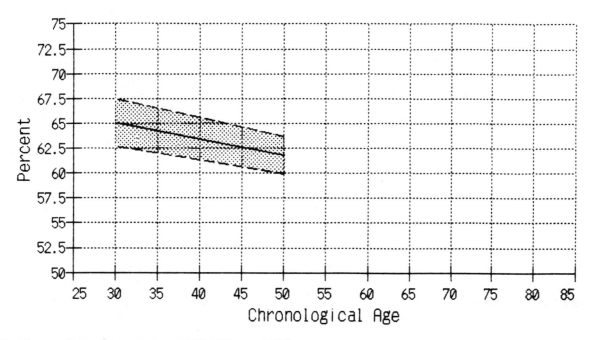

Fig. B. 12-1. **T lymphocyte level (%)** (Dilman, 1985).

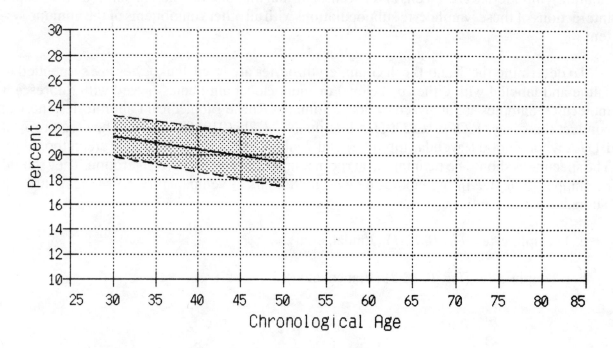

Fig. B. 12-2. **B lymphocyte level (%)** (Dilman, 1985).

12-2. Lymphocyte blast transformation test (response to phytohemagglutinin (PHA)) (*Fig. B. 12-3*): (Toh, et al 1973; Penhale; Hefton and Weksler). Lymphocyte transformation or blastogenesis is an *in vitro* method used to assess the cellular immunity of patients with immunodeficiencies, autoimmune diseases, infectious diseases, cancer, and aging. Because lymphocyte activation measures the functional capability of lymphocytes to proliferate following antigenic challenge, immunocompetence is measured more reliably with this method than when it is estimated only by quantification of lymphocyte types (i.e., T and B lymphocyte quantitation). Immunoenhancement and immunosuppressive therapies can be monitored with these techniques.

This test (*Blastogenic index*) is also performed by Roche Biomedical Laboratories. They require two 10 ml tubes of heparinized whole blood, which must arrive in their laboratory within 24 hours of collection. The specimen should be shipped at ambient temperature, and should not be chilled.

Sub-tests Appendix B

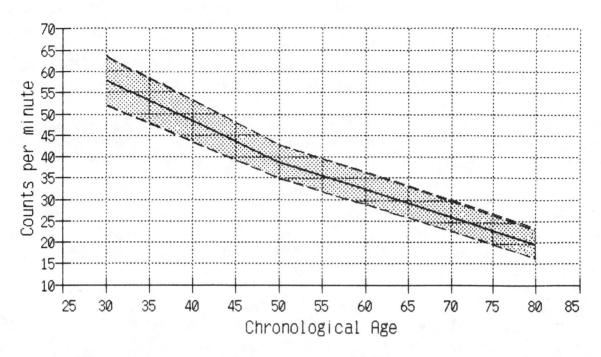

Fig. B. 12-3. **Lymphocyte blast transformation — men**, measured by rate of incorporation of thymidine in counts per minute (Combined data from: Dilman, 1985; and Weksler and Hutteroth).

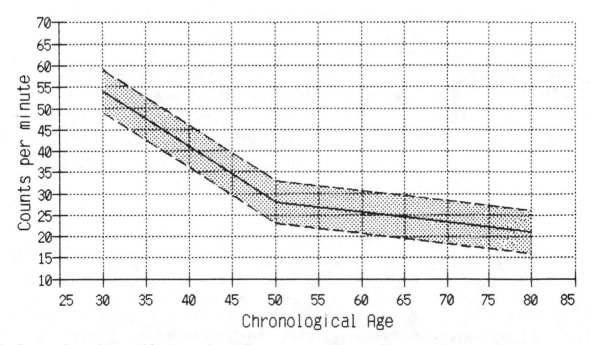

Fig. B. 12-4. **Lymphocyte blast transformation — women**, measured by rate of incorporation of thymidine in counts per minute (Combined data from: Dilman, 1985; and Weksler and Hutteroth).

12-3. Contact sensitization (delayed hypersensitivity) skin tests (*Fig. B. 12-5*) (Fudenberg).

a. Dinitrochlorobenzene (DNCB): Apply 2 mg of DNCB in 0.1 cc acetone to an area of skin of the upper inner portion of the arm circumscribed by a 2 cm diameter plastic ring. At the same time, in order to determine any preexisting sensitivity to the agent, two challenge doses of DNCB (0.1 and 0.05 mg in 0.1 cc acetone) are applied in the same way on areas of the ipsilateral forearm. The site treated with 2 mg of DNCB is occluded by a 1-inch dressing for five days and then left open to the air; the sites treated with 0.1 and 0.05 mg are covered for 48 hrs and observed then and at 72 hrs for signs of delayed hypersensitivity (erythema, edema, vesiculation).

Fourteen days after the application of the 2 mg sensitizing dose the patients are challenged with 0.1 and 0.05 mg DNCB to the contralateral forearm in a manner similar to that of the initial testing. Subjects are considered sensitized to DNCB if the characteristic signs of delayed hypersensitivity appear (Waldorf, et al; Catalona).

b. Candida and tuberculin: 0.1 ml each of candida (Bencard) or tuberculin (Commonwealth Serum Laboratories, Melbourne) are injected intradermally, using a 1-ml syringe with a 26-gauge needle, in the forearm (if both are used, the injections should be 3-4 cm apart). Reactions are read at 48 hr after injection. The reaction is positive when the mean of the maximum and minimum diameters of the area of induration is greater than 0.6 cm (Toh, et al).

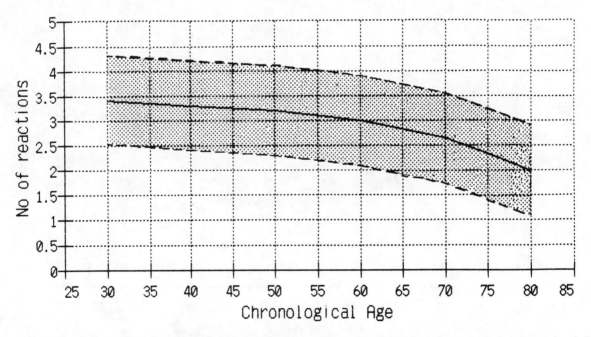

Fig. B. 12-5. **Mean number of positive delayed hypersensitivity reactions**, showing the progressive fall with age in the prevalence of positive reactions to five antigens (Candida, mumps, trychophyton, tuberculin and Varidase) (Toh, et al).

Additional guidance to conduct many of the tests listed in Appendix B can be found in the following books:

A Manual of Laboratory Diagnostic Tests, by Frances Fischbach. J.B. Lippincott Co., 1984.

Cardiovascular Survey Methods, WHO Monograph Series No. 65, Geneva, 1982 (price SFr.22).

Clinical Biochemistry of the Elderly, by Malcolm Hodkinson (ed). Churchill Livingstone, 1984.

The Complete Book of Medical Tests, by Mark A. Moskowitz and Michael E. Osband. W. W. Norton and Co., Inc. 1984.

Designs for Fitness, by Vivian H. Heyward, Burgess, 1984.

Do it Yourself Medical Testing, by Cathey and Edward R. Pinckney. Facts on File, 1983.

Fundamentals of Exercise Testing, by K. L. Anderson, R. J. Shephard, H. Denolin, E. Vearnauskas, R. Masioron, F. H. Bonjer, J. Rutenfranz, and Z. Fejfan. WHO, 1971.

REFERENCES

Abbo, F. E. The 17 ketosteroid/17 hydroxycorticosteroid ratio as a useful measure of the physiological age of the human adrenal cortex. *J Geront*, 1966, 21: 112-114. (in: Wolfson, A. R. *Aging and the adrenals*, pp. 55-79. in: Korenman)

Abraham, S. Total Serum Cholesterol Levels of Adults 18-74 years, U.S., 1974. *Vital and Health Statistics: Series 11, Data from the National Health Survey*, No. 205, DHEW Pub No. (PHS) 78-1652.

Albert, A., Randall, R. V., Smith, R. A., and Johnson, C.E. Urinary excretion of gonadotropins as a function of age. In: *Hormones and the Aging Process*, by E. T. Engle and G. Pincus, (eds), New York, Academic Press, 1956.

Andersen, K. L., et al. *Fundamentals of Exercise Testing*, Geneva, WHO, 1978.

Andres, R., Tobin, J. D. The relationship of standard true creatinine clearance and age. from: Rowe, J.W., Andres, R., Tobin, J.D., Norris, A.H., and Shock, N.W. 1976. The effect of age on creatinine clearance in man: A cross-sectional and longitudinal study. *J Geront*, 31, 155-163.

Arends, J. Old traditional beliefs die slowly. *American Medical Jogger's Association Newsletter*, Dec 1979.

Astrand, I. Aerobic capacity in men and women with special reference to age. *Acta Physiologica Scandinavica* 49 (1960) Supplementum 169: 1-92.

Astrand, P. O., and Rhyming, I. A nomogram for calculation of aerobic capacity (physical fitness) from pulse rate during submaximal work. *JAP*, 1954, 7: 218-221.

Baker, H.W.G., Burger, H.G., deKretser, D. M., and Hudson, B. Endocrinology of aging: Pituitary testicular axis. *Proc 5th Intl Congress of Endocrinology*, pp. 479-483, in: Swerdloff, R. S., and Heber, D., Effects of Aging on Male Reproductive Function, p. 131, in: Korenman, S. G., *Endocrine Aspects of Aging*, New York, Elsevier Biomedical, 1982.

Berkowitz, B. The Wechsler-Bellevue performance of white males past 50. *J Geront*, 1953, 8, 76-80.

Bianco, C., Patrick, R. Nussenzwaig, V. A. A population of lymphocytes bearing a membrane receptor for antigen-antibody complement complexes. I. Separation and characterization. *J Exp Med*, 132, 702-706, 1970.

Bloom, S., Till, S., Sonksen, P., and Smith, S. Use of a biothesiometer to measure individual vibration thresholds and their variation in 519 non-diabetic subjects. *British Medical Journal*, 16 Jun, 1984, 288, 1793-1795.

Borkan, G. A. *The Assessment of Biological Age During Adulthood*, Ph. D. Thesis, 1978. University Microfilms, Int. Doc. No. 7822861.

Burch, P. R. J., Murray, J. J., and Jackson, D. The age-prevalence of arcus senilis, greying of hair, and baldness. Etiological considerations, *J of Gerontol*, 1971, Vol. 26, No. 3, 364-372.

Catalona, W. J., Taylor, P. T., Rabson, A. S., and Chretien, P. B. A method for dinitrochlorbenzene contact sensitization, *NEJM*, Feb 24, 1972, Vol 286, No. 8, pp 399-402.

Comalli, P. E., Wapner, S., and Werner, H. Interference effects of Stroop color-word test in childhood, adulthood, and aging. *J Genetic Psych*, 1962, 100: 47-53.

Damon, A. Seltzer, C. C., Stoudt, H.W., and Bell, B. 1972. Age and physique in healthy white veterans at Boston. *Aging and Human Development*, 3, 202-208.

Davidson, J. M., Chen, J. J., Crapo, L., Gray, G. D., Greenleaf, W. J., and Catania, J. A. Hormonal changes and sexual function in aging men. *J Clin Endoc and Metab*, 57: 1, 71-77

Dehn, M. M., and Bruce, R. A. *JAP*, Vol 33, No. 6, December 1972, 805-807.

Dilman, V. *The Law of Deviation of Homeostasis and Diseases of Aging*, Boston, John Wright.PSG, 1981.

Dilman, V. Personal communication, 15 Feb 1985.

Dirken, R. M. *Functional Age of Industrial Workers*, Netherlands Institute for Preventive Medicine TNO, Wolters-Noordhoff Publishing Groningen 1972.

Duane, A. Studies in monocular and binocular accommodation, *Amer J Ophthal*, (1922) 5, 865-877.

Emmrich, V. R., and Schwarz, J. Die gelenkbeweglichkeit in abhangigkeit vom altern und ihr verhalten bei verschiedenen krankheiten. *Zeitschrift fur Alternsforschung*, Vol 16 No 4, Oct 1963, pp. 297-303.

Engelman, K., and Braunwald, E. Hypertension and the shock syndrome, in: *Principles of Internal Medicine*, 7th ed., by Wintrobe, M.W., et al (eds). New York, McGraw Hill, 1974.

Fordice, M. W. Age and sex effects on plasma analytes for adults. Symposium: Clinical chemistry of aging. Pertinent reference information for the geriatric population. American Aging Association Annual Meeting, 9 October 1985, San Francisco.

Fowler, E. P., and Sabine, P. E. Tentative standard procedure for evaluating the percentage loss of hearing in medicolegal cases, *JAMA*, Vol 133 (1947), pp 396-404.

Friedlander, J. S., Costa, P. T., Bosse, R., Ellis, E., Rhoads, J. G., and Stoudt, H. W. Longitudinal physique changes among healthy white veterans at Boston. *Human Biology*, Dec 1977, Vol 49, No 4, pp. 541-558.

Furukawa, T., Inoue, M. Kayiya, F., Inada, H., Takasugi, S., Fukui, S., Takeda, H., and Abe, H. Assessment of biological age by multiple regression analysis. *J Geront*, 1975, Vol 30, No 4, 422-434.

Furukawa, T. Personal communication, 13 Feb 1985.

Gillibrand, D., Grewal, D., and Blatter, D. P. Chemistry reference values as a function of age and sex, including pediatric and geriatric subjects, in: *Aging--its Chemistry*, by A. A. Dietz (ed.). American Association for Clinical Chemistry, 1979, pp. 366-389.

Goldberg, M. L., et al. Dose-response of lymphocytes to purified, protein-free phytohemagglutinin. *Proc Soc Exp Biol Med*, 1970, Vol 134, No 2, pp 459-461.

Greenblatt, D. J. Reduced Serum albumin concentration in the elderly: A report from the Boston collaborative drug surveillance Program. *J Am Ger Soc.*, 27: 20-22. 1979.

Hall, D. A. *The Biomedical Basis of Gerontology*. Boston, John Wright.PSG, 1984.

Hallock, P. Arterial elasticity in man in relation to age as evaluated by the pulse wave velocity method. *Arch Int Med* 54: 770-798, Oct, 1934.

Halsted, J. A. *The Laboratory in Clinical Medicine*. W. B. Saunders Company, Philadelphia, 1976.

Hamilton, J. B. Patterned loss of hair in man: types and incidence. *Annals of the New York Academy of Sciences*, 1951, 53, 708-728.

Hefton, J. M., and Weksler, M. E. The Study of Immune Function in aged humans, *CRC Handbook of Immunological Methods in Aging Research*. pp 165-202.

Heikkinen, E. Personal communication, 26 June 1985.

Heikkinen, E., Arajarvi, R. L., Era, P., Jylha, M., Kinnunen, V., Liskinen, A. L., Leskinen, E., Massesli, E., Pohjolainen, P. Rahkila, P., Suominen, H., Turpeinen, P., Vaisanen, M., and Osterback, L. Functional capacity of men born in 1906-10. 1926-30, and 1946-50. A Basic Report. *Scand J Soc Med Suppl* 33, 1984.

Hershman, J. M. Clinical application of thyrotropin-releasing hormone. *NEJM*, 886-890, 1974.

Herzberg, H. T. E., Churchill, E., Dupertuis, C. W., White, R.M., and Damon, A. *Anthropometric Survey of Turkey, Greece, and Italy*. (1963) London: Pergamon Press.

Hollingsworth, J.W., Hashizume, A., and Jablon, S. (1965). Correlations between tests of aging in Hiroshima subjects: an attempt to define "physiologic age." Yale J Biol Med, in: Comfort, A. *The Biology of Sensescence*, Elsevier, New York, 1979.

Jenike, M. A. Dexamethasone suppression test as a clinical aid in elderly depressed patients. *J Am Ger Soc*, Jan 1983, Vol 31 No 1, 45-48.

Johnsen, Svend, G. A clinical routine method for the quantitative determination of gonadotrophins in 24 hour urine samples. II: Normal values for men and women at all age groups from pre-puberty to senescence. *Acta Endocrinologica*, Vol 31, 209-227, 1959.

Jondal, M., Hom, G., Wigzell, M. Surface markers on human B and T lymphocytes. I. A large population of lymphocytes forming nonimmune rosettes with sheep red blood cells. *J Exp Med*, (1972) 136, 207-212.

Judd, H. L., and Korenman, S. G. Effects of aging on reproductive function in women, in: Korenman, S. G. (ed), *Endocrine Aspects of Aging*, New York, Elsevier Biomedical, 1982.

Kannel, W. B., and Hubert, H. Vital capacity as a biomarker of aging, in: *Biological Markers of Aging*, by M. E. Reff, and E. L. Schneider (eds). Bethesda, USDHHS, NIH, PHS, 1982.

Keogh, E.V., and Walsh, R. J. (1965) Rate of greying of human hair, *Nature*, 207, 877-878, in: Lamb, M.J. *Biology of Aging*, Blackie, London 1977.

Kenny, R. A., and Fotherby, K. The sex steroids and trophic hormones, in: *Clinical Biochemistry of the Elderly*, by Malcom Hodkinson (ed). Churchill Livingstone, London, 1984.

Korenman, S. G. *Endocrine Aspects of Aging*, New York, Elsevier Biomedical, 1982.

Landowne, M. Characteristics of impact and pulse wave propagation in brachial and radial arteries. *J Appl Physiol*, 12, 91-97 (1958).

Melmed, S., and Hershman, J. M. The Thyroid and Aging, in: *Endocrine Aspects of Aging*, New York, Elsevier Biomedical, 1982.

Mints, A. J., Dubina, T. L., Lysenyk, V. P., Zhuk, E. V. Determination of individual biological age and evaluation of aging degree. *Physiologichiski Zhurnal*, Vol 30, No 1, 1984.

Mints, A. Ya. *Cerebral atherosclerosis*. Kiev, Zdororja, 1970.

Morgan, R. F. and Wilson, J. *Growing Younger*, Toronto, Methunen, 1983.

Morris, J. F., Koski, A., and Johnson, L. C. Spirometric standards for healthy nonsmoking adults. *American Review of Respiratory Disease*, Vol 103, 1971, 57-67.

Moroz, E. V., and Verkhratsky, N. S. Hypophyseal-gonadal system during male aging. *Arch Gerontol Geriatr*, 4 (1985) 13-19.

Muiesan, G., Sorbin, C.A., Grass, V. Respiratory function in the aged. *Bull Physio Path Resp*, 1971, 7, 973-1009.

Nakamura, E. The aged people and its physiological ages in relation to work capacity *Kyoiku Igaku* (Education and Medicine), 1982, 28:1 2-11.

Onrot J., Wood, A. Hypertension in the elderly. *Post-graduate Medicine* (1984; 76 (5): 48).

Ordy, J.M., Brizzee, K. R., Beavers, T., and Medart, P. Age differences in the functional and structural organization of the auditory system in man, in: Sensory Systems and Communication in the Elderly. *Aging*, Vol 10, by Ordy, J. M., and Brizzee, K. (eds), Raven Press, New York, 1979.

Pehnale, W. J. A rapid micro-method for the phytohemagluttinin-induced human lymphocytes in transformation test. *Clin Exp Immunology*, 18, 155-167, 1974.

Peterson, B., Treel, E., Sternby, N.H. *JAMA*, 1981, 245: 2056-2057.

Pinckney, C., and Pinckney, E.R. *Do it Yourself Medical Testing*. Facts on File, NY, 1983, p. 47.

Pincus, G., Romanoff, L.P., and Carlo, J. The Excretion of Urinary Steroids by Men and Women of Various Ages. *J Gerontol*, April 1954, Vol. 9, No. 2, pp. 113-132.

Pitts, D. G. The effects of aging on selected visual functions: dark adaptation, visual acuity, steroeopsis and brightness contrast. In: Sekuler, R., Kline, D., and Dismukes, K. (eds), *Aging and Human Visual Function*, Alan R. R. Liss, New York, 1982, in: Reff and Schneider, p. 227.

Pollock, M. L., Wilmore, J. H., and Fox, S. M. *Health and Fitness Through Physical Activity*. New York. John Wiley and Sons, 1978.

Roberts-Thomsen, I. C., Whittingham, S., Youngchaiyud, U., Mackay, I. R.), Aging Immune Response and Mortality. *The Lancet*, August 17, 1974.

Ross, G. D., Rabellino, E. M., Polley, M. J., and Grey, H. M. Combined studies of complement receptor and surface immunoglobulin-bearing cells and sheep erythrocyte rosette-forming cells in normal and leukemic human lymphocytes. *J Clin Invest.*, Vol 52, Feb 1973, 377-385.

Rubenstein, H. A., Butler, V. P., Jr., Werner, S. C. Progressive decrease in serum triiodothyronine concentration in human aging: Radioimmunoassay following extraction of serum. *J Clin Endocr Metab.* 37: 247-253 (1973).

Russell, A. L. A system of classification and scoring for prevalence surveys of periodontal disease. *J Dent Res*, Jun 1956, 35: 350-359.

Sekuler, R. Vision as a source of simple and reliable markers for aging, in: Reff, M.E., and Schneider, E. L. (eds). *Biomarkers of Aging*, p. 226.

Shephard, R. J., and Kavanagh, T. The effects of training on the aging process. *Physician and Sports Medicine*, 6:33-40, 1978.

Shock, N. W., Systems integration, in: Finch, C. E., and Hayflick, L. *Handbook of the Biology of Aging*, New York, Van Nostrand Reinhold, p. 642.

Shock, N. W., Greulich, R. C., Andres, R., Costa, P. T., Lakatta, E. G., and Tobin, J. D. *Normal Human Aging—The Baltimore Longitudinal Study of Aging*, USDHHS, PHS, NIA, GRC, NIH Pub No 84-2450, 1984.

Siersbaek-Nielsen, K., Molholm Hansen, J., Kampmann, J., and Kristensen, M. Rapid Evaluation of Creatinine Clearance, *The Lancet*, May 29, 1971, pp. 1133-1134.

Stites, D. P. Laboratory methods of detecting cellular immune function, in: Fudenberg, H. H, Stites, D. P., Caldwell, J. L., and Wells, J. V. (eds) *Basic and Clinical Immunology*. Los Altos, Lange, 316.

Suominen, H. Personal communication, 1 April 1986.

Svanborg, A., Bengtsson, C., Lindquist, O., Roupe, S., and Steen, B. Plasma lipid changes in the female in aging and the menopause. Results from three population studies. *Clinica Chimica Acta*, 79 (1977) 299-307.

Taylor, E. M. *Psychological Appraisal of Children with Cerebral Defects*, 1959. Boston, Harvard U. Press.

Toh, B. H., Robertts-Thomson, I. C., Mathews, J. D., Whittingham, S., and MacKay, I. R. Depression of cell-mediated immunity on old age and the immunopathic diseases, lupus erythematosis, chronic hepatitis and rheumatoid arthritis. *Clin Exp Immunol* (1973) 14, 193-202.

Tyroler, H. A. Cholesterol and Cardiovascular Disease. *The American Journal of Cardiology*, Vol 54, Aug 27, 1984, pp. 14c-26c.

Vermeulen, A., Rubens, R., and Verdonck, L. 1972. Testosterone secretion and metabolism in male senescence. *J Clin Endocrinol Metabol* 34: 730-735.

Waldorf, D. S., Willkens, R. F., Decker, J. L. Impaired delayed hypersensitivity in an aging population. *JAMA*, March 4, 1968, Vol 203, No. 10, 111-114.

Weksler, M. E., Hutteroth, T. H. Impaired lymphocyte function in aged humans. *J Clin Invest*, 1974, Vol 53, pp. 99-104.

Wills, M. R., and Havard, B. *Laboratory Investigation of Endocrine Disorders*, 1983, Boston, Butterworths.

Appendix C

RECORD KEEPING
Calculation Sheet and Chart

Aging measurements can be used to determine the Biological Aging Index (BAI). Longitudinal measurements can be used to determine the rate of aging ($\Delta BA/\Delta CA$). The calculation technique and guidelines for interpreting results are discussed in Chapter 23.

The next page contains a calculation sheet and chart that can be photocopied and incorporated into a patient's records. This should be updated each time an aging measurement test is conducted.

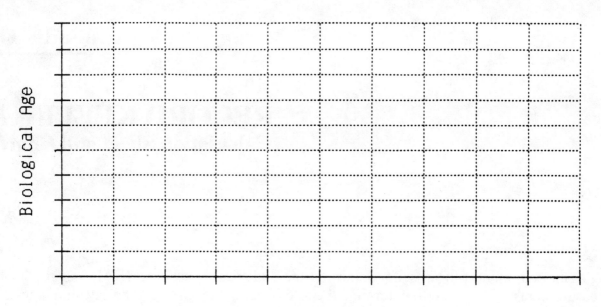

Chronological vs. Biological Age
Calculation Sheet and Chart

Test Battery: _____ Equation No. _____

Test Date .... : _____ _____ _____ _____ _____ _____
Test No. .... (n=): _____ _____ _____ _____ _____ _____

Chronological Age (CA_n) : _____ _____ _____ _____ _____ _____
Biological Age (BA_n) .... : _____ _____ _____ _____ _____ _____
Biological Aging Index ... : _____ _____ _____ _____ _____ _____
($BAI_n = BA_n/CA_n$)
$\Delta BA_n = BA_n - BA_1$ ...... : _____ _____ _____ _____ _____ _____
$\Delta CA_n = CA_n - CA_1$ ...... : _____ _____ _____ _____ _____ _____
Aging Rate .... : _____ _____ _____ _____ _____ _____
($AR_n = \Delta BA_n / \Delta CA_n$)

* In this chart, the Biological Aging Index ($BAI_n = BA_n/CA_n$), change in Biological Age ($\Delta BA_n = BA_n - BA_1$), change in Chronological Age ($\Delta CA_n = CA_n - CA_1$), and Aging Rate ($AR_n = \Delta BA_n / \Delta CA_n$) are calculated in absolute terms; i.e., the most recent value is compared with the first, to reflect change over the entire period of aging measurement. Incremental evaluations can also be made by comparing the two most recent values.

Appendix D

RECOMMENDED READING

Potential age-retarding substances and regimens are being proposed in a growing number of popular life-extension books. Many of the programs recommended by the books are based on the results of animal experimentation, and there is no evidence yet that the regimens are effective in humans. Nevertheless, thousands of people are self-experimenting with many of these regimens.

It is essential for all clinical gerontologists and physicians who care for such patients to be aware of the programs their patients are following, and to understand the rationale behind the use of certain drugs and nutrients their patients might be taking.

However, books relating to aging intervention are not restricted to those for the TV talk show audience. Also included in this appendix are some of the growing number of serious professional/academic books that discuss potential human gerontotherapeutic regimens. Clinical gerontologists and researchers should be aware of the advances in this rapidly growing field outlined in these books.

A list of newsletters and journals primarily focused on gerontological research pertaining to aging intervention is included. Most are directed at a popular audience, but are quite technical and generally well-referenced.

Appendix D — Recommended Reading

Popular:

The Age Reduction System, by Richard C. Kaufman, Rawson Associates, New York, 1986.

Anti-Aging Weight Loss Program, by Hans Kugler, International Academy of Holistic Health and Medicine, 1988.

Growing Younger, by Robert F. Morgan, Methuen, 1982.

Life Extension, by Durk Pearson and Sandy Shaw, Warner Books, 1982.

The Life Extension Companion, by Durk Pearson and Sandy Shaw, Warner Books, 1984.

The Life Extension Revolution, by Saul Kent, Morrow, 1980.

Maximum Life Span, by Roy Walford, Norton, 1983.

The One Hundred and Twenty Year Diet, by Roy Walford, Simon and Schuster, 1986.

Prolongevity II, by Albert Rosenfeld, Alfred A. Knopf, 1985.

Secrets of Life Extension, by John Mann, Bantam, 1982.

Slowing Down the Aging Process, by Hans Kugler, Pyramid Books, 1975.

Your Personal Life Extension Program, by Saul Kent. Morrow, 1985.

Professional/Academic:

Aging and Life Prolonging Processes, by V. V. Frolkis, Springer-Verlag, 1982.

Experimental and Clinical Intervention in Aging, by Richard F. Walker and Ralph L. Cooper, Marcel Dekker, 1983.

Intervention in the Aging Process, Parts A and B, by William Regelson and F. Marot Sinex, (eds.), Alan R. Liss, 1983.

APPENDIX E

SUPPLEMENTAL BIBLIOGRAPHY

The articles in this bibliography discuss the theory and statistical relevance of biological aging measurement systems. As mentioned in the Preface, Part B, these subjects are intentionally not discussed in this book.

This book is intended to be a practical clinical manual. It contains information that is not available elsewhere in any form. It describes practical aging measurement systems that can be used clinically now.

To include the theoretical/philosophical discussions that are available elsewhere (in the below-listed publications) would be interesting but of little practical value, and would detract from the book's usefulness.

I strongly urge those interested in the subject to review the publications in this Appendix for a more eloquent and accurate discussion of these subjects than I could have done. Although a few of these publications have been cited as supporting references in the book, none of the chapters have been based on them.

Bell, Benjamin. Significance of functional age for interdisciplinary and longitudinal research in aging. *Aging and Human Development*, Vol 3, No 2, 1972, 145-147.

Bourliere, F. *The Assessment of Biological Age in Man.* WHO, Geneva, 1970.

Bourliere, F. Indices of physiological age, in: *Aging: A Challenge to Science and Society, Vol 1, Biology*, by D. Danon, N. W. Shock, and M. Marois (eds). Oxford U. Press, New York, 1981, 269-270.

Brown, K. S., Math, B., and Forbes, W. F. A mathematical model of aging processes. *J Gerontology*, 1974, Vol 29, No 1, 46-51.

Brown, K. S., Math, B., and Forbes, W. F. A mathematical model of aging processes, II. *J Gerontology*, 1974, Vol 29, No 4, 301-409.

Brown, K. S., and Forbes, W. F. A mathematical model of aging processes, III. *J Gerontology*, 1975, Vol 50, No 5, 513-525.

Carpenter, D. G. Biological aging of living systems. *Speculations in Science and Technology*, Vol 7, No 4, 1983, 233-255.

Clark, J. W. The aging dimension: A factorial analysis of individual differences with age on psychological and physiological measurements. *J Gerontology*, 1958, 183-187.

Comfort, A. Test battery to measure aging rate in man. *Lancet*, December 27, 1969, 1411-1415.

Conard, R. A. An attempt to quantify some clinical criteria of aging. *J Gerontology*, 1960, Vol 15, 358-365.

Costa, P. T., and McCrae, R. R. Concepts of Functional or Biological Age, in: *Principles of Geriatric Medicine*, by R. Andres, E. L. Bierman, and W. R. Hazzard (eds). McGraw Hill.

Costa, P. T., and McCrae, R. R. Functional age: A conceptual and empirical critique, in: *Proceedings of the Second Conference on the Epidemiology of Aging*, by S. G. Haynes, M. Feinleib (eds), Bethesda, NIA, 1980.

Dempster, A. P. Functional age and age-related measures. *Aging and Human Development*, Vol 3, No. 2, 1972, 195-196.

Duplenko, Yu. P. N. Sokolov and the problem of biological age, in: Tokar, A. V., and Voitenko, V. P. *Biological Age, Heredity and Aging--Gerontology and Geriatrics Yearbook, 1984.* Kiev, AMS, USSR, USSR Gerontological and Geriatrics Society, 1984.

Supplemental Bibliography — Appendix E

Emanuel, N. The principles of biological age determination and human viability, in: Tokar, A. V., and Voitenko, V. P. *Biological Age, Heredity and Aging--Gerontology and Geriatrics Yearbook, 1984*. Kiev, AMS, USSR, USSR Gerontological and Geriatrics Society, 1984.

Fozard, J. L. Predicting age in the adult years from psychological assessments of abilities and personality. *Aging and Human Development*, Vol 3, No 2, 1972, 175-182.

Fozard, J. L, and Thomas, J. C. Jr. Psychology of aging--Basic findings and some psychiatric applications, in: *Modern Perspectives in the Psychiatry of Old Age*, Vol 6, by John Howells, (ed). New York, Bruner/Mazel, 1975, 107-109.

Frolkis, V. V. Individual biological age and its interspecies comparison, in: Tokar, A. V., and Voitenko, V. P. *Biological Age, Heredity and Aging--Gerontology and Geriatrics Yearbook, 1984*. Kiev, AMS, USSR, USSR Gerontological and Geriatrics Society, 1984.

Harrison, D. and Archer, J. R. Physiological assays for biological age in mice: Relationship of collagen, renal function, and longevity. *Exp Aging Research*, Vol 9, No 4, 1983, 245-251.

Heikkinen, E. Assessment of Functional Aging, in: *Lectures on Gerontology, Volume I: On Biology of Aging, Part B*. New York, Academic Press, 1982, 481-516.

Heron, A., and Chown, S. *Age and Function*. Little, Brown and Company, Boston, 1967.

Hofecker, G., Skalicky, M., Kment, A., and Niedermuller, H. Models of the biological age of the rat. I. A factor model of age parameters. *Mech Aging Dev*, 14 (1980) 345-359.

Hofecker, G., Niedermuller, H., Skalicky, M., Kment, A. Revitalization studies in laboratory rats. Biological Age and Aging Risk Factors--International Symposium on Gerontology, Madrid, 1985.

Ingram, D. K. Toward the behavioral assessment of biological aging in the laboratory mouse: Concepts, terminology, and objectives. *Exp Aging Research*, Vol 9, No 4, 1983, 225-238.

Ingram, D. Biological age: Estimation strategy, in: Tokar, A. V., and Voitenko, V. P. *Biological Age, Heredity and Aging--Gerontology and Geriatrics Yearbook, 1984*. Kiev, *IMS, USSR, USSR Gerontological and Geriatrics Society, 1984.

Jalavisto, E., and Makkonen, T. On the Assessment of Biological Age, I-III. *Annales Academiae Scientiarum Fennicae*, Series A. Helsinki, 1963-1964.

Kent, S. Measuring human health and aging, in: *Geriatrics*, June 1978, 108-111.

Ludwig, F. C., and Masoro, E. J. The Measurement of Biological Age. *Exp Aging Research*, Vol 9, No 4, 1983, 219-220.

Ludwig, F. C., and Smoke, M. E. The measurement of biological age. *Exp Aging Research*, Vol 6, No. 6, 1980, 497-521.

Ludwig, F. C. Quantitation of aging: Possibilities and limitations, in: Tokar, A. V., and Voitenko, V. P. *Biological Age, Heredity and Aging--Gerontology and Geriatrics Yearbook, 1984*. Kiev, AMS, USSR, USSR Gerontological and Geriatrics Society, 1984.

Mackay, I. R., White, S., Mathews, J. D., Gladwell, P., and Shepherd, J. Studies on the estimation of aging in man. *J Clin Exp Gerontology*, 1980, Vol 2, No 4, 211-230.

Murray, I. M. Assessment of physiologic age by combination of several criteria--vision, hearing, blood pressure and muscle force. *J Gerontology*, 1051, 120-126.

Ordy, J. M., and Schjeide, O. A. Biological age and its determination: An interdisciplinary study, In: *Proceedings, 9th International Congress of Gerontology, Vol 2*, July 2-7, 1972, Kiev, USSR, pp. 315-318.

Palmore, E., and Jeffers, F. C. *Prediction of Life Span*, Lexington, Heath Lexington Books.

Reff, M. E. and Schneider, E. L. *Biological Markers of Aging*, Washington, USDHHS, NIH, PHS, 1982.

Regelson, W. and Sinex, F. M. (eds). *Intervention in the Aging Process, Part A: Quantitation, Epidemiology, and Clinical Research; and Part B: Basic Research and Preclinical Screening.* Alan R. Liss, Inc., New York, 1983.

Rose, C. L. The measurement of social age. *Aging and Human Development*, Vol 3, No 2, 1972, 153-168.

Shock, N. W. Physiological and chronological age, in: *Aging--Its Chemistry*, by A. A. Dietz and V. S. Marcum, Washington, The American Association for Clinical Chemistry, 1980, 3-24.

Shock, N. W. Indices of functional age, in: *Aging: A Challenge to Science and Society, Vol 1, Biology*, by D. Danon, N. W. Shock, and M. Marois (eds). Oxford U. Press, New York, 1981, 270-286.

Skalicky, M., Hofecker, G., Kment, A., and Niedermuller, H. Models of the biological age of the rat. II. Multiple regression models in the study on influencing aging. *Mech Age Dev*, 14 (1980) 361-377.

Skalicky, M., Niedermuller, H., Hofecker, G. Multivariate methods in the assessment of the biological age. Biological age and aging Risk Factors--International Symposium on Gerontology, Madrid, 1985.

Tobin, J. D. Physiological indices of aging, in: *Aging: A Challenge to Science and Society, Vol 1, Biology*, by D. Danon, N. W. Shock, and M. Marois (eds). Oxford U. Press, New York, 1981.

Tokar, A. V., and Voitenko, V. P. *Biological Age, Heredity and Aging--Gerontology and Geriatrics Yearbook, 1984*. Kiev, AMS, USSR, USSR Gerontological and Geriatrics Society, 1984.

Voitenko, V. P., Polyukhov, A. M., Barbaruk, L. K., Kolodchenko, V. P., and Khodzinsky, A. N. Biological age as a key problem of gerontology, in: Tokar, A. V., and Voitenko, V. P. *Biological Age, Heredity and Aging – Gerontology and Geriatrics Yearbook, 1984*. Kiev, AMS, USSR, USSR Gerontological and Geriatrics Society, 1984.

Young, J. C., and Rickert, W. S. Concerning the precision of age estimates based on biological parameters. *Exp Geront*, 1973, Vol 8, 337-343.

INDEX

A

AAA (American Aging Association) 244

Abbo, F. 248

Abdominal depth 57, 350

Academy of Medical Sciences (Soviet) 147, 157, 171

Acommodation (near vision) .... 28, ... 34, 36, 84, 158, 191, ... 231, 321-322, 324

Acid phosphatase 26

Adrenocorticoprophin releasing hormone (ACTH) 213

Adult Growth Examination (AGE) 33-45

AGE (Adult Growth Examination) 33-45

Aging as a disease .... x, 16-20, 106

Aging, definition 157

Aging, theories
entropic 205
free radical 244

Aging measurement tests 4
criteria for 4

Aging rate 4-10, 150
difference between men and women 151
reduction 265-266

Aging Research Institute 241

AIDS 22

Albumin .... 25, 26, 136, ... 141, 370, 375

Alkaline phosphatase .... 26, 28, ... 191, 369

American Aging Association (AGE) 244

American Longevity Association 247

American Society of Bariatric Physicians 209

Ames, B. N. 247

Anteflexion 191, 354-5

Anthropometric .... 29, 53-58, ... 290, 342-358

Anti-oxidants 244-246

Arterial oxygen tension 178, 314
analyzers 176, 276

Arterial pulse wave velocity..... 158, ... 172, 313
measuring device 158, 172, 275

Atomic Bomb Casualty Commission (ABCC) 93-101, 104

Audiometer 158, 176, 278

Audiometric tests .... 2, 8, 34, 37, ... 61, 104, 112, 158, ... 178, 229, 319-320

Auditory reaction time 179, 229

Aviators 20-21

B

B-cell assay 397, 398

Baldness 56, 190, 357

Baltimore Longitudinal Study of Aging 190, 208

Basal metabolic rate (BMR) 205-210, 214, 386

Basal-Tech, Inc. 209

Berens near-point indicator 110, 158, 279

BHA 244

BHT 244

Bideltoid breadth 56, 349

Bilirubin 25, 26

Biological aging measurement tests 49-51
criteria for 4

Biomechanical force platform 112, 287

Bjorksten, J. .... vii, 240

Bleeding time 27

Block Design Test 112, 289, 335

Blood pressure
diastolic 84, 178, 299-300
maximum systolic 62, 299
systolic .... 34, 38, 72, 73, 84, ... 111, 130, 136, 158, ... 178, 191, 298-299

Body flexibility 353-355

Bogitch light extinction test 288, 338

Borkan, G. 53, 129-132

Bourdon-Wiersma test 61, 283, 328

Bruce, R. A. 259

BSP 27

Index

BUN..................25, 26, 28, 72,
................................73, 136, 191, 368

Butylated hydroxytoluene
(BHT)................................244

Butylated hydroxyanisol
(BHA)................................244

C

Calcium............................73, 372

Calipers
 anthropometric........56, 290, 292
 skin fold..........................56, 292
 sliding............................56, 292

Calorimetry, whole body
................................205-210

Camera..............................56, 293

Candida............................215, 400

Cardiac index............................49

Caries index......28, 35, 42, 190, 360

Categorization....................61, 330

CBC......................................25, 27

Cerebroactive drugs..................265

Cherkin, A. 233

Chlorpromazine test..........214, 221

Choice-reaction time 288,
................................338-340
 four-choice........61, 113, 338, 340
 three-choice..............111, 338-339
 measuring device....................111

Cholesterol...............23, 24, 26, 28
................................73, 136, 172,
................................191, 364-365
 HDL....................26, 28, 191, 365

Clofibrate................................223

Clomiphene test..........214, 216, 220

Coleman, D. L. 236

Color word test.........176, 178, 289,
................................337-338

Concentration test......................61

Contact sensitization skin tests
 Candida..........................215, 400
 Dinitrochlorobenzene
 (DNCB)........................215, 400

Correction factors..........62, 64, 111
................................114, 135, 139, 142, 148

Corticotrophin releasing hormone
................................213

Cortisol.....................217, 218, 395

Counter, hand tally............286, 333

CPK..26

Creatinine..............25, 26, 380-383

Creatinine clearance..........29, 130,
................................380-383

D

Damon, A. 53-58

Dark adaptation test........111, 112,
................................323-324

Dehydroepiandrosterone
(DHEA)........................235-239

Dental tests....28, 176, 190, 358-360
 caries index....28, 35, 42, 178, 360
 periodontal index........28, 35, 41,
................................358-359

Dexamethasone suppression test
................................214, 220, 394

Diabetes............................136, 211

Digit symbol test........158, 289, 334

Dilantin (phenytoin)..................223

Dinitrochlorobenzene
(DNCB)..........................215, 400

Dilman, V. 18, 211-225, 259

Dirken, J. M. 59-68, 134, 148

Dubina, T. L. 147-155, 171

Dutch intelligence test..........61, 283

Dynamometer, handgrip......56, 84,
................................96, 110, 112, 130,
................................172, 176, 190, 290

Dyundikova, V. A. 147

E

Ear
 breadth..........................56, 345
 length............................56, 347

Electrocardiogram....172, 217, 313

Electrocardiograph..........172, 275

Entropic theory of aging...........205

Entropy..................................205

Ergometer, bicycle..............61, 137,
................................272, 302

Erythrocyte sedimentation rate
(ESR)..........................27, 28, 361

Estrogen......214, 216, 223, 389-390

Ethoxyquine............................244

Exercise, effect on aging...105-107,
................................139

F

FAA......................................20-21

Fibrinogen........................191, 377

Finger dexterity........................111

Fitness, effect on aging.....105-107,
................................139

Flexibility....................85, 353-355
 tester........................190, 293-294

Flexometer........................293, 294

Florini, J. 240

Follicle stimulating hormone
(FSH))............213, 214, 388, 390

Forced expiratory volume in
1 second (FEV_1)........28, 72, 130,
................................230, 315

Forced vital capacity.......28, 49, 73,
................................84, 108, 110, 136,
................................158, 178, 191, 230,
................................316-317

Free radical
theory of aging................244-245

Index

Free radicals 244-247
Frequency of testing............260-261
Functional capacity 16-18, 259
Furukawa, T. 81-91, 136

G

G6PD 26, 236
Geromat 176, 177, 341-342
Gerontology Research Center
....129
  tapping test...............130, 333-334
Gerontotherapeutics...........222-223
GIT test cards 61, 283
Glenn, P. 240
Glucose......................25, 26, 28, 34,
...............................35, 39, 215, 367
Glucose tolerance test ...29, 34, 39,
.....................136, 211, 215, 384-385
Glutamic oxaloacetic
  transaminase (SGOT) 25, 26,
.... 141, 374
Glutamic pyruvic transaminase
  (SGPT) 25, 26, 136, 371-372
Gonadotrophins, urinary..........214,
......................................215, 390-391
Goniometer......................176, 293
Gout 378
Grayness........56, 176, 190, 342-343
Growth hormone...............214, 219

H

H-SCAN..............176, 227-231, 259
Hair
  baldness.....................56, 190, 352
  grayness 56, 176, 190, 342-343
Hall, J. 11-14
Handgrip dynamometer 56, 84,
...........................96, 110, 112, 130,
.....................172, 176, 190, 290-291

Handgrip strength 29, 56, 85,
..................................96, 111, 112,
.................................130, 172, 178,
.... 191, 343-344
Hand steadiness measuring
  device 61, 282
Hand tally counter 84, 286, 333
Harman, D. 18, 244-245
Harrison, D. ....xii, 236, 261
Health Hazard Appraisal
  (HHA) 11-14, 255
Health Improvement Company
 241
Hearing loss...............28, 34, 37, 61,
............................104, 112, 158, 178,
.... 229, 319-320
Heart rate
  maximum...................62, 138, 178,
....191, 307
  monitor...............61, 137, 176, 274
  recovery rate.............85, 178, 191,
.... 259, 308-311
  recovery ratio 138, 259, 318
  resting.......................138, 141, 178
Heat stress 241
Height
  sitting................................56, 346
  standing........29, 84, 190, 229, 356
Heikkinen, E. 103-127
Hemoglobin...............28, 136, 362
Hershey, D. 205-210, 259
HIV (Human Immunodeficiency
  Virus) 22
Hochschild, R. 176, 227-231
Hollingsworth, J. W. 93-101
Hypertension......................135, 136
Hyperthyroidism........................208
Hypothalamus 213

I

Immune stimulants
  Dehydroepiandrosterone
  (DHEA) 235-239
Immunoglobulin
  electrophoresis 26
Immunological tests 214, 215,
....397-400
  B-cell assay......................397, 398
  Contact sensitization
  skin tests 215, 398, 399
  Candida 215, 400
  Dinitrochlorobenzene
  (DNCB)..........................215, 400
Immunological tests (cont'd)
  Tuberculin..............................400
  response to phytohemaglutinin
  ....215, 398-399
  T-cell assay.....................215, 397
Immunoglobulin electrophoresis
 26
  Lymphocyte blast transforma-
  tion index................ 158, 398, 399
  Pulmonary macrophage
  sputum test 27
Inframatic 8100 reflective near
  infra-red spectrometer 245
Institute of Gerontology
  (Soviet) 147, 157, 171
Insulin stress test 214, 217-218
International Academy of
  Bariatric Medicine 209

J – K

Jablon, S. 93-101
Karl Marx University................175
Ketosteroid
  17-KS/17-OHCS excretion ratio
  ....214, 215, 395-396
Kiiskinen, A. 109-111
Kohn, R. 259
Krimsky-Prince Rule 279
Kuzuya, F. 189

Index

L

LDH 26
L-dopa test 214, 220
Landolt test 176, 284, 328-329
Law of Deviation of Homeostasis and Diseases of Aging 223
Lecithin 172, 373, 377
Lecithin/cholesterol ratio . 172, 373
Life Extension 25-29
Light extinction device (Bogitch) 95
Light extinction time ..96, 288-289, ... 338, 341
Lipoprotein electrophoresis 26
Lippman, R. 244-246
Logie, A. R. 71
Luteinizing hormone (LH) ..... 213, ... 214, 386-387
  releasing hormone (LHRH) 213, 214, 220
Lymphocyte
  B cell 215, 397, 398
  response to phytohemaglutinin 215, 398-399
  T cell 215, 397-398
Lymphocyte blast transformation test 158, 398-399
Lymphocyte peroxidation test 247

M

Manhattan Project 240
Maximal breathing capacity 49, 62, 317
Maximal oxygen uptake (VO_2 max) .... 28, 112, 137, ... 301-307
Maximum Life Span 51
Maximum heart rate .... 62, 138, ... 178, 191, 307

Maximum respiratory rate .... 49, ... 62, 317
Maximum voluntary ventilation (MVV) 137, 318
Melanocyte stimulating hormone (MSH) 393
Memory 148, 152, 335
Mints, A. Ya. 171-174
Miquel, J. 240
Morgan, R. F. 33-45
Morin, R. 247
Movement time 230
Multiple regression analysis 50

N

Nagoya U. 189
Nakamura, E. 133-146
National Health Information Clearinghouse 13
National Institute on Aging .... 50, ... 129, 190, 259
Near vision .... 28, 34, 36, 84, ... 158, 190, 231, ... 321-322, 324
Neuropsychological tests .. 325-342
Niacin 219
Normative Aging Study 130
Norris, A. 130
Nose breadth 56, 348

O

O'Connor pegboard test ...... 29, 34, ... 43, 281, 325
Occult blood 27
Oral glucose tolerance test ..29, 35, ... 39, 136, 211, ... 215, 384-385
Orentreich, N. 238-240

Oxalate 27
Oxygen removal rate . 138, 309, 312

P

Pattern recognition analysis (PRA) 233-235
Pauling, L. 233-234
Pearson, D. .... xiv, 21
Pegboard tests:
  O'Connor 29, 34, 43, 281, 325
  Purdue .... 29, 110-111, ... 281, 325-326
Periodontal index .... 28, 35, 41, ... 358-359
Phenformin 223
Phensolfonphthalein test (PSP) 84, 379
Phenytoin (Dilantin) 223
Phospholipids 26, 191, 377
Physical fitness, effect on aging .... 105-107, ... 139-140
Physiological monitoring system 137, 272, 273
Picture recognition 61, 327
Pitch ceiling (High Frequency Audiometry) 61, 320
Pituitary 213
Poethig, D. 175
Positioning (hand steadiness) 61, 237
Potassium 25, 26
Prolactin 220, 221, 393
PSP clearance 84, 379
Pulmonary function tests 28, 315-318
Pulmonary macrophage sputum test 27
Pulse pressure 110, 300-301

Pulse wave velocity............ 158, 172, 313-314

Pulse wave velocity measuring device 158, 172, 275

Purdue pegboard test 29, 110, 111, 281, 325-326

Q – R

Radiation Effects Research Foundation (RERF) 93-101, 104

Reaction time............... 61, 179, 229
 auditory............................ 179, 229
 choice.......................111, 338-340
 clock.. 179
 visual 179, 229, 341

Red blood cell count........ 191, 363

Reflective near infra-red spectroscopy 245

Regelson, W. ....viii, xii

Rejuvenation................................7-8

Renal plasma flow 49

Respiratory rate............. 49, 62, 317

Richardson, A. 235

Robbins, L. C. 11

Robinson, A. B. 233-234

Roes, W. 175-187

Risk age 11-14

S

Sanar 238-242

Scale, body weight 137, 295

Schloss, B. 240-244

Schneider, E. .... xiv, 107

Schwartz, A. 235-238

Schmidt, E. 175

Semantic categorization test panel 61, 284-285

Sequential multiple analysis (SMAC)............................... 21

SGOT 25, 26, 141, 374

SGPT 25, 26, 136, 371-372

Shaw, S. 21

Shibata, K. 189

Shimokata, H., ... 189-202

Shock, N. W. .... xii, 259

Skinfold thickness, triceps.......................... 56, 351

Society of Prospective Medicine 13

Sodium 25, 26

Sphygmomanometer..... 34, 83, 108, 110, 136, 158, 176, 271

Spirometer 61, 71, 104, 108, 130, 136, 137, 158, 176, 190, 277

Staircase, Master's 137, 190, 274, 302

Static balance test 112, 158, 191, 336-337

Step test 137, 191, 274, 302

Stopwatch 190, 295

Stroop color word test...... 176, 178, 289-290, 337-338

Suominen, H. 103-127, 133

Sweat rate 241

T

T-cell assay 215, 397

T wave, amplitude of deflection..................... 172, 313

Tape measure 83, 190

Tapping (button) 230

Tapping board............ 128, 286-287

Tapping rate 128, 178, 230, 333-334, 342
 GRC Tapping test . 128, 286-287, 333-334

Tapping rate (cont'd)
 Hand tally counter 286, 333
 Tapping (button).................. 230
 Tapping board 128, 286-287

Tendon extensibility... 178, 357-358

Testosterone 216

Thermoregulatory system......... 241

Thorazine (chlorpromazine) test 214, 221

Thyroid function tests 208
 PBI.................................... 26
 TSH........... 26, 214, 216, 222, 392
 T3 .... 26, 214, 216, 391
 T4 .... 26, 214, 216, 391

Thyroid hormone 26, 222, 223

Tokar, A. V. 157-169

Total protein 191, 376

Treadmill..... 137, 272, 273, 301-302

Triangle, draftsman's 56, 293

Triceps skinfold thickness.. 56, 351

Triglycerides 191, 214, 215, 366

Tuberculin test................... 215, 400

U

U. of Cincinnati 205

Urate...................................... 25, 27

Urea nitrogen 72, 136, 368

Uric acid............................ 191, 378

Urine................................... 25, 26

V

Vaughan, W. 233, 240

Veteran's Administration, Normative Aging Study 129

Vibratory sensitivity 85, 96, 104, 148, 172, 230, 330-332

Vibrometer............ 84, 96, 104, 148, 172, 228, 285

Index

Vision tester 280

Visual accommodation
(near vision) 28, 34, 36, 84
.... 158, 191, 231,
.... 321-322

Visual acuity 28, 61, 136,
.... 178, 323

Visual field analyzer 112, 280

Vital capacity 28, 49, 73, 84,
.... 110, 136, 158, 178,
.... 191, 230, 316-317

Vitamin E 244

Voitenko, V. 157-169

W

Walford, R. 18, 51

Webster, I. W. 71-79, 136

Wechsler
  Block Design 112, 289, 335
  Digit Symbol Test ... 158, 289, 334
  Weight 29, 84, 158, 190,
.... 215, 217, 357

X – Z

Zhuk, E. V. 147

Notes

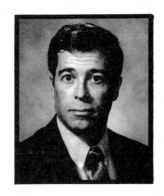

ABOUT THE AUTHOR

Dr. Dean is a graduate of the U.S. Military Academy, West Point, New York, and received his M.D. degree from Han Yang University, Seoul, Korea, and M.S. degree (physiology) from Kyung Buk University, Taegu, Korea. He received post-graduate training at Letterman Army Medical Center in San Francisco, the U.S. Navy Aerospace Medical Institute, Pensacola, FL, and the U.S. Air Force School of Aerospace Medicine, San Antonio, TX.

Dr. Dean is a parachutist, a skilled SCUBA and hard-hat diver, is fluent in Korean, Vietnamese and Spanish, has been a steamship company executive, a member of the Army Pentathlon Team, a U.S. Army Ranger Instructor, and was an advisor to the Vietnamese Rangers in combat.

A former U.S. Army Flight Surgeon and Diving Medical Officer, Dr. Dean spent 3 years as the Flight Surgeon for America's top-secret counterterrorist unit, the Delta Force, where he participated in a number of classified missions.

He has been actively engaged in gerontological research for over 10 years, and has published over 50 articles and reviews in professional journals. He was on the Board of Directors of the American Aging Association, and is a member of the Gerontological Society of America, the American Geriatrics Society, the Association of Military Surgeons of the U.S., American Physiological Society, and an Associate Fellow, Aerospace Medical Association.